Nursing Care
of the
Older Adult

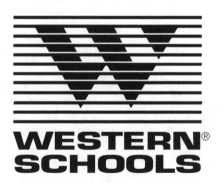

WESTERN® SCHOOLS

By
Suzanne Fitzsimmons, MSN, ARNP

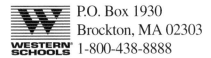

P.O. Box 1930
Brockton, MA 02303
1-800-438-8888

ABOUT THE AUTHOR

Suzanne Fitzsimmons, MSN, ARNP, is a faculty member in the College of Health Professions at Florida Gulf Coast University in Fort Myers, Florida. She is both a geriatric nurse practitioner and a recreational therapist. She is currently involved in numerous dementia-care research projects and teaches courses in gerontology, recreational therapy, and health promotions for older adults with mild cognitive impairments. Her research has been published in many healthcare journals and she is the co-author of the *Dementia Practice Guideline for Recreational Therapy: Treatment of Disturbing Behaviors*. Ms. Fitzsimmons is a regular speaker at the National Alzheimer's Association, the Geriatric Society Association, and the National American Therapeutic Recreation Association yearly conferences. On a local level she is a board member of many organizations that provide services to older adults, does trainings for professional and family caregivers, and gives workshops for community-dwelling older adults on various aspects of aging.

Suzanne Fitzsimmons has disclosed that she receives research grants pertaining to older adults, from Florida Gulf Coast University.

ABOUT THE SUBJECT MATTER REVIEWER

Meredith Wallace, Ph.D., APRN, has been a nurse since she completed her BSN degree Magna Cum Laude at Boston University in 1988. Following this, she earned an MSN in medical-surgical nursing with a specialty in geriatrics from Yale University and a Ph.D. in nursing research and theory development at New York University (NYU). During her time at NYU she was awarded a pre-doctoral fellowship at the Hartford Institute for Geriatric Nursing. In 2001, she won the *Springer Publishing Company* Award for Applied Nursing Research. She is the author of several journal articles and book chapters. Dr. Wallace recently published *Prostate Cancer: Nursing Assessment Management and Care*, in April 2002, which won the *American Journal of Nursing* Book of the Year Award. Preceding this, she was the Associate Editor of *The Geriatric Nursing Research Digest*, which also won the *American Journal of Nursing* Book of the Year Award in 2002. She is currently an Assistant Professor of Nursing at Fairfield University.

Meredith Wallace has disclosed that she has no significant financial or other conflicts of interest pertaining to this course book.

Copy Editor: Arlene Miller, Carole Kenner
Indexer: Sylvia Coates

ISBN: 1-57801-097-7

P0206SH

IMPORTANT: Read these instructions *BEFORE* proceeding!

Enclosed with your course book you will find the FasTrax® answer sheet. Use this form to answer all the final exam questions that appear in this course book. If you are completing more than one course, be sure to write your answers on the appropriate answer sheet. Full instructions and complete grading details are printed on the FasTrax instruction sheet, also enclosed with your order. Please review them before starting. *If you are mailing your answer sheet(s) to Western Schools, we recommend you make a copy as a backup.*

ABOUT THIS COURSE

A "Pretest" is provided with each course to test your current knowledge base regarding the subject matter contained within this course. Your "Final Exam" is a multiple choice examination. **You will find the exam questions at the end of each chapter.**

In the event the course has less than 100 questions, leave the remaining answer boxes on the FasTrax answer sheet blank. **Use a black pen to fill in your answer sheet.**

A PASSING SCORE

You must score 70% or better in order to pass this course and receive your Certificate of Completion. Should you fail to achieve the required score, we will send you an additional FasTrax answer sheet so that you may make a second attempt to pass the course. Western Schools will allow you three chances to pass the same course…*at no extra charge!* After three failed attempts to pass the same course, your file will be closed.

RECORDING YOUR HOURS

Please monitor the time it takes to complete this course using the handy log sheet on the other side of this page. See below for transferring study hours to the course evaluation.

COURSE EVALUATIONS

In this course book you will find a short evaluation about the course you are soon to complete. This information is vital to providing the school with feedback on this course. The course evaluation answer section is in the lower right hand corner of the FasTrax answer sheet marked "Evaluation" with answers marked 1–21. Your answers are important to us; please take five minutes to complete the evaluation.

On the back of the FasTrax instruction sheet, there is additional space to make any comments about the course, the school, and suggested new curriculum. Please mail the FasTrax instruction sheet, with your comments, back to Western Schools in the envelope provided with your course order.

TRANSFERRING STUDY TIME

Upon completion of the course, transfer the total study time from your log sheet to question #21 in the Course Evaluation. The answers will be in ranges; please choose the proper hour range that best represents your study time. You MUST log your study time under question #21 on the course evaluation.

EXTENSIONS

You have 2 years from the date of enrollment to complete this course. A six (6) month extension may be purchased. If after 30 months from the original enrollment date you do not complete the course, *your file will be closed and no certificate can be issued.*

CHANGE OF ADDRESS?

In the event you have moved during the completion of this course, please call our student services department at 1-800-618-1670 and we will update your file.

A GUARANTEE TO WHICH YOU'LL GIVE HIGH HONORS

If any continuing education course fails to meet your expectations or if you are not satisfied in any manner, for any reason, you may return it for an exchange or a refund (less shipping and handling) within 30 days. Software, video and audio courses must be returned unopened.

Thank you for enrolling at Western Schools!

WESTERN SCHOOLS
P.O. Box 1930
Brockton, MA 02303
(800) 438-8888
www.westernschools.com

Nursing Care
of the Older Adult

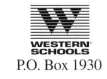

WESTERN SCHOOLS

P.O. Box 1930

Brockton, MA 02303

Please use this log to total the number of hours you spend reading the text and taking the final examination (use 50-min hours).

Date	Hours Spent
7-12-06	2
8-19-06	2

TOTAL

Please log your study hours with submission of your final exam. To log your study time, fill in the appropriate circle under question 21 of the FasTrax® answer sheet under the "Evaluation" section.

Nursing Care of the Older Adult

WESTERN SCHOOLS
CONTINUING EDUCATION EVALUATION

Instructions: Mark your answers to the following questions with a black pen on the "Evaluation" section of your FasTrax® answer sheet provided with this course. You should not return this sheet. Please use the scale below to rate the following statements:

A Agree Strongly   **C Disagree Somewhat**
B Agree Somewhat   **D Disagree Strongly**

The course content met the following education objectives:

1. Identify factors that influence older adults and the aging process as it pertains to health.

2. Discuss aging theories and describe some of the normal aging changes.

3. Discuss basic principles for working with older adults and the nursing skills required for optimal interactions specific to this population.

4. Discuss physiological changes that affect medication disposition and the various problems associated with drug therapy in the older adult.

5. Discuss clinical problems that are prevalent in the older adult.

6. Discuss clinical problems that are related to cognitive changes and dementia as a part of the aging process.

7. Discuss the implications of, and strategies for, management and coping with common chronic diseases and conditions in the older adult.

8. Discuss the implications of, and strategies for, management and coping with problems related to the aging sensory system.

9. Discuss the common mental health problems and the impact these have on the older adult population.

10. Discuss how social factors affect an older adult's psychological well-being.

11. Discuss the implications of prevention on the health of older adults and how rehabilitation and various therapies assist in returning to or maintaining maximum levels of functioning.

12. Understanding of how select special issues – sexual orientation, driving, and smoking – impact the rights and quality of life of older adults.

13. Discuss the various aspects of different care settings of the older adult.

14. Discuss legal issues that are pertinent to the older adult.

15. The content of this course was relevant to the objectives.

16. This offering met my professional education needs.

17. The objectives met the overall purpose/goal of the course.

18. The course was generally well-written and the subject matter explained thoroughly? (If no, please explain on the back of the FasTrax instruction sheet.)

19. The content of this course was appropriate for home study.

20. The final examination was well-written and at an appropriate level for the content of the course.

21. **PLEASE LOG YOUR STUDY HOURS WITH SUBMISSION OF YOUR FINAL EXAM.** Please choose which best represents the total study hours it took to complete this 30-hour course.

A. less than 25 hours

B. 25–28 hours

C. 29–32 hours

D. greater than 32 hours

CONTENTS

FIGURES AND TABLES

PRETEST

Note: You will not find this pretest in the exam section, and you will not be able to select your answers in this document. This is for your own personal assessment.

Begin by taking the pretest. Write your answers down on a separate piece of paper. Compare your answers on the pretest to the answer key (located in the back of the book or in the reference file). Circle the items that you missed. The pretest answer key indicates the course chapters where the content of that question is discussed.

Next, read each chapter. Exam questions are provided at the end of each chapter so that you can assess your progress and understanding of the material. Focus special attention on those items you answered incorrectly.

1. A summary measurement of the overall health status of a population is

   a. infant mortality.
   b. life expectancy.
   c. chronic disease.
   d. fertility rate.

2. An aging theory based on the instability of cells to reproduce themselves after approximately 50 divisions is called

   a. Hayflick phenomenon.
   b. cellular degeneration.
   c. exchange theory.
   d. activity theory.

3. A primary risk factor for strokes in older adults is

   a. dementia.
   b. marital status.
   c. hypertension.
   d. age.

4. A nurse desiring to understand a patient is displaying

   a. tolerance.
   b. kindness.
   c. sensitivity.
   d. empathy.

5. The process of the passage of a medication from the administration site into the systemic circulation is called

   a. absorption.
   b. distribution.
   c. elimination.
   d. metabolism.

6. Older adults frequently take herbal remedies and supplements. These products usually

   a. are safe for older adults.
   b. do not interact with medications.
   c. do not have FDA approval.
   d. have adequate research to support their medicinal claims.

7. Unintentional harmful incidents or conditions that result from diagnostic, prophylactic, or therapeutic interventions or omissions are called

    a. idiopathic.
    b. iatrogenesic.
    c. intentional.
    d. intrinsic.

8. The medium in which all the body's metabolic activities take place, and an essential structural component of every cell is

    a. water.
    b. sodium.
    c. lipids.
    d. nucleus.

9. The onset of Alzheimer's disease is

    a. preceded by a stroke.
    b. gradual and insidious.
    c. the same in each person.
    d. sudden and profound.

10. A risk factor for disturbing behaviors in older adults with dementia is

    a. female gender.
    b. self-ambulatory.
    c. male gender.
    d. age.

11. A musculoskeletal condition that may not become apparent until a fracture occurs is

    a. spinal stenosis.
    b. osteoarthritis.
    c. rheumatoid arthritis.
    d. osteoporosis.

12. A factor that affects older adults' tolerance of daily physical activity is

    a. gender.
    b. personality.
    c. pain.
    d. blood pressure.

13. A confusional state characterized by acute onset of cognitive impairment with disturbances of consciousness and attention is

    a. delirium.
    b. depression.
    c. dementia.
    d. delusions.

14. A client whose behavior is fearful, suspicious, and overly sensitive to criticism is displaying the following personality

    a. narcissistic.
    b. paranoid.
    c. compulsive.
    d. schizoid.

15. Ignoring or isolating an older adult and excluding them from daily activities is considered

    a. psychological abuse.
    b. exploitation.
    c. psychological neglect.
    d. physical neglect.

16. An older adult who is expressing concerns with the meaning of life and death or their belief system is displaying signs of

    a. depression.
    b. low self-esteem.
    c. emotional abuse.
    d. spiritual distress.

17. An intervention designed to restore physical, emotional, or cognitive function is

    a. rehabilitation.

    b. preventative.

    c. motivation.

    d. assistive.

18. The older adult should consider giving up driving if he/she is

    a. able to use public transportation.

    b. getting lost in familiar surroundings.

    c. over the age 80.

    d. dependent on an assistive device.

19. A form of supportive housing designed for those who need extra help but do not require 24-hour skilled nursing is

    a. a sub-acute unit.

    b. a special care unit.

    c. an assistive living center.

    d. a rehabilitation center.

20. The process by which a fully informed patient can participate in choices about his/her healthcare is

    a. informed consent.

    b. conservatorship.

    c. surrogate decision making.

    d. self-determination.

INTRODUCTION

Nursing care of the older adult is a challenging task requiring knowledge, skill, and a desire to work with this population. As a youth-loving society, aging is sometimes viewed as undesirable yet demographics show increasing numbers of older adults with an increasing life span. The older adult may be found in a number of care settings ranging from the community-dwelling elder to an older adult with dementia on a special care unit. Many older adults have numerous chronic diseases and conditions requiring complex care. The accumulated years of an older adult also provides rich life experiences with diverse personalities and methods of coping. As people age, disease labels are less important than are the responses to disease. The responses are what determine the quality of life. Promotion of functional abilities and independence is of utmost importance no matter what the care setting is.

The purpose of this course is to provide nurses with the basic principles, knowledge, skills, and attitudes required to provide nursing care to older adults and their families. The broad range of topics in this course is offered to educate nurses on issues affecting older adults and to view the patient as a holistic individual. It is also hoped that it will dispel some of the common myths of aging such as:

- *Exercise and diet are useless.*

- *The damage is already done.*

- *Older adults are no longer interested in nor could they perform sexual acts.*

- *If you live long enough you will end up in a nursing home.*

- *Older adults are not able to learn new information or perform new tasks.*

- *Older adults are boring, slow, and similar in their abilities.*

Clinical nursing knowledge is advancing at a tremendous rate, so this course should not be considered all a nurse needs to know. This course touches briefly on the major concerns and issues facing older adults, such as chronic conditions, common clinical problems and psychosocial issues, and methods for nurses to handle these concerns.

CHAPTER 1

HEALTH CARE AND OLDER ADULTS

CHAPTER OBJECTIVE

After studying this chapter, the reader will have an overall impression of the factors that influence older adults and the aging process as it pertains to health.

LEARNING OBJECTIVES

After studying this chapter, the learner will be able to

1. discuss the impact of demographic trends on healthcare delivery to older adults.

2. identify the goals of Health People 2010 related to the nursing care of older adults.

3. relate how the health behaviors of older adults are formed and influenced.

4. describe the importance of cultural considerations for health care providers.

5. identify the impact of poverty on the older adult population.

6. explain concepts that define successful aging and strategies for promotion.

INTRODUCTION

For much of the fifty or so thousand years of human history the average life expectancy was less than 30 years. This gradually increased. By 1900 this average was 48 years for persons in the United States. In the 20th century an unprecedented event unfolded and nearly 30 years of life was added to the average life expectancy. In one small slice of history, a stunningly swift change occurred that added an entire new normative stage to the life cycle (Lee, 1997). The addition of longer lives and older people altered demographics and culture in a tremendous way. Most of the social policies and cultural norms that define our society were placed into practice when American life was very different than it is today. Three decades ago life expectancy was short, divorce rates lower, lifetime marriage was the norm, the average number of children born to a woman was greater than today, and children grew up and stayed near their birthplace. Pneumonia, influenza, and tuberculosis were the leading causes of death, life expectancy was short after retirement, and most Americans were Caucasian (Carstensen, 2002). With declining infant mortality, falling fertility rates, and increasing life expectancy, we are now faced with an aging society (Friedland & Summer, 1999). Despite the predicted growth in the older population, the United States is a relatively young country compared to other developed nations where older adults already account for 15% or more of the population, compared to our 13%. There are many grave warnings today of the growing older adult population and the need to be prepared and ready to provide the types of health care needed. Much of this is described in terms that indicate that this is bad news. Consider that Americans 65 and older constitute the largest number of cognitively impaired individuals, yet this same group includes the wisest, richest, and most psychologically resilient people in our society (Gatz, Kasl-Godley, & Karel, 1996). There is no reason to expect that our aging society will cause a series of problems unless society is not prepared to understand the complexities of older adults and make educated and wise choices in providing health care to them. This chapter will provide a snapshot of who the older adults of today are and some of the individual and societal factors that impact health, health behaviors, and positive aging.

DEMOGRAPHICS

Population

In 2000, an estimated 35 million people were age 65 or older, accounting for almost 13% of the population in the United States. Starting in 2011, the "baby boomers" will begin to turn 65. By 2030 it is projected that 20% of the population, 70 million people, will be over the age of 65. Women account for 58% of the population over the age of 65 and 70% of those over 85. In 2000 there were about 65,000 people over the age of 100 and it is estimated that this group will grow to 381,000 by the year 2030 (AOA, 2000). The states with the highest proportion of older adults are Florida, West Virginia, Pennsylvania, Iowa, and North Dakota.

As society grows older, it will become more diverse and programs and services will require greater flexibility to meet the demands of a diverse population. Ethnically an estimated 84% of people over the age 65 are non-Hispanic white, 8% African American, 6% Hispanic, 2% Asian and Pacific Islander, and .04% American Indian and Alaskan native. Education attainment influences socioeconomic status with higher levels of education associated with higher incomes, standards of

living and above-average health status. In 1950 only 18% of all older adults had a high school education, compared to 67% in 1998. For ethnic minorities the percentages are much lower: 44% African American, 65% Asian, and 29% Hispanic (AOA, 2000).

Marital status can strongly affect an older adult's emotional and economic well-being by influencing living arrangements and availability of caregivers for those with an illness or disability (AOA, 2000). (See Table 1-1.)

TABLE 1-1: MARITAL STATUS						
	Age 65–74		Age 75–84		Age 85 & older	
	Men	Women	Men	Women	Men	Women
Never Married	4%	4%	3%	5%	5%	6%
Divorced	8%	9%	4%	5%	4%	4%
Widowed	9%	32%	20%	56%	42%	77%
Married	79%	55%	74%	34%	50%	13%

(AOA, 2000.)

Living Arrangement

Over half (55%) of older, non-institutionalized persons lived with their spouse in 2000. The proportion living with their spouse decreases with age, especially for women. Only 28.8% of women 75+ years old, lived with a spouse. About 30% (9.7 million) of all non-institutionalized older persons in 2000 lived alone (7.4 million women, 2.4 million men). The proportion living alone increases with advanced age. Relatively small numbers (1.56 million) and percentages (4.5%) of the 65+ population lived in nursing homes in 2000. This ranged from 1.1% for persons 65–74 years to 4.7% for persons 75–84 years and 18.2% for persons 85+ (AOA, 2000).

Health Status

Life expectancy is a summary measurement of the overall health status of a population. Current life expectancy for males is 81.3 and females 84.2

years. The leading causes of death for persons 65 and older are heart disease, cancer, stoke, chronic obstructive pulmonary disease (COPD), pneumonia and influenza, and diabetes. (See Table 1-2.) Chronic health conditions are long-term illnesses that are rarely cured. These conditions may become

a significant health and financial burden to the older adult, their families, and the health care system. These conditions affect quality of life, contribute to decline in functioning, and cause the need for residential placement. For older adults, over the age 70, the presence of a chronic disease has actu-

TABLE 1-2: LEADING CAUSES OF DEATH

MALES AGE 65 or OLDER by RACE

	White	African American	Asian & Pacific Islander	American Indian & Alaskan Native	Hispanic
1.	Heart Disease	Heart Disease	Heart Disease	Heart Disease	Heart Disease
2.	Cancer	Cancer	Cancer	Cancer	Cancer
3.	Stroke	Stroke	Stroke	Diabetes	Stroke
4.	COPD	COPD	Pneumonia & Influenza	Stroke	Diabetes
5.	Pneumonia & Influenza	Pneumonia & Influenza	COPD	COPD	Pneumonia & Influenza
6.	Diabetes	Diabetes	Diabetes	Pneumonia & Influenza	COPD
7.	Unintentional injuries	Nephritis	Unintentional injuries	Unintentional injuries	Unintentional injuries
8.	Nephritis	Unintentional injuries	Nephritis	Liver Disease	Liver Disease
9.	Alzheimer's Disease	Septicemia	HTN	Nephritis	Nephritis
10.	Septicemia	HTN	Septicemia	Septicemia	Septicemia

FEMALES AGE 65 or OLDER by RACE

	White	African American	Asian & Pacific Islander	American Indian & Alaskan Native	Hispanic
1.	Heart Disease	Heart Disease	Heart Disease	Heart Disease	Heart Disease
2.	Cancer	Cancer	Cancer	Cancer	Cancer
3.	Stroke	Stroke	Stroke	Diabetes	Stroke
4.	COPD	Diabetes	Pneumonia & Influenza	Stroke	Diabetes
5.	Pneumonia & Influenza	Pneumonia & Influenza	Diabetes	Pneumonia & Influenza	Pneumonia & Influenza
6.	Diabetes	COPD	COPD	COPD	COPD
7.	Alzheimer's Disease	Nephritis	Unintentional injuries	Unintentional injuries	Unintentional injuries
8.	Unintentional injuries	Septicemia	Nephritis	Nephritis	Liver Disease
9.	Nephritis	HTN	HTN	Septicemia	Nephritis
10.	Athero-sclerosis	Unintentional injuries	Septicemia	Liver Disease	Alzheimer's Disease

MALES AGE 85 or OLDER by RACE

	White	African American	Asian & Pacific Islander	American Indian & Alaskan Native	Hispanic
1.	Heart Disease	Heart Disease	Heart Disease	Heart Disease	Heart Disease
2.	Cancer	Cancer	Cancer	Cancer	Cancer
3.	Stroke	Stroke	Stroke	Stroke	Pneumonia & Influenza
4.	Pneumonia & Influenza	Pneumonia & Influenza	Pneumonia & Influenza	Pneumonia & Influenza	Stroke
5.	COPD	COPD	COPD	COPD	COPD
6.	Unintentional injuries	Nephritis	Diabetes	Diabetes	Diabetes
7.	Diabetes	Diabetes	Unintentional injuries	Unintentional injuries	Unintentional injuries
8.	Nephritis	Septicemia	Nephritis	Nephritis	Nephritis
9.	Alzheimer's Disease	Unintentional injuries	HTN	Septicemia	Alzheimer's Disease
10.	Athero-sclerosis	HTN	Alzheimer's Disease	HTN	Septicemia

FEMALES AGE 85 or OLDER by RACE

	White	African American	Asian & Pacific Islander	American Indian & Alaskan Native	Hispanic
1.	Heart Disease	Heart Disease	Heart Disease	Heart Disease	Heart Disease
2.	Stroke	Cancer	Stroke	Stroke	Cancer
3.	Cancer	Stroke	Cancer	Cancer	Stroke
4.	Pneumonia & Influenza	Pneumonia & Influenza	Pneumonia & Influenza	Pneumonia & Influenza	Pneumonia & Influenza
5.	COPD	Diabetes	COPD	Diabetes	Diabetes
6.	Alzheimer's Disease	Septicemia	Diabetes	COPD	COPD
7.	Diabetes	Nephritis	Unintentional injuries	Unintentional injuries	Alzheimer's Disease
8.	Unintentional injuries	HTN	HTN	Alzheimer's Disease	Athero-sclerosis
9.	Athero-sclerosis	COPD	Septicemia	Septicemia	Nephritis
10.	Nephritis	Alzheimer's Disease	Nephritis	Athero-sclerosis	Unintentional injuries

COPD = Chronic Obstructive Pulmonary Disease, HTN = Hypertension
Note. From U.S. Census Bureau, 2000.

ally increased, whereas disability has decreased (Manton & Gu, 2001). (See Table 1-3.) Explanations for this include improved management and treatment, change in health behaviors, and use of assistive devices (AOA, 2000).

TABLE 1-3: SELECT CHRONIC DISEASE IN PERSONS OVER 70 YEARS OF AGE

	Male	Female
Arthritis	50%	64%
Diabetes	13%	12%
Cancer	23%	17%
Stroke	10%	8%
Hypertension	41%	48%
Heart disease	25%	19%
(AOA, 2000.)		

HEALTHY PEOPLE 2010

Healthy People 2010 (U.S. Department of Health and Human Services, http://www.healthypeople.gov) is a set of health objectives for the nation to achieve over the first decade of the new century. Healthy People is the prevention agenda for the nation. It is a statement of national opportunities, a tool that identifies the most significant preventable threats to health and focuses public and private sector efforts to address those threats. Healthy People offers a simple but powerful idea: Provide the information and knowledge about how to improve health in a format that enables diverse groups to combine their efforts and work as a team. It is a road map to better health for all that can be used by many different people, states and communities, businesses, professional organizations, and groups whose concern is a particular threat to health, or a particular population group. Two overarching goals, increasing quality and years of healthy life, and eliminating health disparities, served as a guide for developing objectives that will actually measure progress. The objectives are organized in 28 focus areas, each representing an important public health area. (See Table 1-4.)

Each objective has a target for improvements to be achieved by the year 2010. An example of this might be a Healthy People target goal of 60% of those over 65 to have had an influenza vaccine in the past year. A limited set of the objectives, known as the Leading Health Indicators, are intended to help everyone more easily understand the importance of health promotion and disease prevention and to encourage wide participation in improving

TABLE 1-4: HEALTHY PEOPLE 2010 FOCUS AREAS

1. Access to Quality Health Services
2. Arthritis, Osteoporosis, and Chronic Back Conditions
3. Cancer
4. Chronic Kidney Disease
5. Diabetes
6. Disability and Secondary Conditions
7. Educational and Community-Based Programs
8. Environmental Health
9. Family Planning and Sexual Health
10. Food Safety
11. Health Communication
12. Heart Disease and Stroke
13. HIV
14. Immunizations and Infectious Diseases
15. Injury and Violence Prevention
16. Maternal, Infant, and Child Health
17. Medical Product Safety
18. Mental Health and Mental Disorders
19. Nutrition
20. Occupational Safety and Health
21. Oral Health
22. Physical Activity and Fitness
23. Public Health Infrastructure
24. Respiratory Diseases
25. Sexually Transmitted Diseases
26. Substance Abuse
27. Tobacco Use
28. Vision and Hearing

Note. From U.S DHHS, http://www.healthypeople.gov

health in the next decade. These indicators were chosen based on their ability to motivate action, the availability of data to measure their progress, and their relevance as broad public health issues. Each of the indicators depends to some extent on:

- The information people have about their health and how to make improvements.

- Choices people make (behavioral factors).

- Where and how people live (environmental, economic, and social conditions).

- The type, amount, and quality of health care people receive (access to health care and characteristics of the healthcare system).

Improvements for the set of indicators will require effective public and private sector programs that address multiple factors. Many nurses working with older adults will be using these indicators to determine if their programs and services are meeting the Healthy People 2010 goals.

The Leading Health Indicator Categories

1. Physical Activity
2. Overweight and Obesity
3. Tobacco Use
4. Substance Abuse
5. Responsible Sexual Behavior
6. Mental Health
7. Injury and Violence
8. Environmental Quality
9. Immunization
10. Access to Health Care

Detailed information on specific goals are available from the Office of Disease Prevention and Health Promotion, U.S. Department of Health and Human Services. Extensive information is available at: http://www.healthypeople.gov.

HEALTH BEHAVIORS

Many models have been developed to try to explain why older people behave as they do, especially regarding their health. Health behaviors are the actions that a person does, or does not take, that have great impact on their health at any age. Diet, exercise, vaccinations, smoking, alcohol consumption, and safety issues such as wearing a seat belt are examples of health behaviors.

The Health Belief Model (Janz & Becker, 1984) proposes that people will take action to prevent or cope with a problem only if they believe themselves at significant risk of harm and that the proposed action will reduce the harm at less personal cost than the problem itself.

The Locus of Control Model (Wallston & Wallston, 1978) proposes that people who believe they can control what happens to them will do better in systems where they maintain that control, whereas people who feel controlled by outside forces will manage better in systems where they are not forced to make decisions.

The Model of Motivation (Loeb, O'Neill, & Gueldner, 2001) has many components that incorporate the parts of the two above models with other factors such as social and spiritual support and self-determination. This model is based on the belief that older adults are a heterogeneous group with diverse life differences. Factors that facilitate motivation in one individual, may not work as effectively for another (Loeb, O'Neill, & Gueldner, 2001).

Current State of Health Behaviors

Based on Healthy People 2000 guidelines, many of the health behaviors for older adults did not reach goals set for 2000. This included indicators of preventative health issues such as physical activity, optimal weight, healthy diet, and safety issues. The role of nursing is to assist patients in understanding their health and support them in making the changes necessary for health improvements. Exercise programs, stress management techniques, and dietary restrictions are examples of some common interventions that require patient motivation. Patients may easily understand lifestyle modifications but consistent, life-long behavior changes are difficult. Recommendations for nurses helping patients to change include the "just do it" approach, extensive office or home visits, behavior modification, record-keeping suggestions and fol-

low-up telephone calls. Patients may view nurses who use a confrontational approach as being critical rather than supportive. Relapse during any treatment program is sometimes viewed as a failure by all involved. A feeling of failure, especially when repeated, may cause patients to give up and avoid contact with their healthcare providers or avoid treatment altogether. After investing time and energy in promoting change, patients who fail are often labeled "noncompliant" or "unmotivated."

TABLE 1-5: TRANSTHEORETICAL STAGES OF CHANGE

Precontemplation Stage: During this stage, patients do not even consider changing. For example, smokers do not consider quitting, or patients with high cholesterol levels may feel "immune" to the health problems that strike others. *Nursing Role:* Starting with brief and simple advice about the health change. The goal for patients at this stage is to help them begin to think about changing a behavior. Empathy has been found to help engage patients in contemplating a change. Patients may become argumentative, hopeless, or in "denial," and the natural tendency is to try to "convince" them. This is viewed as a confrontational style, which is not often effective. Resistance is evidence that the nurse has moved too far ahead of the patient in the change process. It often takes weeks, months, or perhaps years to get a patient beyond this stage. Develop and maintain a positive relationship, personalize the risk factors, and pose questions that provoke thoughts about patient risk factors and the perceived benefits.

Contemplation Stage: During this stage, patients are ambivalent about changing. Giving up an enjoyed behavior causes them to feel a sense of loss, despite the perceived gain. During this stage, patients consider barriers as well as the benefits of change. *Nursing Role:* Education is required, focusing on the benefits of the specific change, various methods of changing, and the difficulties that might arise.

Preparation Stage: During this stage patients prepare to make a specific change. They may experiment with small changes as their determination to change increases, such as cutting down on smoking. They make specific plans such as the type of diet to go on, and they set a date. *Nursing Role:* Assist the patient in goal setting and when to start the change, and define a specific plan on how it will be done. Assist in providing services and information needed. An example is a patient who decides to stop smoking. Help her to set a date, make the decision to go to a smoking cessation group, and use a nicotine replacement patch. Provide information on smoking cessation meetings and make certain transportation is available. Also make certain she has the nicotine replacements prior to the "quit" date.

Action Stage: This stage is the one that most nurses are eager to see patients reach. *Nursing Role:* Any action taken by patients should be praised because it demonstrates the desire for lifestyle change. Assess for any difficulties that the patient is having, and determine what can be done to help overcome these.

Maintenance and Relapse Prevention: This stage involves incorporating the new behavior "over the long haul." Discouragement over occasional "slips" may halt the change process and result in the patient giving up. However, most patients find themselves "recycling" through the stages of change several times before the change becomes truly established. *Nursing Role:* Keep in touch with patients to encourage maintenance. For patients who experience relapses, the nurse should restart with them at stage two.

(Prochaska, 1979)

Labeling a patient in this way places responsibility for failure on the patient's character and ignores the complexity of the behavior change process. Research into smoking cessation and alcohol abuse has advanced the understanding of the change process. The Transtheoretical Stages of Change Model (Prochaska & Norcross, 2003) is useful for selecting appropriate interventions. (See Table 1-5.) It shows that for most persons, a change in behavior occurs gradually, with the patient moving from being uninterested, unaware, or unwilling to make a change (precontemplation), to considering a change (contemplation), then to deciding and preparing to make a change. Genuine, determined action is then taken and, over time, attempts to maintain the new behavior occurs. Relapses are almost inevitable and become part of the process of working toward life-long change. By identifying a patient's position in the change process, the nurse individualizes the intervention, usually with skills they already possess. The focus of the selection of an intervention is how to best facilitate the patient to move to the next stage of change.

CULTURAL INFLUENCES

According to Samovar and Porter (2003), culture refers to the cumulative deposit of knowledge, experience, beliefs, values, attitudes, meanings, hierarchies, religion, notions of time, roles, spatial relations, concepts of the universe, material objects, and possessions acquired by a group of people in the course of generations through individual and group striving. This is just one of many different definitions. A culture may be any group. A person can actually belong to more than one culture such as a male African American, who is a veteran and deaf. The greatest influence on culture is ethnicity while the sub-cultures take on a secondary role for most people. The role of ethnicity in health care is extremely important as the United States becomes more diverse and minorities gain in population percentages. In 2000

for persons over the age 65, 83.5% were white, 8.1% African American, 5.6% Hispanic, 2.4% Asian and Islanders, and 1.4% American Indian and Alaska Natives. These numbers are projected to continue to increase, with Hispanics being the fastest growing minority (U.S. Census Bureau, 2000). Research for the most part has looked at primarily white participants; therefore, much of the knowledge we have is specific to this population. Assessment instruments and tools have mostly been supported on white subjects. Medications have been tested for efficacy and side effects on mostly white subjects. It is very difficult to attempt to generalize about any population until more specific research is performed. The Hispanic culture has had some research attention. It has been found that this group tends to use more herbal medicines, is more likely to live in poverty, tends to hold onto traditional gender roles, views physical touch as a vital form of communication, and considers religion as a central element in their lives (Loera, Black, Markides, Espino, & Goodwin, 2001). From this information it may be concluded that there is a basis for understanding the Hispanic culture. However, some people feel that the term Hispanic makes a mockery out of diversity, by portraying Hispanics as a monolithic racial group with common heritage, culture, values, and interests. The term Hispanic encompasses at least three races, 18 nationalities, and scores of ethnic subgroups. A Hispanic may be an aristocrat from Spain, a Black from communist Cuba, or an Indian peasant from Mexico. In spite of this diversity Hispanics are continually lumped together as if they are of one race or from one nation. In examining the Native American culture, including Indians and Alaskans, another geographically diverse group is seen. The Native American population consists of over 500 different recognized tribes, each having their own culture, traditions, beliefs, and distinctions (Lowe & Struthers, 2001). Culture has an extensive impact on health behaviors, and nurses must realize that within each ethnic group are great numbers of sub-groups. Determining how a person's culture affects heath and health behaviors must be determined individually, by asking patients their particular beliefs, lifestyles, customs, and common practices.

POVERTY

The number of older adults living in poverty has declined steadily over the past several years. The official measurement of poverty is based on a family's annual income with different criteria based on family size and composition. Persons identified as living in poverty are at risk of having inadequate resources for food, housing, utilities, health care, clothing, transportation, and other basic needs. Poverty thresholds for an individual over age 65, living alone is $8,628 and for 2 persons is $10,874. Based on this, 10.1% of persons over 65 lived in poverty in 2001, with the highest rate being for those age 85 or over. Older women had higher poverty rates (12.8%) than men (7.2%), non-married (17.4%) versus married (4.9%). For ethnic groups, the poverty rates are white 8.2%, African Americans 26.4%, Asian & Pacific Islander 16% and Hispanics 21% (Social Security Administration, 2000). Nurses working with older adults need to be aware of any economic hardships of their patients. The addition of just one medication may cause an older adult to have to choose between the drug, food, or heat. Special diets may be difficult for a patient to afford, and lack of good health insurance may reduce a patient's access to health care. Lack of transportation, telephone service, or a low educational level may make it difficult for an older adult to arrange needed services. Nurses must be aware of the local, state, and federal programs available to help older adults and provide assistance in setting these services in place.

SUCCESSFUL AGING

Definitions and standards to measure successful aging abound. Some consider successful aging not just a long life span but a longer healthy life span. Chronological age tells us less about the circumstances, needs, or chance for successful aging of an individual. Many definitions of successful aging use quantitative data as criteria, that is, variables that can be counted and compared. Examples of these are measuring successful aging by being free of disabilities, the absence of disease, the maintenance of mental and physical functioning, or not losing any Activities of Daily Living (ADL) functioning. Still, some count the number of chronic illnesses or active engagement in life, or a complicated measurement of something in-between. When measured in any of these methods, less than half of older adults are aging successfully and for some methods, success is achieved by fewer than 20% (Strawbridge, Wallhagen, & Cohenet, 2002).

So what is successful aging? Perhaps asking older adults to self-rate their own health provides a good indicator of successful aging. This method gathers qualitative data, things that cannot easily be counted. When asked this way, 77% of older Caucasian adults (65–74), 69% of Hispanics, and 60% of African Americans rated their health as excellent. For the over 85 group, those that rated their health as excellent were 66.5% Caucasian, 53% Hispanic, and 50% African Americans (AOA, 2000). These figures are much more promising and serve to remind healthcare professionals that health and successful aging is much more than physical health. It is also about feeling needed, loved, and a sense of belonging within a community. It is about having a sense of perceived control over one's life (Kunzmann, Little, & Smith, 2002). It is about having basic needs met and some sense of financial security. It is about having opportunities, freedom, and being respected. It is about having events in one's life that bring joy and happiness. For nursing, assisting patients to age successfully means attending to all of their needs in a holistic manner and allowing the patient to determine success.

SUMMARY

Older adults of today are a vastly diverse group whose healthcare behaviors have a great impact on their quality of life and health. With diversity comes the need for nurses to have a wide variety of "tools" with which to help these individuals achieve, what they consider to be, successful aging. Knowing the who, what, and where of this population is the first step in developing a custom set of "tools" for the nursing trade.

EXAM QUESTIONS

CHAPTER 1

Questions 1-6

1. For the older adult, higher levels of education are usually associated with

    a. higher incomes and below-average health status.

    b. more stability in marital relationships.

    c. higher incomes and above-average health status.

    d. early retirement due to chronic diseases.

2. A healthcare setting that targets health promotion and disease prevention for Healthy People 2010 is

    a. an influenza vaccination clinic.

    b. a special care unit.

    c. a surgical unit.

    d. an emergency room.

3. Healthy behaviors are ones that are

    a. not amenable to change.

    b. not important to health outcomes after age 70.

    c. important to health outcomes at any age.

    d. only important in childhood.

4. When working with a Hispanic patient you will best communicate with her if you

    a. read about the Hispanic culture ahead of time.

    b. ask her how her beliefs and culture affect her health behaviors.

    c. only speak Spanish.

    d. ask her husband to answer any questions.

5. Your patient is an older man who lives with his wife in subsidized senior housing. For them to be considered above the poverty level, their yearly income must be at least

    a. $8,628.

    b. $10,874.

    c. $4,800.

    d. $9,875.

6. Successful aging can be measured by examining quantitative and qualitative data. A qualitative method of measuring successful aging is the

    a. number of chronic illnesses.

    b. chronological age.

    c. self-rating ones own health.

    d. amount of annual income.

CHAPTER 2

AGING:
THEORIES, PROCESS, AND MODELS

CHAPTER OBJECTIVE

After studying this chapter, the reader will be able to discuss aging theories and describe some of the normal aging changes.

LEARNING OBJECTIVES

After studying this chapter, the learner will be able to

1. recognize that aging has multiple causes, involving biological, psychological, and social causes.

2. discuss the implications that aging has on the needs of older adults according to Maslow.

3. describe the Chronic Illness Model and how this applies to older adults.

4. describe the cellular cause of physiological changes.

5. discuss the components of risk and their relationship to physiological changes of aging.

6. relate anatomical alterations in the cardiovascular system that impact decreased activity levels.

7. explain why older adults are at risk for the development of respiratory failure during stressful situations.

8. specify physiological changes of the musculoskeletal and nervous systems.

INTRODUCTION

It is generally agreed that there is no single known factor that causes aging or prevents the process. A very obvious feature of an aged population is the range of function. The rate of aging among different body systems within one individual may vary, with one system showing marked declines, while another may demonstrate no significant changes. A variety of degrees of physiological changes, capacities, and limitations can also be found within a given age group. These changes and losses demand multiple adjustments for the elderly and they are important for the healthcare provider to consider as a foundation for assessment and a framework for care. Aging is said to begin at conception and is a complex, multidimensional, natural phenomenon. Chronological age alone is not a predictor of individual performance or appearance. Lifestyle variables like physical activity, eating, drinking, smoking, and personality characteristics have an effect on the aging process. Some factors that predispose a person to disease also influence that person's response to aging. They include heredity, culture, race, nutritional status, and environmental factors. Experts sometimes have difficulty distinguishing changes that occur with normal aging and those that are caused by disease processes. In the past, considerable decline in major body systems was attributed to normal aging. It is now known that in addition to normal aging, disease, and disuse also play a significant role in functional decline. Consider the rule of thirds when working with older adults:

"Aging Changes" =
Disease + Disuse + Normal Aging

THEORIES OF AGING

Most individual theories about the causes of aging, like early theories about child development, center on a particular environmental or hereditary factor. There is growing opinion, however, that aging cannot be explained by an individual theory but rather that many different factors cause aging. Some of the biological and environmental theories of aging are summarized here, including a discussion of how some of them are interrelated.

At the cellular level, human aging shows the buildup of biological and chemical waste materials, which reduce the efficiency of the cell, until it loses ability to function. Cellular degeneration can result from environmental influences, such as damage caused by free radicals, radiation, viral cross-linking, or lipofuscin, or it can come from an intrinsic genetic influence, such as the inability to eliminate waste products. Free radicals are highly charged ions that damage many cellular structures, including DNA (Droge, 2002). Environmental radiation, which includes the solar radiation that everyone is exposed to every day, also can damage cells and their DNA. Viral cross-linking occurs when viruses borrow DNA strands from host cells and scramble the strands before giving them back. The scrambled DNA cannot work properly in making the cellular components it made before. As one ages, lipofuscin, a by-product of metabolism, accumulates, especially in the liver, heart, ovaries, and neurons. The exact function of lipofuscin is unknown (Brunk & Terman, 2002).

An intrinsic limit to aging was proposed by Hayflick, which is now called the Hayflick limit or Hayflick phenomenon (Hayflick, 1984). His proposal was that cells lose the ability to reproduce after approximately 50 divisions. This limit may parallel the gradual accumulation of nonfunctional cells that is also considered a part of aging. Interestingly, cancer cells do not have this limit and instead continue to grow indefinitely. However, if an old cell is combined genetically with a cancer cell, the new cells will no longer be able to divide indefinitely. In the interactions between cells, both environmental stress and genetics have an effect. For instance, environmental stress causes activation of the sympathetic nervous system, known as the fight-or-flight response, which, in time, causes the calcification of cells. But genetic factors also influence both the severity of the stress reaction and the amount of cellular change it causes. Environmental factors such as poor diet, inadequate exercise, and smoking can decrease respiratory and circulatory function, leading to many kinds of chronic disease. Intrinsically, the immune system loses its specificity as one ages. Simultaneously, humans lose their immunity to foreign antigens, called isoimmunity, and acquire an increasing immunity to one's own changing cells, called autoimmunity. A decrease in the size of the thymus occurs with age and causes a diminished number of newly formed T lymphocytes and a decreased capability of T lymphocytes to proliferate. It is apparent that a cell can change quite a bit before it loses its ability to function, but a very small change can result in a cell's being seen as an intruder to be attacked by one's own immune system. This immune response may cause many of the problems that occur in people as they get older, such as arthritis, diabetes, heart disease, cancer, and even tooth loss. There is also a theory that an intrinsic aging hormone begins to be produced at adolescence and increases over time, causing many of the changes of aging. These theories of biological aging may help us to understand the physical process of aging, but they do not begin to explain the interpersonal behavior that occurs as a person ages. To understand interpersonal interactions, several social theories of aging have been proposed.

SOCIAL THEORIES OF AGING

Several theories have evolved to explain the social interaction of people as they age. The old theory of **disengagement** was that the elderly and society withdraw from each other in a mutually sought and satisfying separation (Bell, 1978). This theory has not been able to explain why seniors who are not withdrawn are generally healthier and happier. The **activity theory** proposes that there is a connection between activity and life satisfaction (Lemon, Bengtson, & Peterson, 1972). Both interpersonal activity and physical activity contribute to a persons sense of well-being as he or she becomes older. A **socioenvironmental theory** was developed that proposed that senior citizens living with others of their own age would have increased social interaction and therefore have increased life satisfaction (Stone, 1996). This theory fits in with surveys that indicated that, on the average, the elderly would rather live with others of their own age, and near, but not with, their children. But the social interaction theory could not explain why many satisfied elderly lived in age-integrated communities, or why many elderly living in age-segregated communities were not happy or healthy.

An **exchange theory**, adapted from political science, explained that people tend to maximize rewards of social interaction while minimizing costs: PROFIT = REWARD – COST (Dowd, 1975). Therefore, two people will continue to interact if it is to the social profit of each. When one person receives more social profit from an interaction, that person gains power over the person who receives less profit. In our society, in which youth and modernization are valued, the elderly may lose more and more power as they become more dependent on the young. Seniors can restore this power

through three mechanisms: (1) withdrawing, which decreases their cost; (2) developing alternative skills that will be valued by others and increase the others' reward; or (3) forming social and political coalitions that increase the seniors' power directly.

The **continuity theory** is a psychosocial theory of aging that states that as individuals strive to cope with aging and achieving their goals, their past experiences, decisions, and behaviors will form the foundation for their present and future decisions and behaviors (Lifton, 1973). This may serve as a useful framework for nurses to use to understand how an individual adapts to aging, illness, and disability.

As people age, the basic needs as defined by Maslow remain intact. **Maslow's Hierarchy of Needs** is a holistic look at what motivates people and that certain lower needs must be satisfied before higher needs can be met (Maslow, 1954). Aging has an impact on the ability to meet these needs just as the inability to meet these needs contributes to the aging process. This theory defines people as basically trustworthy, self-protecting, and self-governing with tendencies toward growth and love. As long as a person is motivated to satisfy these cravings while aging, there is movement towards growth, and ultimately self-actualization. Satisfying these needs is healthy. Blocking gratification makes people physically or emotionally sick. The needs as defined by Maslow (1954) are:

Physiological Needs: These are very basic needs such as air, water, food, sleep, or sex. When these are not satisfied the older adult usually feels sickness, irritation, pain, or discomfort. These feelings motivate individuals to alleviate them as soon as possible to establish homeostasis. Until these needs are met, it is difficult to focus on anything else. For older adults with dementia, it may be difficult for them to satisfy these basic needs on their own.

Safety Needs: These have to do with establishing stability and consistency in a chaotic world. These needs are mostly psychological in nature. The older adult needs the security of a home, friends, and family on whom to rely on and financial stability. The older adult may also have a fear of being abused, driving, pain, the future, becoming injured or not having a reliable person to assist them to remain in their home. Safety needs sometimes motivate people to be religious. Religion comforts with the promise of a safe secure place after one dies and leaves the insecurity of this world.

Love Needs: Love and belongingness come from the human desire to belong to groups such as clubs, work groups, religious groups, family, or gangs. It is the need to feel loved (non-sexual) and to be accepted by others. An older adult who is unable to get out may become socially isolated and depressed as their needs for belonging are unmet.

Esteem Needs: There are two types of esteem needs. First is self-esteem, which results from competence or mastery of a task. Second, there is the attention and recognition that comes from others. This is similar to the belongingness level; however, wanting admiration has to do with the need for power. For the older adult, this need becomes satisfied by their lifetime achievements, be it in a career, a mastery, or though satisfaction from their children. When nurses show older adults respect and take the time to find out who their patients are, the nurses are acknowledging patients as people and helping to satisfy the patients' esteem needs.

Self-Actualization: The need for self-actualization is the desire to become more and more what one is and to become everything that one is capable of becoming. When this occurs individuals are able to find knowledge, peace, esthetic experiences, and/or self-fulfillment. This can bring peace to an older adult at the end of life. Nurses can assist in this process by helping patients perform a life review, which is a structured way of looking back, re-experiencing, and sharing with others important life experiences, decisions, and relationships.

CHRONIC ILLNESS MODEL

Very few older adults manage through the aging process without having any chronic illness or condition. Mismanagement of the condition by the older adult contributes to the aging process; therefore, an understanding of this chronic illness model is important.

A chronic disease model creates a basis for the underlying care of older adults. The Corbin and Strauss Trajectory Model (Corbin & Strauss, 1991) is based on the premise that a chronic illness course can be shaped and managed over time, even if the course of the disease cannot be modified. This model defines chronic illness as the irreversible presence, accumulation, or latency of disease states or impairments that involve the total human environment for supportive care and self-care, maintenance of function, and prevention of further disability. "Trajectory" implies a multidimensional course or unfolding of chronic illness that profoundly affects an individual and those around him or her in all aspects of life. Illness, characterized by symptoms, influences a person's life, and aspects of life influence a person's ability to manage their illness. This model details various stages that occur for a patient with a chronic illness. The management of all phases of most chronic illness, except for acute and deteriorating, takes place in the home. Part of the model is the understanding that an illness is not just experienced as part of life, it must be managed and requires work. Healthcare providers, family, friends, or the ill person can do this work. Within the context of home and family life, the central feature of illness management is the establishment and maintenance of arrangements. These arrangements enable the illness work to be more or less effective. Most arrangements involve organizing the time and efforts of the ill person in conjunction with those of family, friends, relatives, and perhaps neighbors. These arrangements are almost always revised and reorganized in accordance with changes in illness phases. The major concern of the ill and their families is not merely managing an illness, but maintaining quality of life, as defined specifically by them, despite the illness. The goal of nursing within this model is to assist those afflicted to shape their course while maintaining quality of life. Nursing care centers on health promotion and collaboration with the individual, family, or community and self-care or management of the chronic condition. (Corbin & Strauss, 1991).

PHYSIOLOGICAL CHANGES

In order to stay alive, the body must live on the wings of change. The skin replaces itself once a month, the stomach lining every five (5) days, and the skeleton every three (3) months. As one ages, overall physiological changes can be traced to basic cellular changes. It is estimated that an older person possesses 30% fewer cells than when they were younger. This is partially due to generalized slowing of cell division. This loss of cells accounts for substantial weight reduction in a number of body organs. Cells also change in their ability to perform specialized integrated functions and combine in irregular patterns. These changes may be attributed to cellular changes including lipofuscin accumulation; decreased cytoplasmic RNA; and cell nucleus changes, with DNA not being replaced after final developmental mitosis or cell division. An additional overall change is a decrease in both intracellular and extracellular fluids. This total body fluid decrease makes an elder more susceptible to dehydration and affects the dilution ability of the body when certain kinds of drugs are used. These cellular changes contribute to the fact that physiological changes are universal, progressive, decremental, and intrinsic. These changes do not hinder an elder in the task of daily living under normal, nonstressful conditions. A person adapts to needs and functional ability, and special considera-

tion may be necessary in times of stress, illness, and overexertion. Major physiological aging can be analyzed through parameters such as cardiac output, pulmonary function, and glomerular filtration or through physiological changes by body systems. In both cases, it is important to consider the person as a whole and to consider the whole as more than the sum of its parts.

RISK: A FRAMEWORK

A risk is a condition that may compromise a person's health or longevity (Hill & Smith, 1990). One may conclude that a major difference exists between morbidity and mortality in the young and old because of differences in risks. These risks are related to situations in which an individual is exposed to an increased possibility of emotional, social, or physical injury. Risk factors may be actual, potential, or perceived. They threaten a person's health or well-being. From a physiological perspective, risks may be due to structural and functional changes of aging. They may decrease a person's ability to maintain homeostasis. The conceptual model for risk reduction proposed by Blum (1980) provides a good beginning to determine the needs of individuals and groups of older adults. Nurses have an important role in fostering a level of self-care, self-responsibility, and self-determination in decreasing risk, adapting to change, and promoting wellness. This role is important in all settings: hospitals, nursing homes, community, and other sites that provide health care to the elderly. Effective nursing care planning recognizes potential risks and strategic ways to intervene rationally to reduce these risks. It is important to note that risks are not an all-or-none situation, and nurses must consider degrees of risk.

Risk Factors Contributing to Impaired Functional Status

Many evaluate their health state in relation to their functional ability or activity status. Society tends to translate a person's value and worth into what the person does and contributes. For an elderly person, what is done and contributed might differ than when they were a younger adult. As one ages, functional status is affected by capabilities and limitations, as well as external factors mandated by society. Successful aging is often evaluated by the ability of the person to stay active, maintain activities, and continue to be involved in life. Maintaining independence is a major goal for an elderly person, and a major issue is the fear of becoming a burden or dependent. For nurses, the inclusion of functional status as part of an assessment shifts the delivery of care from a curing-of-disease focus to improving or maintaining function. Such an approach has an indirect and a direct impact on a person's daily quality of life.

As a group (a macro perspective), one in five persons 65 years or older have mild degrees of functional impairment. These mild limitations affect basic activities of living (ADL) needs, such as eating, dressing, toileting, grooming, ambulating, and bathing. Some persons may also have difficulties in maintaining themselves in the community. This might be reflected as an inability to do instrumental activities of daily living (IADL) such as shop, clean house, do laundry, handle fiances, or use transportation. As one advances in age, the probability of multiple or severe functional impairment develops.

As a group, the elderly are a microcosm of society. Overall, many in our country live sedentary lives, which make it increasingly difficult to remain or become active. It is estimated that only 8% of the elderly are regularly active. Regularly active is defined as engaging in activities lasting at least 20 minutes, three times per week. This regular activity requires motivation. The pace must be adjusted to avoid fatigue, muscle pain, and cramping. Less efficient management may cause shortness of breath, muscle weakness, severe fatigue, and decreased range of motion. It is important to note that regular, ongoing activity facilitates the functioning of the respiratory, circulatory, and musculoskeletal systems. Impaired functioning of these systems may affect a person's ability to stay actively involved and cognitive abilities.

Activity can be compromised because of physiological changes. Under normal circumstances, a person's activity level progressively slows, and he or she exhibits a methodical manner that allows him or her to engage in normal activity while conserving energy, preventing undue fatigue, and providing balance. Persons with insufficient physiological energy to ensure or complete required or desired daily activities may be experiencing activity intolerance.

According to Bowles (1991), the following are common contributing factors to activity intolerance:

- Compromised oxygenation
- Neuromuscular limitations
- Progressive decreased activity
- Bed rest and immobility
- Generalized weakness or fatigue

From a systems perspective, the following may be risks to maintaining an active state and may cause potential activity intolerance:

- Decreased cardiac output
- Decreased breathing capacity and efficiency
- Decreased muscle mass, strength, and movement
- Demineralization of bone; deterioration of cartilage and surface of joints
- Altered neurological functioning inhibiting regulating activities, such as skeletal movement

What physiological changes may contribute to each of these?

PHYSIOLOGICAL CHANGES OF THE CARDIOVASCULAR SYSTEM

As one ages, the heart and blood vessels change in several ways. From middle age, the prevalence of cardiovascular disease continues to be the major cause of death. Because normal changes occur independently of pathological processes and because of a high incidence of cardiac disease, it is often difficult to determine which changes are age-related and which are associated with disease. As with other bodily changes, cardiovascular changes are slow and insidious (Cheitlin, 2003). Major influences on these changes in the cardiovascular system are arteriosclerotic changes, which increase with aging and are considered by many a normal aging process, because it develops in everyone to some extent. The cardiovascular system adapts to these processes and most exhibit no related health problems. Arteriosclerotic changes begin soon after birth and are characterized by progressive thickening of the arterial lumen and collagen and calcium accumulation. The term "arteriosclerosis" encompasses the pathologic processes of atherosclerosis, arteriolosclerosis, and Monckeberg's medial calcific sclerosis. Monckeberg's sclerosis (Chaudhry, 2003) is a form of arteriosclerosis that is characterized by calcific deposits in the media of small to medium-sized muscular arteries. Because the intima is not involved, the lumen is not compromised, and there is little clinical consequence to the pure form of this abnormality. Arteriolosclerosis affects small vessels (arterioles) and is best demonstrated in the renal arterioles. Atherosclerosis is the presence of plaque composed primarily of fat on the artery walls and is a major cause of cardiovascular disease. In general, the arteries, which are pliable and elastic when young, become less elastic, dilated and elongated. These physiological changes make the heart work harder to push blood into the less elastic arteries. It is important to note that research studies demonstrate that sodium intake has an effect on arterial elasticity (Barenbrock, Kosch, & Hausberg, 2003). Overall arterial changes appear to be widespread and result in diminished circulation to all organs and tissues. A major impact is the reduced circulation to the brain and kidneys, but adaptive responses contribute to age-related normal functioning. Factors such as stress and exercise increase cardiovascular workload on this stabilized, maintained system. It is estimated that cardiovascular workload increases as much as four or five times during stress.

The impact of aging on the heart influences the total cardiovascular system. The heart, as a muscular organ, changes as muscle fibers are replaced by fibrous tissue. Collagenous buildup can almost encase the heart in a collagen matrix. These anatomical changes lead to diminished contractibility and filling capacity (Burgess, McCrea, & Hedrick, 2001). Heart valves tend to increase in thickness, and calcium salt deposits may occur on certain valves. These changes may modify the normal closing of the valves, causing murmurs or abnormal heart sounds. An overall adaptive response may be myocardial hypertrophy. This response is made in an attempt to maintain normal heart volume and pump function. Considerations must be given to cardiac strength, efficiency, and the decreased stroke volume. Despite these adaptations, cardiac output does decrease. It is estimated that the cardiac output decreases as much as 50% by the age of 80. The normal average output of 5 liters/minute decreases below 3 liters/minute. This diminished cardiac output again becomes significant when an elderly person is physically or mentally stressed by illness, disability, activity, worry, loss, or excitement.

A frequent cardiovascular measure is blood pressure. It is debatable as to how aging and these physiological changes affect this measure of cardiovascular status. Some believe normal blood pressure for older persons is in the range of 140mm Hg systolic and 90mm Hg diastolic. Older and younger adults have similar blood pressure. The definition of hypertension is a systolic pressure at or above 140mm Hg and a diastolic pressure at or above 90mm Hg. Three quarters of women and one half of men over the age 75 have hypertension (Samraj & Kuritzky, 2002). Some think systolic increases are due to decreased aortic elasticity, and others believe that peripheral resistance in the vessels causes an increase in both systolic and diastolic pressure. Whatever the belief, it is importance to establish a baseline normal for each patient. Hypertension can be a major health problem for the elderly because it is the primary risk factor for strokes and is a contributing factor for myocardial infarctions (Samraj & Kuritzky, 2002). The usefulness of treating hypertension in the elderly is still being studied. Most elderly people will want to be treated if it is relatively inexpensive and the side effects of the treatment not too bothersome. Lifestyle and dietary changes should continue along with drug therapy.

Another measure of cardiovascular evaluation is the electrocardiogram (ECG). The ECG may reveal changes in heart functioning as affected by exercise. For example, during exercise, S-T segment shifts may point to inadequate oxygen metabolism possibly due to partial coronary occlusion. Extra beats of the ventricles may be precipitated by exercise. The frequency of an abnormal exercise ECG increases with age and is present in about 30% of persons 65 and older. Conduction is also affected by a decrease in the total number of pacemaker cells in the sinoatrial node. Alterations may include blocks or irregular discharges. The baroreceptors in the aortic and carotid arteries also become less sensitive to pressure changes with aging. This results in low response to postural changes, and changes in position may cause dizzi-

ness or syncope. Elderly persons who are taking vasodilators, diuretics, or beta-blockers should be observed for this orthostatic response in the form of hypotension.

In summary, with advancing years, the physiological changes of the cardiovascular system affect and alter the function of the whole body. Under normal circumstances, the cardiovascular system adapts and allows the person to maintain a "normal" level of functioning, but the effect of these changes may alter activity level. Table 2-1 is a summary of the contributing cardiovascular changes.

TABLE 2-1: FACTORS CONTRIBUTING TO CARDIOVASCULAR CHANGE

The Heart

Elasticity decreases.

Rate at rest and maximum achievable rate declines.

Decrease in rate is compensated for by an increase in stroke volume to maintain cardiac output.

The conduction system loses cells and fibers and becomes infiltrated with fat.

Intrinsic contractile functioning declines.

Diastolic murmurs increase (more than 50% of older adults have such a murmur).

Vascular

Compliance decreases due to changes in proliferation and fibrosis, decreased elasticity, and calcification.

Peripheral resistance increases.

Systolic blood pressure increases, with lower rate if increase in diastolic pressure.

PHYSIOLOGICAL CHANGES OF THE RESPIRATORY SYSTEM

Respiratory health is vital to the elder's ability to maintain a physically, mentally, and socially active life style. It can make the difference between whether or not a person will maximize opportunities to live life to the fullest or be too fatigued and uncomfortable to leave the confines of his or her home. Often the frightening and anxiety-producing feeling of breathlessness is accepted as a situation associated with growing old. To prevent this subjective feeling, a person may diminish activity (Stanley & Beare, 1995). Breathlessness, or activity intolerance, is the most common physiologic response to exercise of a sedentary person. It is estimated that the maximum oxygen consumption rate during stress and moderate exercise can increase nine times for an older adult. For older adults whose physiological changes of the respiratory system are both structural and functional, respirations tend to be shallower and more frequent, and control becomes less precise. Maximum breathing capacity is diminished 50% by age 60, and actual air flow is reduced 20–30%. Older men and women have a lower total lung capacity and vital capacity. A 20-year-old man has a vital capacity of 5.20 liters compared with 4.00 liters for those 60 years old. Women's values are 4.17 and 3.29 liters, respectively. This change requires the elderly to move 50% more air than younger persons. By age 90, most lungs have enough alveolar destruction to meet the strict criteria for a diagnosis of emphysema. These changes are related to loss of elasticity in the chest wall, calcification of cartilage in rib joints and vertebrae, destruction of the alveoli, and general wasting of muscles, including those required for respiration.

Respiratory system changes, as in other body systems, are gradual. Problems develop more easily and are more difficult to manage. Immobility, due to fractures, depression, weakness, a fear of falling, and a multitude of other reasons, is a major threat to pulmonary health. Pulmonary health becomes even more compromised when a person becomes bedridden, even for a short period. This problem is due to the fact that although lung capacity is not significantly altered, redistribution occurs with lung expansion and inflation at the lung base, which is dramatically decreased. A loss of cough strength reduces mucus transport, which also complicates the situation. In addition to evaluating the respiratory status of patients who are bedridden or immobile, healthcare providers need to be concerned about medications that patients may be taking. Many medications cause problems and affect the somewhat compromised respiratory system. Cough suppressants and analgesics may cause depression of respirations and sputum retention. Sedatives and tranquilizers may also depress respirations. These potential drug responses reinforce the fact that a drug history, including over-the-counter drugs, is essential.

Under normal circumstances, the elderly can engage in activities of daily living without evidence or concern for the changes in the respiratory system. It is important to note that these changes have been affected by an accumulation of environmental factors such as air pollution, tobacco smoking, and infection. The prevalence of respiratory abnormalities tends to be much higher in the elderly population than in other segments (Manda & Rennard, 2002).

Respiratory status can be assessed best from interview, observation, and auscultation. Keep in mind that respiratory system limitations may not be apparent when the patient is at rest.

The following are some of the questions that should be asked during the initial assessment:

- Do you have wheezing, chest pain, coughing, phlegm, a heavy feeling in your chest, or shortness of breath after a walk?

- Do you frequently get a cold or flu? How often during the season?

- How many pillows do you use?

- Do you or have you ever smoked? How long and how much?

- Have you ever worked in a job that may have caused you to be short of breath or caused you to cough? What kind of job was this? Were you ever exposed to asbestos?

Respiratory system changes can be categorized into four aspects: airway clearance, immunity or defense mechanism alteration, physical properties, and respiratory control. Analyses of important changes include structural and functional changes as well as defense mechanism changes. These changes include alterations to those organs directly related to the respiratory system as well as supportive and facilitating associated organs. Cardiac output is also directly related to pulmonary function, endorsing and supporting the interrelationship of body systems.

Structural changes reduce maximum breathing capacity. Some of these changes include changes in the thoracic cage, reduced lung elasticity, and pulmonary artery changes as in the cardiovascular system. Lung expansion is altered by configuration changes of the thorax, calcification of the costal cartilages, and changes in posture and abdominal girth. The chest diameter from anterior to posterior may increase and the transverse measure decreases. This alteration is called kyphosis. Reduced lung elasticity is another major structural change associated with a cross-linkage in collagen and elastin fibers around the alveolar sacs. The primary fibrous connective tissue proteins of the lungs are collagen, elastin, and reticulum. With aging, the ratio of elastin to collagen is increased (Hampton, 1991). This causes a reduction in elasticity, altering the alveolar ducts and stretching the alveoli, which decreases the amount of surface available for oxygen diffusion.

TABLE 2-2: FACTORS CONTRIBUTING TO RESPIRATORY CHANGES

Decreased pulmonary elasticity as a result of collagen and elastin changes

Accessory muscle atrophy of pharynx and larynx

Decreased respiratory muscle strength

Decreased chest wall compliance, due to stiffness of chest wall and costal cartilage calcification

Increased anteroposterior diameter of chest

Alveolar duct and sac enlargement and less total alveolar surface for gas exchange

Fewer alveoli in lungs and thickening of the alveolar membranes

Decreased diffusion

Decrease in ciliary hair movement

Increased trapping of air

Decreased blood flow in pulmonary circulation

Increase in residual volume and functional residual capacity

Decrease in vital capacity and expiratory flow rates

Decrease in arterial PO2

The main functional respiratory problems in the elderly who do not have pulmonary disease are reduced ventilation of all alveoli, especially at the bases of the lungs, and reduced oxygen postural pressure in the arterial blood. From a physiological perspective, these changes are seen as alterations in supportive or ancillary function as well as altered lung mechanics and ventilatory function. The major functional changes are alterations in respiratory muscle functioning, associated loss or decreased elastic recoil, and alterations in lung volumes and breathing patterns. Although total lung capacity does not dramatically change, residual volume increases, and a decrease in vital capacity also occurs. The older person's response may be noticed as incomplete exhalation, inhibiting lung inflation and promoting secretion collection. Table 2-2 summarizes the physiological changes of the respiratory system.

These alterations place the elderly at risk for impaired functional status. It is also important to note that the maintenance of respiratory functioning is enhanced by the maintenance of functional status at the highest level possible.

PHYSIOLOGICAL CHANGES OF THE MUSCULOSKELETAL SYSTEM

The general integrity of the musculoskeletal system is related to its physiological functions of protection of internal organs, body shape, mobility, stability, coordination, and balance. Maintenance requires an appropriate level of activity, adequate rest of its parts, and adequate nourishment. The decrease of muscle mass, loss of strength, skeletal inflexibility, loss of equilibrium, and limited ability to provide movement are most often seen as the major contributors to impaired functional status. The physiological changes of the musculoskeletal system are among the earliest and most obvious to the person affected. Posture and structural changes occur primarily because of calcium loss from bone and atrophy of cartilage and muscles.

Alterations are affected by circulatory and respiratory function. The changes affect mobility and may force an elderly person to become more dependent on others and may diminish his or her life span.

An analysis of the physiological changes that occur in the musculoskeletal system must consider each component that contributes to a healthy sys-

tem. These three components are muscle, bone structure, and joints. These three form an integrated system, adapting to meet the needs of a person.

Muscle

Muscle change during aging is an individualized process with a high degree of variability. The muscles undergo a great amount of atrophy with age, and there is a gradual decrease in both the number of muscle fibers and their individual bulk. This muscle mass reduction may make it more difficult to control movement. A diminished storage of muscular glycogen may cause a loss of energy reserve, which contributes to a rapid onset of fatigue. Patterns of adaptation to this physiological change include taking frequent rest periods and taking and allowing more time to go somewhere or to do something. As noted, muscle fibers decrease and atrophy as age progresses. This process begins by age 40, and fibrous tissue gradually replaces muscle tissue, because muscle cells do not regenerate. This process is influenced by diet, especially potassium and ineffective oxygenation. Cellular changes occur in the muscles. Muscles are composed of postmitotic cells, and these cells are dependent on the inclusion of neural components. These cells become depositories for lipofuscin, the refuse of cellular function. Muscle mass is altered by extracellular increases in fat, collagen, and interstitial fluid. Extracellular water, chloride, and sodium are increased in the muscles of the elderly. Regular exercise, even if started in later life, improves muscle strength, tone, and stamina. Generally, it is speculated that a man of 70 has 50% the strength of a man of 30. By 80 years of age, strength and stamina decrease to 65–85% of the maximum strength that a person had at his or her peak of 25 years of age.

Bone Structure

Around the age of 40, bone mass and density shift and begin to decline. In addition to affecting mobility, these changes also predispose the elderly to accidents. Bone mass changes are associated with age, sex, and race. Other influencing factors include nutrition; sedentary life style; alcohol abuse; immobilization; and diseases such as diabetes, chronic renal disease, hyperthyroidism, and adrenal hyperactivity. Women are more vulnerable to bone loss; men have approximately 50% of the age-related bone loss than women do. This bone loss in women occurs especially in the decade following menopause. Ethnic differences have also been seen. Blacks have a higher peak bone density than whites, and Hispanic women have lower bone density than black women, but higher than white women.

The changes of bones are gradual and are due to reabsorption of the interior matrix of the long and flat bones. The external surface of the bones also begins to thicken. These changes are not observable but are evident by alterations in posture and stature. A human being loses 1.2 cm of height every 20 years. The decrease in height occurs in both men and women but is greater in women. It presents itself in the characteristic short trunk and long extremities and is caused by osteoporotic vertebral narrowing. Two additional factors contributing to this shortening of stature are kyphosis and osteoporosis. It is important to note that this change alters a person's center of gravity. Reaching and climbing may become more difficult. Stooped posture may also cause a decrease in the visual field.

Joints

Joints are the articulating surfaces of adjoining bones. Deterioration of these surfaces begins at age 30 and is exaggerated by injury, obesity, and excessive use. By age 70, an evaluation of the joints reflects a lifetime of wear and tear. Overall, the joints become less mobile, because the cartilage tends to lose water and the joints fuse at the cartilage surfaces. In summary, the musculoskeletal changes can be analyzed by looking at changes in muscles, bone structure, and joints. A summary of these changes is outlined in Table 2-3.

Five characteristics may be seen in various degrees. These are muscle wasting, lack of strength, lack of endurance, lack of agility, and complaints of fatigue. Assessment of these characteristics should include consideration of the following:

- Posture, stance, gait (length of stride), and pace
- Speed when walking
- Difficulty sitting and standing
- Ability to climb and descend stairs

These elements may give clues to musculoskeletal integrity and its relationship to a person's level of physical activity.

TABLE 2-3: FACTORS CONTRIBUTING TO MUSCULOSKELETAL CHANGES

Decrease in muscle weight and lean muscle mass in addition to muscle cell atrophy

Decrease in muscle strength and endurance due to decrease in muscle fibers

Shortening of trunk due to intervertebral space narrowing

Bone loss (universal and highly variable, more rapid in women after menopause)

Decrease in water content in hyaline cartilage lining joint surfaces

Hardening of ligaments, tendons, and joints, leading to an increase in rigidity and a decrease in flexibility

Decrease in muscular glycogen storage, causing loss of energy reserve

PHYSIOLOGICAL CHANGES OF THE NERVOUS SYSTEM

It is difficult to identify with accuracy and exactness the impact of aging itself on the nervous system, due to the dependence of this system's function on other body systems. This relationship

FIGURE 2-1: AGING CHANGES IN THE BRAIN

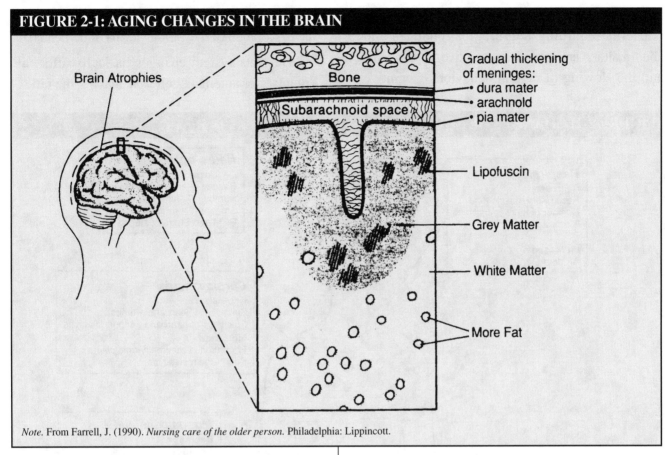

Note. From Farrell, J. (1990). *Nursing care of the older person.* Philadelphia: Lippincott.

and the complexity of function of the nervous system make it difficult to differentiate changes that are caused by aging or disease. The changes that do occur in the nervous system may be unnoticed and nonspecific and progress slowly. They may be vague, abstract complaints, and alterations in thinking, feeling, reasoning, and remembering. Alterations of the nervous system can affect activities of daily living, contribute to impaired functional status, and modify the quality of life.

The cells of the nervous system do not regenerate, and they are never replaced. This loss of cells begins at birth, is not uniform throughout the system, and has little impact on the functioning of that system. The changes in the nervous system are primarily the result of two things: diminished blood flow to the brain and loss of nerve cells (neurons). It is estimated that a person loses several thousand neurons a day. Dendrite branches decrease, and the rate of nerve impulse conduction decreases about 10%. It has also been found that with aging, glucose

and protein synthesis decreases in the neurons, causing loss of neurons. The total system of brain, nerves and spinal cord exhibits decreased vascularity and fibrotic changes.

Accompanying aging is a slow, progressive loss in brain size. Over a normal life span, a 10% or greater loss of brain weight can be anticipated. Losses occur in both gray and white matter, more so in gray matter, which is thought to contribute to the development of Alzheimer's Disease. Cerebral cortical cell loss is notable after age 50, and by age 90, the loss in some cortical zones (frontal and superior temporal regions) is about 50%. The coverings of the brain, dura mater, arachnoid, and pia mater gradually thicken and become more fibrous. These changes are summarized in Figure 2-1.

A person interacts with the environment through his or her nervous system. It is an organizing and communication interaction, composed of receiving, processing, and responding. These functions occur through a complex system of connections and interconnections of neurons. Two major concerns regarding neurological changes and abnormalities are related to cognitive impairments and the slowing of certain behaviors. Cognitive impairments are addressed in another chapter with the exploration of the various forms of dementia.

Nervous system changes basically affect all voluntary or automatic reflexes, making the reflex-

FIGURE 2-2: CHANGES OF AGING AT A GLANCE

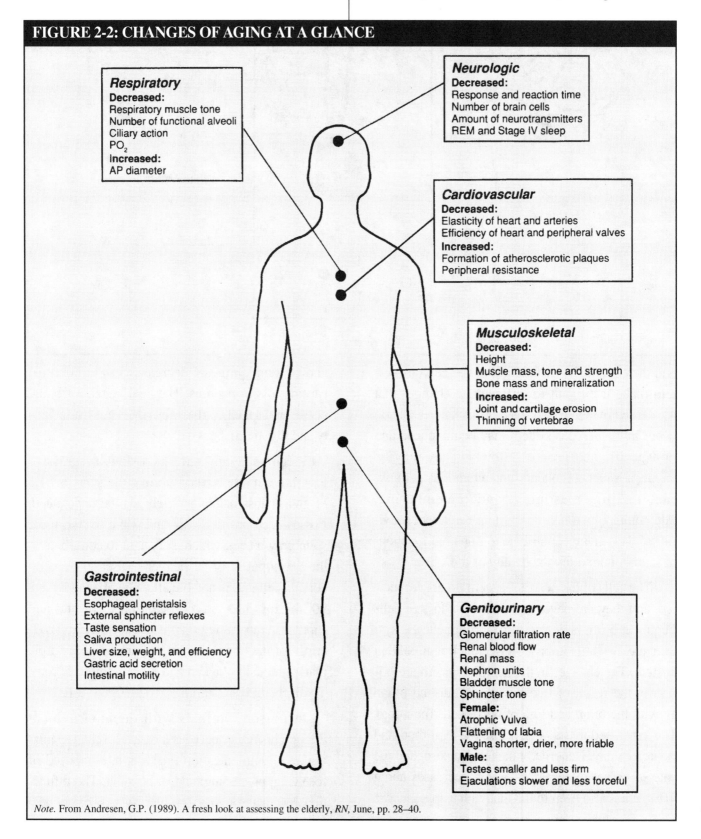

Respiratory
Decreased:
Respiratory muscle tone
Number of functional alveoli
Ciliary action
PO_2
Increased:
AP diameter

Neurologic
Decreased:
Response and reaction time
Number of brain cells
Amount of neurotransmitters
REM and Stage IV sleep

Cardiovascular
Decreased:
Elasticity of heart and arteries
Efficiency of heart and peripheral valves
Increased:
Formation of atherosclerotic plaques
Peripheral resistance

Musculoskeletal
Decreased:
Height
Muscle mass, tone and strength
Bone mass and mineralization
Increased:
Joint and cartilage erosion
Thinning of vertebrae

Gastrointestinal
Decreased:
Esophageal peristalsis
External sphincter reflexes
Taste sensation
Saliva production
Liver size, weight, and efficiency
Gastric acid secretion
Intestinal motility

Genitourinary
Decreased:
Glomerular filtration rate
Renal blood flow
Renal mass
Nephron units
Bladder muscle tone
Sphincter tone
Female:
Atrophic Vulva
Flattening of labia
Vagina shorter, drier, more friable
Male:
Testes smaller and less firm
Ejaculations slower and less forceful

Note. From Andresen, G.P. (1989). A fresh look at assessing the elderly, *RN,* June, pp. 28–40.

es slower. The slowing of certain behaviors is viewed as one of the most significant age-related functional changes of the nervous system. It is composed of both slower reflexes and delayed responses to multiple stimuli. These changes can make reflexes needed for tasks such as driving, writing, or dressing slower. These changes, or slowing down of movement, can be frustrating to a hurried healthcare provider who may find it easier and faster to do for patients rather than to have them do it for themselves. Table 2-4 summarizes factors that contribute to nervous system changes.

TABLE 2-4: FACTORS CONTRIBUTING TO NERVOUS SYSTEM CHANGES

Slowing of voluntary or automatic reflexes with a decreased ability to respond to multiple stimuli

Moderate cortical atrophy

Lower nerve conduction velocity

Loss of neurons in neocortex, substantia nigra, and limbic system

Decrease in number and size of peripheral nerve fibers with a decrease in motor and sensory nerve conduction

Less kinesthetic sense

Accumulation of lipofuscin

Decrease in binding sites for dopamine and serotonin

Decreased blood flow to the brain

SUMMARY

This chapter explored many different theories on aging including biological and social theories. It also explored a multitude of physiological changes that occur with aging. Not all body systems are included in this chapter as a number of other systems are addressed in other chapters. Figure 2-2 summarizes a number of these changes.

It is important to know the distinction between normal aging changes and a disease process.

EXAM QUESTIONS

CHAPTER 2

Questions 7-14

7. The most accurate statement concerning the cause of aging is

   a. genetic changes are solely responsible for the aging process.

   b. environment is stronger than heredity.

   c. disengagement explains the isolation of older people.

   d. aging is probably caused by multiple factors.

8. A physiological need as defined by Maslow (1954) would be an older adult who

   a. can no longer go to her Women's Club.

   b. lives with an abusive spouse.

   c. does not have enough money to buy food.

   d. has no means of transportation.

9. According to Corbin and Strauss (1991), the major concern of chronically ill persons is

   a. maintaining quality of life despite an illness.

   b. the successful curing of the illness.

   c. maintaining hope for a cure.

   d. modifying the course of the disease.

10. Overall physiological changes of aging can be traced to

    a. basic cellular level changes.

    b. heredity factors.

    c. body system changes.

    d. the environment.

11. A risk can be best defined as

    a. any event that involves stress.

    b. a condition that may compromise health or longevity.

    c. a condition that threatens activities of daily living.

    d. alterations in functional or cognitive ability or activity status.

12. It is estimated that by age 80, cardiac output has decreased as much as

    a. 5%.

    b. 10%.

    c. 25%.

    d. 50%.

13. By age 90, most lungs have enough alveolar destruction to meet the criteria for a diagnosis of

    a. black lung disease.

    b. cancer.

    c. emphysema.

    d. pneumonia.

14. A physiological change of the musculoskeletal system involves

    a. increased muscle mass.

    b. decreased muscle mass.

    c. increased bone density.

    d. lengthening of the trunk.

CHAPTER 3

NURSING CARE OF OLDER ADULTS

CHAPTER OBJECTIVES

After studying this chapter, the reader will be able to discuss basic principles for working with older adults and the nursing skills required for optimal interactions specific to this population.

LEARNING OBJECTIVES

After studying this chapter the learner will be able to

1. identify nursing qualities that enhance the relationship with older adult patients.

2. describe person-first language usage when referring to older adults.

3. specify the various roles of nurses pertaining to research with older adults.

4. recognize the need for being an advocate when working with older adults.

5. list the rights of older adults in various health care settings.

6. specify strategies to promote communication with older adults.

7. choose teaching methods to enhance learning in older adults.

INTRODUCTION

As a population, older adults are a remarkably diverse group with a broad range of abilities and needs in all domains. Their long and rich lives and medical history require highly individualized nursing care. Nursing care of older adults differs from that of younger patients for many reasons. Some of these differences can be traced to changes that occur during the aging process, to multiple diseases and chronic health conditions, and to psychosocial losses. Some of these differences are the results of the way older adults are treated by society. Nursing of the older adult is a complex specialty that requires special qualities and methods. The nurse needs to possess clinical alertness to catch subtle changes in status so an anticipatory approach is achieved and emerging problems are identified early. The qualities required consist of a good sound basis of knowledge, appropriate approach and attitude, and personal warmth.

Nurses are involved in all phases of health care for older adults by preventing illness, promoting healthy behaviors, assisting in coping with chronic and acute conditions, and caring for persons who cannot care for themselves. To provide the highest quality of care, the nurse must demonstrate certain qualities.

QUALITIES NEEDED BY THE GERIATRIC NURSE

Nurses who work with older adults need to be stable and mature and demonstrate sincere interest and affection for the patient. Insincerity is quickly noticed in this population, as the older adult has had a lifetime to gain wisdom and understanding of other people. Nurses should also be kind, tolerant, and patient. Being patient requires allowing sufficient time and not acting rushed or in a hurry. Only when a nurse has gained a true respect for him or herself, can the nurse show true respect for others.

Empathy involves understanding. To have empathy for a patient, a nurse must act from a desire to understand the patient as much as from a desire to help. One model of human interaction that explains this need to act from a desire to understand is that all human interaction is directed either by the desire to protect oneself or by a desire to understand the other person. Whenever people act out of a desire to protect themselves — and most human interaction is of this type — they increase the barriers between themselves and the people with whom they are communicating. Only when separation and isolation become painful do people switch to a desire to understand. Behavior motivated by the desire to understand another person increases sharing and respect between people. Nurses need to nurture the ability to approach patients not with a protective attitude, but with a desire to understand the patient's problems from the patient's point of view. Since nurses usually work in settings where they are responsible for accomplishing a specific set of tasks, the need to protect themselves by "completing" the assigned work may become the main motivating force. Providing care that does not fit the patient's perception of his or her needs, however, will not contribute to the well being of that patient in the long run. All the care that nurses provide should be given with an underlying desire to understand that patient, in other words, with empathy.

SENSITIVE TERMINOLOGY

Communicating positive attitudes towards patients with disabilities or other health conditions through sensitive terminology should be incorporated into all written and oral forms of communication. It is recommended that all nurses break away from words that convey insensitivity, stereotyping, and discrimination, and instead use terminology that signifies dignity, respect, and positive attitudes (Folkins, 1992).

When using person-first language, the nurse defines the person first, then the disability or condition whenever charting and during verbal communication. Example: The demented often cannot remember the names of their children. This would be better stated as: Older adults with dementia often cannot recall the names of their children.

Emphasize the individual's abilities rather than focusing on limitations. Example: Mrs. Smith is wheelchair-bound. This would be better stated as: Mrs. Smith uses a wheelchair for mobility.

Avoid using terminology that reflects concepts of helplessness and dependency. Phrases such as "afflicted with…", "suffers from…", "stricken with…", "a victim of…" sensationalizes a person's disability or condition. Example: Mrs. Smith suffers from dementia. This would be better stated as: Mrs. Smith has dementia.

These methods of communication will not only portray a positive attitude towards the patients, but also help in the development of a trusting relationship. These techniques should be considered for both verbal and written communication.

RESEARCH AND NURSING

By examining examples of successful aging, research-based guidelines for preventive practices may be developed that minimize health problems and maximize health and function in the older adult. Nurses play a critical role in this research. Nurses may become involved in research by implementing research interventions or collecting data for a project designed by nurse researchers at local universities and other organizations. Nurses may become indirectly involved in research by assisting a patient to determine what clinical trials are available for his or her particular condition. For patients who are involved in research projects the nurse may assist them by assuring the patients rights of informed consent are not being violated. If directly involved in a research project, the nurse must attempt to follow the research protocol exactly, as research results become a part of nursing knowledge and impact future research and care directions.

Keeping up with the latest research requires reading journals, attending conferences, and other training workshops. It also requires an understanding of the different types of research that are reported in articles. Descriptive studies attempt to define a problem as it pertains to variables of a population. Longitudinal studies examine groups of people and how they change over a period of time. Researchers examine these data to find correlations between demographics, health behaviors, practices, and outcomes. From this, clinical trials are designed to examine the effects of various interventions on older adults to determine which ones have statistically significant results. Well-designed clinical trials, using randomization and a control group, provide strong research evidence. Meta-analysis research is a method of statistically analyzing the results of many research studies together and is the strongest form of research evidence. Case studies report what occurred with usually one or a few subjects. They are designed as a detailed example of using specific interventions to positively impact on health. In addition to participation in research, nurses are responsible for putting research into practice (research utilization) by changing nursing care protocols when new information is disseminated. Nurses should always use evidence-based practice and protocols specific to older adults when available.

ADVOCACY

Advocacy is the process of acting or speaking on the behalf of a patient. Advocacy for older adults is particularly important, as the older population is often vulnerable, has numerous health care needs, and lives in a society that tends to have diminished respect for older adults. Advocacy requires that the nurse understands the perspective of the patient and that strategies of care be adopted that are flexible and accommodate variations in a range of sociocultural factors. As an advocate, the nurse is responsible for safeguarding, promoting, and supporting the patient's lifestyles, values, and decisions. Processes and skills needed to successfully advocate for patients include: accountability, ethical analysis and decision-making, awareness and adherence to clinical standards and legal definitions of nursing practice, health teaching, health counseling, leadership, collaboration, communication, and ability to implement change.

RIGHTS OF OLDER ADULTS

Many federal, state, and local laws and regulations affect the lives of older adults. Often, older adults depend on the government for such things as housing, basic income, and health care. They find it confusing dealing with government agencies. Older adults living at home can be victims of dishonest door-to-door and telemarketers.

Rights may also be violated by age and other types of discrimination. For an older adult with a disability, access to public places and services are protected by the Americans for Disabilities Act (U.S. Department of Justice, 2003). As grandparents, older adults may have rights over maintaining a relationship with their grandchildren. Nurses come into intimate contact with older adults in a variety of settings and are often the ones to spot rights violations. As an advocate, the nurse should assist the older adult by contacting appropriate local government agencies to handle the violation. Protecting the rights of older adults requires great sensitivity to the vulnerability of this population and an ability to be honest with oneself when rights are abridged in the name of efficiency or beneficence.

Older adults as patients in hospitals have rights that are adapted from the American Hospital Association (AHA) recommendations (AHA, 1992). Every hospital has their own wording of these rights, which must be given to new patients upon admission. These cover how a patient is treated, how information is delivered, rights of decisions, and privacy issues.

In a long-term care setting, the residents have all the same rights and protections of all United States citizens. Nursing home residents have certain rights and protections under the law that may vary from state to state. Nursing homes must provide residents with a written description of their legal rights. At a minimum, Federal law specifies that a nursing home resident's rights include the following: (U. S. Department of Health & Human Services, 2002a).

Freedom from Discrimination: Nursing homes do not have to accept all applicants, but they must comply with Civil Rights laws that do not allow discrimination based on race, color, national origin, disability, age, or religion under certain conditions. If you believe a patient has been discriminated against, call the Department of Health and Human Services Office of Civil Rights at 1-800-368-1019.

Respect: The right to be treated with dignity and respect. As long as it fits into the care plan, residents have the right to make their own schedule, including when to go to bed, rise in the morning, eat their meals, and choose the activities in which to participate.

Freedom from Abuse and Neglect: The right to be free from verbal, sexual, physical, and mental abuse, and involuntary seclusion by anyone. This includes, but is not limited to, nursing home staff, other residents, consultants, volunteers, staff from other agencies, family members or legal guardians, friends, or other individuals. If you feel a resident has been abused or neglected, file a complaint with the nursing home, the local Long-Term Care Ombudsman, or State Survey Agency. It may be appropriate to report the incident of abuse to local law enforcement or the Medicaid Fraud Control Unit. These numbers should be posted in all nursing homes.

Freedom from Restraints: Physical restraints are any manual method, or physical or mechanical device, material, or equipment, attached to or near a patient's body so that the patient cannot move the restraint easily. These restraints prevent freedom of movement or normal access to one's own body. A chemical restraint is a drug used to limit freedom of movement and is not needed to treat medical symptoms. It is against the law for a nursing home to use physical or chemical restraints, unless it is necessary to treat a medical symptom. Restraints may not be used to punish nor for convenience of the nursing home staff. The resident has the right to refuse restraint use except if the resident is at risk of harming themselves or others.

Information on Services and Fees: The resident must be informed in writing about services and fees before moving into the nursing home. The nursing home cannot require a minimum entrance fee as condition of residence.

Money: The right to manage their own money or to choose someone they trust to do this for them. Residents must sign a written statement if they desire the nursing home to manage their personal funds; however, the nursing home must allow the resident access to their bank accounts, cash, and other financial records. The nursing home must protect the funds from any loss by buying a bond or providing similar protection.

Privacy, Property, and Living Arrangements: The right to privacy and to keep and use personal belongings and property as long as they do not interfere with the rights, health, or safety of others. Staff should never open residents' mail unless specifically requested. The resident has the right to use the telephone and talk privately. The nursing home must protect the residents' property from theft. This may include a safe in the facility or cabinets with locked doors in residents' rooms. If a resident and his or her spouse live in the same nursing home, they are entitled to share a room, if they both agree.

Medical Care: The right to be informed about medical conditions, medications, and to see their own doctor. They also have the right to refuse medication and treatments and to take part in developing their care plan. They have the right to look at their medical record and reports when they ask.

Visitors: The right to spend private time with visitors at any reasonable hour. The nursing home must permit family to visit as long as the resident wishes to see them. Residents do not have to see any visitor they do not wish to see. Persons who provide health or legal services may visit at any reasonable hour.

Social Services: The nursing home must provide any needed social services, including counseling, help solving problems with other residents, help in contacting legal and financial professionals, and discharge planning.

Leaving the Nursing Home: Living in a nursing home is the residents' choice and they may choose to move to another place. Nursing homes may have a policy that requires residents to inform the nursing home prior to moving to another place.

Complaints: The right to make a complaint to the staff of the nursing home, or any other person, without fear of punishment. The nursing home must resolve any issue promptly.

Protection Against Unfair Transfer or Discharge: Except in emergencies, nursing homes must give 30-day written notice of any plan to discharge or transfer a resident. A resident cannot be sent to another nursing home, or made to leave the nursing home unless 1) it is necessary for the welfare, health, or safety of the resident or others, 2) the resident's health has declined to the point that the nursing home cannot meet the care needs, 3) the resident's health has improved to the point that nursing home care is no longer necessary, 4) the nursing home has not been paid for the services, or 5) the nursing home closes.

Family and Friends: Family members and legal guardians may meet with the families of other residents and may participate in family councils. By law, nursing homes must develop a plan of care for each resident. Residents have the right to take part in this process, and family members can help if the resident gives permission. Relatives who are legal guardians have the right to look at all medical records and to make decisions.

INTERVIEW/ COMMUNICATION METHODS WITH OLDER ADULTS

To communicate is to send, receive, or interchange messages. Interviewing is a process of communication that is patient-oriented and when effectively done, is the basis of a therapeutic health care relationship. An interview has three phases: orientation, working and termination. Communication with the older adult requires distinct methods and skills in order for information to be effectively and accurately sent and received. The following factors should contribute to effective communication and interviewing:

- Allow plenty of time for the interaction. Slow down or the patient may feel that they are not important.

- Set up the environment. Use a well-lit room with comfortable seating. Avoid placing barriers such as a desk or table between you and the patient. Eliminate background noises by turning off any radio or television and telephone ringer. Try to avoid areas where others are talking or walking through. Know if the patient is visually, cognitively, or hearing impaired. Be aware of patients' primary spoken language, culture, and level of education.

- Obtain all necessary equipment ahead of time. This could be an amplifier for those with hearing impairments, an interpreter, a message board, or tape recorder. Also have all the forms, papers, and records needed. It is disturbing to a patient to wait for the nurse to gather his or her things after initially meeting.

- If family members or friends are present ask them to answer only when directly questioned or ask them to step out of the area until you are finished. Oftentimes meaningful family members respond for the older adult, whose voice then does not get heard.

- Introduce yourself by name and role, state the purpose for the communication, and how much time has been allotted for it. Determine how the patient would like to be addressed. Call the patient by name — never honey, dear, or other such terms — and extend your hand to shake gently and smile.

- Be aware of personal beliefs, values, attitudes, and stereotypes related to the older adult.

- Face the patient directly at eye level, sitting somewhat close. If the patient is hearing-impaired, sit slightly towards whatever side the patient hears best. Lower your voice but do not shout.

- Do not cover the face with your hands or other objects as the patient may use lip reading to assist in understanding what is being said. Do use hand gestures if they help clarify information.

- Slow your rate of speech, avoid jargon, and use simple and exact language to make certain all communication is understood.

- Do not talk down to the patient or lose affect in the process of simplifying speech.

- Body language should match the message. Avoid crossing arms, or tapping or shaking your foot, leg, or pen. Leaning slightly forward shows interest.

- Maintain eye contact and remain silent when the patient is speaking. Pay attention for non-verbal communication. Do not minimize the older adults concerns.

- Touch can be useful to convey understanding, warmth, and caring. Use this only if you know your patient and he or she is receptive to it. Your initial handshake starts the process of using touch and may give clues as to how receptive the patient is to touch.

- Rephrase messages if the patient does not understand what has been said.

- Obtain feedback to make certain the patient has understood what has been said and to avoid misunderstandings. Provide information in writing whenever possible.

- If using a screening instrument that requires a yes/no or some specific response, make certain the patient is aware of this to avoid long drawn-out answers that require interpretation of code.

- Ask open-ended questions when detail is needed.

- Nearing the end of the interaction, repeat important points in different words, and summarize the conclusion. Always ask if there are any questions.

- When interacting with older adults with cognitive impairment, do not assume they cannot understand or make simple choices.

EDUCATION AND THE OLDER ADULT

Education is crucial for helping older adults maintain good health and independent functioning. It is a fundamental role of nursing to educate the patient and family in order for the older adult to live longer and healthier and to achieve the highest quality of life possible. Nurses are on the forefront of providing appropriate education and are challenged to do so with proper teaching methods. Nurses use education in all settings for a variety of reasons from health prevention learning to how to take medications. The educational method may be one-on-one or a small-to-large group. The ability to learn new information remains intact during the aging process, but the time it takes to learn increases. Prior to attempting to educate the older adults, it is important to determine their current knowledge on the subject matter and perceived benefits and barriers to learning new material. Assessing older adults' past learning style can be the key to successful new learning now. In general, older adults prefer educational sessions with formal structure and sound, interaction with peers, an authority figure present, formal seating design, cooler room temperature, ability to move about, and sessions held in the late afternoon (VanWynen, 2001).

Keeping in mind that each patient and setting is unique, the following strategies should be considered useful:

- Environment should be friendly, warm, and comfortably lit.

- Provide fluids for all sessions and snacks if appropriate.

- Focus on topics that are useful and practical.

- Use short presentations with concise summaries.

- Use visual aides.

- Allow time for questions and encourage participation.

- Avoid abstract concepts and anything that requires rote memory.

- Provide clearly written handouts that the patient may keep.

- Use praise and rewards.

SUMMARY

Nurses who work with older adults are special people requiring special qualities and versatility. From being an advocate, an educator, or a skilled communicator, the nurse can help the older adult gain the highest quality of life. The challenge comes from trying to meet the patient's emotional needs as well as the physical needs, and to provide support and encouragement along the way. The intrinsic rewards the nurse receives from meeting this challenge are significant.

EXAM QUESTIONS

CHAPTER 3
Questions 15-21

15. Nursing qualities that would most likely enhance the relationship with older adult are

    a. leadership, efficiency, knowledge, and humor.

    b. stability, maturity, interest, and affection.

    c. control, ability, thoroughness, and sympathy.

    d. superiority, competence, disassociation, and cost-effectiveness.

16. A statement that most accurately communicates a positive attitude through sensitive terminology would be written as

    a. resident is an 89-year-old demented female who is mobile by self-propelling a wheelchair.

    b. resident is an 89-year-old female suffering from dementia who is mobile by self-propelling a wheelchair.

    c. resident is an 89-year-old female with cognitive impairment who is mobile by self-propelling a wheelchair.

    d. resident is an elderly female with cognitive impairment confined to a wheelchair.

17. A nurse working on a skilled nursing unit is involved with patients who are subjects of a research study for a new treatment procedure for the prevention of skin breakdown. When giving this treatment to patients the nurse should

    a. follow the protocol exactly every time.

    b. go back to the old treatment if it appears it is not working.

    c. follow protocol when time is available to do so.

    d. follow protocol only when the researchers are around.

18. An appropriate nursing action demonstrating patient advocacy for an older adult living at home is

    a. conducting nutrition screenings at a Senior Citizens Center.

    b. taking control of the patient's financial assets.

    c. encouraging older adults to participate in research studies.

    d. lobbying local officials for free public transportation for older adults.

19. Residents in any long-term care facility have the right to

    a. have their own personal belongings and pets with them in the facility.

    b. refuse having restraints used on them, even if they pose a risk of harm to themselves.

    c. non-discrimination based on race, color, national origin, disability, age, or religion.

    d. spend private time with family and visitors at any hour in their own room.

20. A strategy used to improve effective communication and interviewing with the older adult is

    a. lower background noises by turning down the television and/or radio.

    b. request that the family answer for the patient.

    c. assume the patient with dementia cannot understand you.

    d. slow your rate of speech and shout loudly.

21. A teaching method most likely to result in the presented material to be understood is to

    a. use short presentations with concise sum- maries.

    b. use a variety of teaching methods in each session.

    c. do not teach groups of more than 12 parti- cipants.

    d. do pre- and post-testing of knowledge.

CHAPTER 4

MEDICATIONS
AND THE OLDER ADULT

CHAPTER OBJECTIVE

After studying this chapter, the reader will be able to discuss physiological changes that affect medication disposition and the various problems associated with drug therapy in the older adult.

LEARNING OBJECTIVES

After studying this chapter the learner will be able to

1. specify the physiological changes that occur with aging that affect the disposition of medications.

2. discuss the various reasons why older adults are at risk for adverse drug reactions.

3. discuss the effects of over-the-counter, home remedies, herbal drug, and alcohol usage on the older adult.

4. state common reasons why older adults do not adhere to prescribed medications and nursing strategies to overcome this.

5. list medications to be avoided in the older adult.

6. explain common issues of medication usage in long-term care facilities.

INTRODUCTION

One of the challenges of healthcare professionals in the care of older adults is to balance the professionals' own concepts of quality of life with what is important to the older adult. In the area of geriatric pharmacology, this is particularly difficult because the professional has the ever-present desire to cure and treat with useful, yet potentially dangerous, drugs. The older adult, however, must incorporate the use of these medications into a lifestyle that maximizes function and independence and balances other aspects of life, including financial security and psychological well-being.

To develop an understanding of how great an impact medications have on older adults consider the following information. Older adults, constitute only 12.3% of the total population yet account for 34% of all prescriptions dispensed and 42% of all prescription spending. The average number of prescriptions for this group, including refills, are 28.5 per year for a total of about $40 billion dollars, with almost half being paid out of pocket (Ihara, 2002). There are approximately 9 million reported adverse reactions each year. One out of every six drug administrations in hospitals are incorrect (SMARxT Coalition, 2003). About 25% of nursing home admissions and 17% of hospital admissions are due to adverse medication reactions (Neafsey & Shellman, 2002). If the list of leading causes of death for the United States included adverse drug reactions and medication errors, it would rank as fourth or fifth. This dramatic effect of medications has not, unfortunately, been accompanied by adequately prioritized mandatory education at the undergraduate, graduate, and postgraduate levels of healthcare education. Only recently, the awareness of the physiological changes that occur with the natural aging process has influenced the approach to clinical drug trials and utilization reviews. More research is needed on the effects of age, dose adjustments, and drug response for this age group. The frail elderly and very old patients, over 85 years of age, in particular, must be included in more investigational drug trials to make medication usage safer.

Appropriate drug use is one of the most important determinants of quality of life. In addition, nurses are being named in an increasing number of malpractice suits with as many as 30% of all suits being filed as a result of drug-related injuries (DrugIntel, 2003). As a nurse striving for health promotion, it is important to be alert to the potential dangers of any medication taken and always have a current drug reference book available.

AGE-RELATED PHYSIOLOGICAL CHANGES: PHARMACOKINETICS

Several basic principles highlight the physiological changes that occur with aging that affect how a drug is utilized in the body and the response to the drug. The path of a drug may be traced from absorption to elimination.

Absorption

Absorption involves the passage of a medication from the administration site into the systemic circulation. Bioavailability is the percentage of the drug that actually reaches the systemic circulation. Whereas a drug may be administered by many

TABLE 4-1: ROUTES OF ABSORPTION	
• Inhalation	• Otic
• Intramuscular	• Rectal
• Intranasal	• Subcutaneous
• Intravenous	• Sublingual
• Ophthalmic	• Topical
• Oral	• Vaginal

routes (see Table 4-1), the oral route of absorption is best studied, and the most frequent route for older adults. Drug absorption may be delayed or hastened by many factors, including co-administration of food or other drugs, gastric pH, lipid or water solubility of the drug itself, stomach emptying time, enteric coating, and vomiting for oral products; local conditions such as edema, abrasions, and presence of hair for topical administration; and retention time for enemas. The bioavailability of the medication is usually unaltered with aging (Luisi, Owens, & Hume, 1999). This is true for most drugs that passively diffuse into the circulation. The rate of absorption, therefore, may be affected by age, but the extent of absorption is usually not changed for drugs taken by mouth. Some drugs, however, such as propranolol (Inderal), are extensively metabolized by the liver before they reach the systemic circulation. This process of absorption from the gastrointestinal tract directly into the portal system and subsequent metabolism, called the first-pass effect, appears to be decreased in the elderly, making more of the drug available for systemic circulation.

Distribution

Once a drug has been absorbed into the systemic circulation, it is distributed throughout body tissues. Distribution is highly dependent on how lipid soluble or water soluble a particular drug is. Distribution also depends upon factors such as blood flow, plasma protein binding, and body composition. An increase in fat-to-muscle ratio occurs gradually with age. Fat content is approximately 15% in a younger person's body, and increases to more than 30% in the elderly. In addition to this increase in total body fat, a decrease occurs in total body water as well as a decline in lean body mass. These changes are reflected in corresponding variations in drug distribution. As expected, water-soluble drugs, with less water to distribute into, become highly concentrated in older adults who receive the same dose per kilogram as younger patients. High plasma concentrations are reflected in higher drug blood levels when monitored, but more importantly, reflected in increased prevalence of drug side effects and toxic reactions. Lipophilic drugs distribute into the fatty tissues of the body and may accumulate over time. Even after a medication is discontinued, patients may experience prolonged evidence of the presence of the drug or toxic effects as the stores are slowly eliminated.

The distribution of drugs is also influenced by the concentration of plasma proteins, the affinity of the proteins for the drug, and the presence of other substances that compete for binding. Many drugs bind to protein in plasma making the bound portions pharmacologically inert. Only unbound portion of the drugs are active. Drugs, such as phenytoin (Dilantin®) or furosemide (Lasix®), are highly bound to plasma proteins. It does appear that the concentration of albumin, one of the primary binding proteins, decreases with age; therefore, there are fewer binding sites and greater concentrations of free drugs. This increase in the unbound, active portion of the drug may result in a greater prevalence of adverse side effects or toxic effects if drug doses are not lowered accordingly. Drug-drug interactions can occur if two or more highly-protein bound drugs are administered. When this occurs, the two drugs compete for the binding sites and results in an increase in free drugs with enhanced effects and increased risk of toxicity.

Metabolism

The primary organ for metabolic biotransformation is the liver. Through enzymatic activity, the liver attempts to convert foreign substances such as drugs and alcohol to products that are more easily eliminated. Metabolism may be influenced by several factors, including diet, exercise, smoking, other drugs, altered blood flow to the liver, and disease states such as congestive heart failure and age. Although liver function test results do not appear to change as patients become older, interpretation of the results in the elderly should include consideration of age-related alterations in metabolism (biotransformation). Medications enter the liver prior to entering the general circulation and the target tissue. During this first pass the liver metabolizes much of the drug before it reaches the site of action. In the older adult, reduced liver blood flow may account for a decrease in first-pass metabolism, which allows more drugs to reach the systemic circulation. Age-related changes in the liver are variable and because of this variability, it is difficult to predict the need to alter a drug dose for patients without overt liver disease. Monitoring serum drug levels can be useful for several drugs with toxic potential, such as phenytoin, that are used by older adults. Although further studies are needed in the area of metabolism, it seems that drugs that are metabolized via oxidation pathways, such as many psychotropic drugs, anticonvulsants, oral anticoagulants, and oral antidiabetic agents, require the "start low and go slow" approach. Drugs such as isoniazid, procainamide, and hydralazine, which are biotransformed in the liver, may not require dose adjustment.

Elimination

Renal excretion is the primary route of elimination for many drugs. Age-related reductions in glomerular filtration and renal blood flow can significantly impair the excretion of water-soluble drugs. Disease, urinary pH, and the presence of other drugs may also affect renal elimination. It is well known that a physiological decline in renal function occurs with aging. An age-related decline of approximately 1–2% per year of age is seen after maturity. Even in the absence of active intrinsic kidney disease, renal clearance is decreased in the elderly to about half that of a younger person. This decline is reflected in a corresponding decrease in creatine clearance. Clinicians do have a method of assessing renal function based on easily accessible information. One of the most commonly used methods for determining clearance, formulated by Cockcroft and Gault (1976), for men is:

$$(\text{men}) \quad \frac{(140 - \text{age}) (\text{lean body weight in kg})}{(72) (\text{serum creatinine})}$$

For women, multiply the results by 0.85 to account for gender differences in muscle mass. This formula can be used for adjusting dosages of drugs according to manufacturer recommendations for patients with decreased renal function.

AGE-RELATED PHYSIOLOGICAL CHANGES: PHARMACODYNAMICS

Drug pharmacodynamics, defined broadly, are the effects that medications have on the body. More specifically, it is the pharmacological effect that results from the interaction of the drug at the actual receptor site of the target tissue. Little information is available on the changes that occur at the receptor and post-receptor levels with aging. The aging organ system can cause changes in a drug's effect and cause many receptors to function less efficiently. Certain drugs such as beta-blockers and beta-antagonists exhibit decreased pharmacodynamics resulting in a diminished response to drugs. Aging also produces a decline in parasympathetic control, which enhances the effects of anticholinergics and reduces the number of neurotransmitters,

making the older adult more sensitive to central nervous system drugs.

ADVERSE DRUG REACTIONS AND MEDICATIONS TO BE AVOIDED

An adverse drug reaction (ADR) can be something as mild as minor sedation to a reaction that is serious and fatal. It is not surprising that the elderly are at particular risk. Advanced age, body composition, excessive number of medications, multiple disease states, development of renal or hepatic dysfunction, and the presence of a high-risk medication all contribute to the increased possibilities of an ADR. It is estimated that over 350,000 ADRs occur in U.S. nursing homes each year (Gurwitz, et al, 2000).

REASONS FOR ADR'S

Newly Released Medications

Most new drugs are approved with an average of 1,500 patient exposures and usually for only relatively short periods of time on young subjects (Center for Drug Evaluation, 2002). A drug that is tested in a few thousand people may have an excellent safety profile; however, when administered to several thousand older adults, rare ADR may arise. That means for drugs that cause rare toxicity, their toxicity can only be detected after, not before, marketing. Administration of relatively new medications to the older adult should be done with caution and close evaluation. Any suspicion of an ADR should be reported. A nurse does not have to be absolutely certain that a drug caused a reaction. All reports contribute to the heightening of the awareness of Food and Drug Administration (FDA) safety scientists as they monitor all of the evidence to evaluate the potential for drug-related toxicity.

Reports are made through the FDA program, MedWatch, which is intended to make it easier for health professionals to report adverse reactions to drugs, medical devices, and other FDA regulated products (Kessler, 1993). This reporting may save many individuals from death or serious adverse reactions that will be acted upon sooner by the FDA. To report online go to www.fda.gov/ medwatch/ and follow the instructions for submitting a report electronically. By mail download a form to print from the website or call 1-800-332-1088, and one will be sent by mail or fax.

Side Effects

Almost all medications have the potential to cause a variety of side effects ranging from minor, clinically insignificant reactions, to severe, debilitating reactions that require immediate medical attention. The most common drugs prescribed to older adult that produce ADRs include warfarin, digoxin, prednisone, psychotropic agents, diuretics, anti-hypertensive, insulin, and even aspirin. These drugs have narrow therapeutic windows. The toxic levels are not too far from levels required for clinical efficacy. Undesirable side effects from antidepressants are seen more frequently in the elderly. In particular, anticholinergic effects such as urinary retention, dry mouth, constipation, and mental confusion are common. In addition to causing obvious inconvenience to the geriatric patient who may have decreased mobility, the use of diuretics may lead to serious electrolyte imbalances. Of particular concern is the loss of potassium. As diuretics are often prescribed along with digoxin for the treatment of congestive heart failure, drug-induced hypokalemia may contribute to the risk of digoxin-induced arrhythmias. Adequate monitoring of electrolyte and digoxin levels is crucial to effective and safe treatment with these agents.

Drug-Drug Reactions

As the older adult is often on multiple medications, they are vulnerable to drug-drug reactions.

Polypharmacy is the use of many medications at the same time. Other definitions include prescribing more medication than is clinically indicated, a medical regimen that includes at least one unnecessary medication, or the empiric use of five or more medications (Michocki, 2000). It can be hard to determine if an individual drug caused a reaction in a complicated patient receiving multiple medications. Any change in condition for an older adult patient should first begin with a review of the current drug regimen to determine if a drug-drug reaction is the cause. This is a particular problem with community-dwelling patients who often receive prescriptions from multiple providers.

Drug-Disease Reaction

These include interactions between certain drugs and specific disease states. Severe liver disease, renal disease, heart failure, acute viral infection, and changes in thyroid function have been associated with altered clearance for some drugs. Review all the medication precautions if a drug-disease reaction is suspected.

Drug-Food Reaction

Several drugs are known to interact with foods, such as tetracycline when taken with milk products; warfarin with dietary sources of vitamin K, such as spinach or broccoli; and grapefruit juice, which can block the metabolism of many drugs (Kane & Lipsky, 2000). Review all the medication's special considerations to determine the feasibility of drug-food reaction.

Over-the-Counter (OTC) Medications

Older adults purchase 25% of the 5 billion OTC medications sold each year and have little knowledge of the harm OTC drugs can cause (Crutchfield, 2002a). Often the product information is printed in a size and language that is difficult for older adults to effectively understand. Older adults often use OTC drugs to self-treat conditions in place of seeing a physician or use OTC drugs to

TABLE 4-2: TEACHING ABOUT COMMON OTC DRUG USAGE

Acid Reducers: (Prevent/relieve heartburn associated with acid indigestion and sour stomach). For products with cimetidine, ask before using if on theophylline, warfarin, or phenytoin.

Antacids: (Acid indigestion, heartburn and/or sour stomach): Calcium and aluminum products may constipate. Magnesium causes diarrhea. Ask before use if patient is allergic to milk, taking a prescription drug, or has kidney disease. These do not protect the stomach from pain relievers or alcohol. Take 2 hours apart from other medications.

Antiemetics: (Motion sickness) Ask before use if taking sedatives or tranquilizers, have a respiratory diagnosis, glaucoma, or enlarged prostate gland. Avoid alcohol.

Antihistamines: (Runny nose, sneezing, itchy nose, throat, or eyes due to hay fever or other respiratory problems). Ask before use if on sedatives or tranquilizers, anti-hypertensive, antidepressant, have glaucoma, an enlarged prostate gland, or a respiratory diagnosis. When using this product: alcohol, sedatives, and tranquilizers may increase drowsiness. Some of these products may increase confusion, urinary retention, drowsiness, dizziness, and unsteady gait.

Antitussives Cough Medicine: (Cough due to minor throat and bronchial irritation as may occur with a cold) Ask before use if taking sedatives or tranquilizers, have glaucoma or difficulty in urination due to an enlarged prostate gland.

Bronchodilators: (Relief of shortness of breath, tightness and wheezing due to bronchial asthma). Ask before use if have heart or thyroid disease, hypertension, diabetes, enlarged prostate gland, ever been hospitalized for asthma, or currently on a prescription drug for asthma.

Laxatives: (Constipation) Ask before using if have stomach pains, nausea or vomiting, or have kidney disease and the laxative contains phosphates, potassium, or magnesium.

Nasal Decongestants: (Relief of nasal congestion due to a cold, hay fever, or other upper respiratory allergies) Ask before use if have heart disease, high blood pressure, thyroid disease, diabetes, or enlarged prostate gland. May cause insomnia.

Nicotine Replacement Products: (Drugs that reduce withdrawal symptoms associated with quitting smoking) Ask before use if have high blood pressure not controlled by medication, heart disease, a recent heart attack, irregular heartbeat, or taking a prescription drug for depression or asthma. Do not use while smoking, using chewing tobacco, or using snuff.

Nighttime Sleep Aids: (Relief of occasional sleeplessness) Ask before use if taking sedatives or tranquilizers, have a respiratory diagnosis, glaucoma, or enlarged prostate gland. Avoid alcohol.

Pain Relievers: (Relief of minor body aches, pains, and headaches) Ask before taking if consume 3 or more alcohol drinks per day. The following ingredients are found in different OTC pain relievers: acetaminophen, aspirin, ibuprofen, ketoprofen, magnesium salicylate, and naproxen. Ibuprofen and other NSAID increase blood pressure. Tylenol® and Ibuprofen can cause liver damage. Aspirin and other NSAID may cause GI bleed. Different OTC drugs may contain the same active ingredient as other OTC or prescribed drugs.

Stimulants: (Restore mental alertness or wakefulness) When using this product limit the use of foods, beverages, and other drugs that have caffeine. Too much caffeine can cause nervousness, irritability, sleeplessness, and occasional rapid heartbeat. Be aware that the recommended dose of this product contains caffeine equivalent to a cup of coffee.

treat side effects of prescription drugs. Many of the drugs that have been switched from prescription to OTC, such as pain relievers, antacids, H2 blockers, and antihistamines are of particular concern due to potential drug-drug interactions and side effects that frequently effect the older adult (Neafsey & Shellman, 2002). Acetaminophen (Tylenol®) is viewed by older adults as a safe drug, yet many become liver toxic if used regularly, particularly if they are on other medications that contain Tylenol®. Healthcare providers do not always ask about OTC medication usage, and those that do ask frequently neglect to include this information in the patients' chart. Nurses should instruct patients to use the same pharmacy for both OTC and prescription medications and to become accustomed to speaking with the pharmacist. Educate patients on common OTC precautions using the material provided in Table 4-2.

TABLE 4-3: POSSIBLE PROBLEMS WITH HERBAL PRODUCTS

Chamomile: Avoid with anticoagulants.

Chondroitin: Avoid with anticoagulants.

DHEA: Increased risks of heart disease stoke and prostrate and breast cancers. May cause fatigue and insomnia. Not be used with patients with cancer or enlarged prostate.

Echinacea: Can depress the immune system. Do not use for longer than 8 weeks.

Ephedra: Contraindicated in those with hypertension, diabetes, glaucoma, thyroid disease, and prostatic hypertrophy. Interacts with Monoamine Oxidase Inhibitors (MAOIs). Increases blood pressure (BP), cardiac output, and heart rate (HR).

Garlic: Avoid with peptic ulcer disease or reflux disease. May decrease blood glucose. May potentate blood-thinning effects of anti-coagulants, antihypertensive, and aspirin.

Ginger: Avoid with anticoagulants.

Ginkgo biloba: May potentate aspirin, warfarin, MAOIs. Avoid with history of seizures.

Ginseng: Overstimulation and insomnia may occur. Avoid use with other stimulants. Caution in patients with uncontrolled hypertension, cardiac disorders, diabetes, or on steroids. Avoid with MAOI's. Avoid with anxiety, manic, psychoses, or estrogen-dependent malignancies.

Glucosamine: May interfere with insulin secretion. May cause bronchopulmonary complications. Also results in anticoagulation. Avoid use with anticoagulants.

Goldseal: Large doses are toxic. Symptoms of toxicity include nausea, nervousness, exaggerated reflexes, hypertension (HTN), convulsions, paraesthesia, paralysis, and death from respiratory failure.

Kava: Long-term use causes yellowing of the skin. Large doses may cause dizziness or muscle weakness. Avoid with barbiturates, antidepressants, and other central nervous system (CNS) drugs. Use with levodopa will increase Parkinsonian symptoms. Use with alprazolam may cause coma.

Melatonin: Contraindicated with hepatic insufficiency, cardiovascular accidents (CVA), cardiovascular risks, gall bladder problems, depression, kidney disease, and any CNS disorder.

Peppermint: Overuse may cause heartburn and lower esophageal sphincter relaxation.

Saw Palmetto: May affect hormone therapy. May cause headaches and diarrhea.

St. John's Wort: Adverse effects include GI distress, allergic reaction, and photosensitivity. Avoid with antidepressant medication and patients with hallucinations or suicide ideation. Avoid with protease inhibitors or other anti-viral drugs and with cyclosporin.

Herbal and Nutritional Supplements

Over 2 million older adults regularly take herbal remedies. An estimated 40% of older adults have used some form of dietary supplement within the past year (Heinrich, 2001). Yet, of that group 57% do not disclose usage to their physicians (Foster, Phillips, Hamel, & Eisenberg, 2000). Many older adults do not view herbs and other supplements as drugs, and believe they are natural and harmless. One herb commonly used by older adults, St. John's Wort, has significant interactions with many medications including digoxin (Johne et al., 1999). See Table 4-3 for potential problems with these products. Plant substances contain hundreds, sometimes thousands of bioactive compounds, and with them comes the risk of potential ADRs. This may be from the herb itself or from a drug-herb interaction. Often called alternative therapies when used alone or as complimentary therapy when used in conjunction with traditional health care, herbs and other supplements lack quality control and are not regulated by the FDA. Of the more than 1,400 herbs sold commercially only five, considered laxatives, have been FDA approved (Stupay & Sivertsen, 2000). An important factor to consider is that herbal remedies have limited, mixed, or no research supporting their claims.

Vitamins and Minerals

Vitamins and minerals may also cause problems for the older adult, especially when taken in large doses. Fat-soluble vitamins, A, D, E, and K, are stored in the body. Mega-doses of vitamins A and D causes toxic reactions. Vitamin E can interfere with blood clotting especially for patients already on a blood-thinning agent. Synthetic forms of vitamin K can cause hemolytic anemia and liver damage. The water-soluble vitamin C and the B complexes are not stored in the body. Although considered nontoxic, excess amounts of vitamin C may cause excess iron absorption, nausea and vomiting and false-positive glucose urine tests. Vitamin B6

may interact with levodopa and reduce phenytoin levels and large doses of folic acid interfere with anticonvulsant agents. The mineral calcium, decreases the absorption of tetracycline. Iron, iodine, and zinc are well-known trace minerals and each is potentially toxic when consumed in excess quantities. Iron supplements taken with antibiotics can reduce or stop the ability of the antibiotics to fight infection. The chemicals in the supplement and the antibiotic bind together in the stomach instead of being absorbed into the bloodstream. Salt substitutes can interact with diuretics or blood pressure medications to increase blood potassium levels.

Alcohol and Medications

Alcohol interacts negatively with up to one-half of the 100 most commonly prescribed drugs for older adults, leading to increased risk of illness, injury, or death (Simon, 2003). For example, alcohol with antihistamines will increase the drowsiness that the medication causes, making driving or operating machinery even more hazardous. Acetaminophen usage with drinking alcohol increases the risk of serious liver damage. (See Table 4-4.) The American Medical Association (AMA) estimates that about 3 million Americans over age 60 have a drinking problem. A survey of 5,000 adults over 60 reported that 15% of men and 12% of women were hazardous drinkers and 9% of men and 3% of women were alcohol dependent (Simon, 2003).

Miscellaneous

Tobacco, caffeine, and recreational drug usage such as marijuana, heroine, or cocaine may cause ADRs. Home remedies are abound and gaining in popularity. These alternative medicines may be an old family recipe or something purchased at a health food store. Remedies may be eaten, inhaled, smoked, placed on the skin, or given as a enema. Some contain alcohol, various oils, salts, vinegar, witch hazel, or even lead. Research has identified 600 instances that these remedies could potentially

Chapter 4–
Medications and the Older Adult

TABLE 4-4: EFFECTS OF ALCOHOL ON MEDICATION

Antibiotics: With acute alcohol consumption, some antibiotics may cause nausea, vomiting, headache, and possibly convulsions; Furoxone®, Grisactin®, Flagyl®, and Atabrine™.

Isoniazid: Acute alcohol consumption decreases the availability of isoniazid in the bloodstream.

Rifampin: Chronic alcohol use decreases the availability of rifampin.

Anticoagulants: Acute alcohol consumption enhances warfarin's availability, increasing risk for life-threatening hemorrhages. Chronic alcohol consumption reduces warfarin's availability, lessening the patient's protection from the consequences of blood-clotting disorders.

Antidepressants: Alcoholism and depression are frequently associated with each other leading to a high potential for alcohol-antidepressant interactions. Alcohol increases any sedative effects of antidepressants. Tyramine, found in some beers and wine, interacts with Monoamino Oxidase Inhibitors (MAOIs) to produce dangerous increase in blood pressure.

Oral Antidiabetic Medications: Acute alcohol consumption prolongs, and chronic alcohol consumption decreases, the availability of tolbutamide (Orinase®). Alcohol also interacts with some drugs of this class to produce symptoms of nausea and headache.

Antihistamines: Intensifies the sedation caused by some antihistamines such as Benadryl®. May also cause excessive dizziness.

Antipsychotic Medications: Alcohol consumption increases the sedative effect of these drugs, resulting in impaired coordination and breathing difficulties. The combination of chronic alcohol ingestion and antipsychotic drugs may result in liver damage.

Antiepileptic Medications: Acute alcohol consumption increases the availability of phenytoin (Dilantin®) and the risk of drug-related side effects. Chronic drinking may decrease phenytoin availability, significantly reducing the patient's protection against seizures.

Anti-ulcer Medications: The commonly prescribed antiulcer medications cimetidine (Tagamet®) and ranitidine (Zantac®) increase the availability of a low dose of alcohol under some circumstances.

Cardiovascular Medications: May cause dizziness or fainting upon standing up. These drugs include nitroglycerin, reserpine, Aldomet®, Apresoline®, Ismelin®, and others. Chronic alcohol consumption decreases the availability of propranolol (Inderal®).

Narcotic Pain Relievers: The combination of opiates and alcohol enhances the sedative effect of both substances, increasing the risk of death from overdose.

Non-Narcotic Pain Relievers: Aspirin and similar nonprescription pain relievers may cause stomach bleeding and inhibit blood from clotting; alcohol can exacerbate these effects. Mixing alcohol with large doses of aspirin to self-medicate for pain presents a high risk for gastric bleeding. Chronic alcohol ingestion activates enzymes that transform acetaminophen (Tylenol® and others) into chemicals that can cause liver damage, even when acetaminophen is used in standard therapeutic amounts.

Sedatives and Hypnotics: Excessive sedation. Lorazepam (Ativan®) and alcohol may result in depressed heart and breathing functions.

result in drug interactions, disease interactions, or adverse reactions. Garlic, when applied to the skin as a poultice, can cause skin burns (Fugh-Berman, 2002). Folk or home remedies for various ailments may also contain lead. These are often bright yellow, white, or red powders. Azarcon and Greta are sometimes used by Mexicans and Mexican-Americans while Caypah is used by Laotian or

Hmong refugees. These are generally used for "empacgo," intestinal illnesses and contain almost 100% lead. Folk medicines containing lead are extremely dangerous and should not be used (Neff, 2002). Aside from toxic effects, other remedies may be potentially dangerous due simply to ineffectiveness and delay in receiving proper treatment. A good method of determining safety of a supplement is the Consumer Lab website [http://www.ConsumerLab.com/index.asp]. The mission of this organization is to identify the best quality health and nutritional products through independent testing. This site has a database of vitamins, herb and supplements that can be used to check safety and effectiveness of a product. It also contains many article with government warnings about various products.

One can see that generalizing medication and possible adverse effects is difficult for this age group. When administering any new medication to a patient, it is paramount for the nurse to assess how the drug fits into the patient's current medication regiment, if the drug is safe given health history and status, and what therapeutic effects should be expected. Lastly, to detect adverse drug reactions, assess the patient based on the specific medication guideline recommendations. Assume that any new symptom the patient develops is caused by a medication until proven otherwise (Hanlon, Shimp, & Semla, 2000).

MEDICATION ADHERENCE ISSUES

Medication adherence is the extent to which a patient follows medical instructions. Taking the right medication, in the right method, at the right time, every time, is a difficult yet vital task for older adults. Medications are the mainstay of disease control in this population (Beers, 2000). Taking medications is a complex task, requiring both mental and physical functioning combined with patient characteristics. A patient may intentionally or unintentionally deviate from the drug regimen prescribed by the physician. These deviations may be trivial, or they may be clinically significant, compromising the ideal therapy outcome.

Types of Noncompliance or Non-Adherence

Patient Psychosocial Characteristics: Education level, culture, demographics, social support, personal self image, perceptions, tolerance, and availability of economic resources all play an important factor in medication adherence. Education level affects the ability to understand complex or even simple medication regimens. For example, a medication may be prescribed to be taken only at bedtime, placed under the tongue for sublingual absorption, not be swallowed or chewed, or not be taken with milk products. Medications that are to be taken "as needed" compound the innate difficulties of prescription taking. Confusion can be caused by brand/trade name, and similar sounding or spelled medications. A patient might stop taking the medication altogether when they feel better, not realizing the medication is for a chronic condition. Patients often share medications with or use medications prescribed for others. Culturally the role of family members may influence medication usage. Demographic characteristics of the patient, such as those living in a rural area with limited access to a pharmacy, have an impact. Social support may be in the form of family or friends who influence or assist in the medication regimen. Personal beliefs play a factor, such as a patient who views him or herself as being 'weak' if too many drugs are needed or if a medication affects sexual performance. Overall perception of the benefits of medications, and trust in healthcare providers and the healthcare system itself has an influence on medication adherence. This not only results in the patient not taking enough or any of the medications but also in the "If one is good, two is better" problem. Individual tolerance for side effects or simply for having to incorporate medications into one's lifestyle contributes to non-adherence. The ability to afford medications, especially when on multiple medications, and limited income and insufficient insurance are common causes of non-adherence. This can prohibit filling a prescription, taking smaller or less frequent doses, sharing medications, or saving some to use at another time.

Patient Cognitive Characteristics: In some situations, memory loss or poor cognitive function may make it difficult for the patient to recall all the information given by the physician or pharmacist. It can also affect the patient's daily ability to remember to take the correct medication, at the correct time, and in the correct manner. It may contribute to forgetting to refill prescriptions or taking extra medications. Patients with dementia may have language difficulties making it hard for them to ask questions or even to ask for assistance. Those with dementia and agnosia may not recognize the medication to be taken. Patients with dementia and paranoia, delusions, or other behavioral disturbances may be resistant to taking any medication. Mood may also affect adherence, as the depressed older adult may not be motivated to take medications.

Patient Physical Characteristics: Physical functioning also plays a major role in medication management. Hearing loss may cause lack of understanding instructions and information. Visual acuity affects the ability to read labels, instructions, and warnings. Arthritis, tremors, pain, dexterity, and fatigue may make opening bottles, splitting tablets, administering eye drops, reaching the back of the body or even getting to where the medication is located, painful, difficult, or impossible to perform.

Consequence of Non-Adherence: It is estimated that medication adherence in chronic disease management is approximately 50%. About 10%–25% of older adults either take their prescription med-

ications partially or forget to take them at all (Durso, 2001). Potential repercussions of noncompliance include worsening or recurrence of illness, transfer to nursing home care, transmission of communicable disease, unnecessary hospitalization, increased number of lost workdays, increased morbidity and mortality, and increased healthcare costs to the individual and society.

Strategies to Overcome Non-Adherence: It is essential to develop a positive trusting relationship with the patient. Effective communication skills and devotion of sufficient time and effort is cardinal to the nurse-patient relationship. Determine if any of the patient psychosocial characteristics impact medication usage. If a patient is personally biased against medications or has no economic means of obtaining a medication, there is no use in one being prescribed until these issues are resolved. An integral part of communication is determining the patient's cognitive and physical abilities that affect the understanding and administration of medications. Knowing what social support a patient has is also important to know at this time, as the medication teaching may have to be directed at this person. Medication instructions should be explicit and delivered both verbally and in writing. Medications that are "as needed" (PRN) should be specific as to their usage. In addition to the time, dose, route, and special considerations, include what the medication is treating, common side effects, and any side effects that warrant attention.

Determine what, if any, compliance aides are currently in use, such as a calendar, a pill container, an electronic alarm reminder, reminders by caregivers or others, or telephone reminders. Assistance may be needed in setting up a compliance aide for patients (Kane, Ouslander, & Abrass, 1999). To encourage continued compliance, especially with medications requiring long-term treatment, follow-up phone calls and/or visits should reinforce instructions. Ask the patient how they are taking each of their medications, if they have been started on any other new medications (prescribed or over-the-counter) by themselves or other providers, and whether they have missed doses of the drug. These questions must be asked with a nonjudgmental approach or patients are most likely to respond with answers they think the clinician wants to hear! A good approach is to ask the patient to bring all of the medications they take, including OTC and others, in a bag for each visit. This will provide the opportunity to see how much the patients know about each medication and give some idea if they are taking them correctly based on the date of filling and the number of doses remaining in the bottle. Home visits to the patient by a nurse professional often disclose interesting and previously unknown drugs and drug-use behavior. During these visits, if prescriptions no longer required by the patient or outdated medications are found, it is best to ask that they be disposed. With permission, this should be done at the home, in front of the patient, while explaining the goal of improved safety. In any setting, make certain to ask the patient how they feel the medication is working and any side effects that they may be experiencing. Also assess for any difficulties with swallowing or administering medications.

MEDICATIONS AND LONG-TERM CARE FACILITIES

At the heart of care to the older adult living in long-term care facilities (LTC) is the nurse. Unlike an acute setting, LTC nurses must often act autonomously with little support. With early discharges from acute settings, care to the older adult in sub-acute long-term care settings is becoming more and more like acute care. Unlike the home health nurse, providing care to one patient at a time, a nurse working in Extended Care Facilities (ECF) often have a medication pass for 50 or more patients.

The typical LTC resident is prime for an adverse drug reaction. The average resident is 85 years of age, has 3–5 medical diagnoses, and takes 6–8 medications daily. Residents on five different medications have a 50% risk of potential drug reactions and of those taking 8 or more medications the risk is nearly 100% (Cadieux, 2002). Two-thirds of LTC residents have a diagnoses of dementia, with up to 90% of them having, at some point in time, behavioral problems. Seventy-five percent of the residents are impaired in 3 or more activities of daily living. This complex, frail population requires specially trained health care professionals that are not always available. Despite the efforts of the American Geriatric Society and its allies nationwide, the number of geriatricians specially trained to care for the rising number of older adults is shrinking. According to testimony made at a session of the Senate Special Committee on Aging (www.senate.gov/index.cfm?), only three of the country's 125 medical schools have geriatric departments. Less than 1 percent of all nurses in the United States are certified in geriatrics, and less than 9,000 of the country's 650,000 physicians are geriatricians — a figure expected to drop to about 6,000 in the next two years. To keep up with America's aging population, the country will need 36,000 geriatricians by 2030. Of the nearly 200,000 pharmacists in the United States, only 720 have geriatric certifications (Advisory, 2002). To make matter worse the Joint Commission for Accreditation of Health Care Organizations (JCAHO, 2002) states that 90% percent of long-term care organizations lack sufficient nurse staffing to provide even the most basic of care. Added to this is a shortage of any type of physician willing to provide care in ECFs and overwhelming amounts of paperwork due to being highly regulated by state and federal governmental agencies.

The geriatric-trained advanced practice nurse (APN) is well-positioned to play a central role in improving the health of the nation's older adults now and in the future. Geriatric nurse practitioners and clinical specialists have been shown to improve care to older adults in the community, in hospitals, and in long-term care facilities (Mezey and Fulmer, 2002). Despite these advances, the number of geriatric nurse practitioners (GNPs) remains small, with only 4,200 certified specialists, about 3%, of the over 88,000 trained NPs (Spratley, Johnson, Sochalski, Fritz, & Spencer, 2000). Of these over 1,300 work full-time in long-term care facilities. Sixty-three master's programs now prepare advanced practice geriatric nurses but face a serious shortage of geriatric nursing faculty. There is a trend of encouraging preparation of more nurses with specialization in geriatrics as compared to encouraging geriatric preparation among nurses whose major field of study is outside geriatrics (Mezey, Fulmer, & Fairchild, 2000). As physician acceptance of advanced practice nurses continues to grow, the role of the advanced practice nurse in LTC will expand. It may be said that the geriatric-trained APN can best address the challenges and complex needs of the older adult.

Oversight by OBRA

The federal government became deeply involved in the oversight of nursing home care with the passage of the Nursing Home Reform Amendments of the Omnibus Budget Reconciliation Act (OBRA) of 1987. OBRA '87 specifies that residents shall be free from unnecessary drugs. The word "unnecessary" is given a fairly broad meaning and includes drugs that are given in excessive doses, for excessive periods of time, or in the absence of a diagnosis or reason for the drug. Unnecessary drugs also include medications for which monitoring data or the presence of adverse side effects indicates that the dose is reduced or the drug eliminated entirely. More specifically, OBRA '87 outlines the appropriate indications for the use of antipsychotic agents. Residents who have not previously used psychotropic drugs, must not be given these agents unless thera-

py is necessary to treat a specific condition. Residents who are currently receiving antipsychotic drugs should receive gradual dose reductions or drug holidays in an effort to discontinue the medications, unless it is documented that this is clinically contraindicated. The appropriate conditions, or diagnoses, that warrant antipsychotic drug usage and unacceptable uses are specified by OBRA '87 (see Table 4-5). More recent revisions in OBRA also target sedatives, hypnotics, and anxiolytics. The rules state that residents should not be prescribed long-acting benzodiazepines unless a shorter acting benzodiazepine has been tried and has failed. The rules go on to say that sedatives and short-acting benzodiazepines should not be used until a thorough assessment has elicited possible causes of disturbing behavior and that environmental manipulation, interdisciplinary teamwork, care planning, and so on, has be attempted. Interestingly, OBRA has made some exceptions to the rules. For example, if diazepam is prescribed for muscle pain rather than anxiety, the rules do not apply. Another example is if diphenhydramine HCl is prescribed for sleep, the thorough assessment must be done and other non-chemical factors must be implemented first. If diphenhydramine HCl is prescribed as an antihistamine, the rules do not apply (Health Care Financing Administration, 1992).

Reasons for the regulation of psychoactive medications is clear, the potential for adverse drug reactions is great. Beers and colleagues (1991) developed explicit criteria to identify inappropriate medications, including psychoactives, for the frail older adult (see Table 4-6). These criteria, developed through literature and consensus methodology, were based on the potential risks and benefits of medications. The Beers' criteria, or a modified version of it, is most often used by researchers and regulators. Higher rates of falls, loss of function, hip fractures, decreased cognition, and premature institutionalization have all been documented

TABLE 4-5: OMNIBUS BUDGET RECONCILIATION ACT (OBRA) INDICATIONS FOR ANTIPSYCHOTIC DRUG USE

Acceptable

- Management of documented psychotic disorder:
    - Schizophrenia.
    - Schizoaffective disorder.
    - Delusional disorder.
    - Psychotic mood disorder, including mania and depression with psychotic features.
    - Acute psychotic episodes.
    - Brief reactive psychosis.
    - Schizophreniform disorder.
    - Atypical psychosis.
    - Continuous crying or screaming.
- Tourette's syndrome.
- Huntington's chorea.
- Organic mental syndromes with associated psychotic and/or agitated features, in which documented behaviors include the following:
    - The patient is a danger to him or herself.
    - The patient is a danger to others.
    - The patient's behaviors interfere with staff's ability to provide care.

Unacceptable

- Simple pacing.
- Wandering.
- Poor self-care.
- Restlessness.
- Crying out, yelling, or screaming.
- Impaired memory.
- Anxiety, nervousness, or fidgeting.
- Depression.
- Insomnia.
- Unsociability or uncooperativeness.
- Indifference to surroundings.
- Any indication for which the order is on an as-needed basis.

Note. From Centers for Medicare & Medicaid Services, (n.d.). *Psychotropic drug use in skilled nursing facilities (SNF).* Retrieved December 10, 2003, from http://www.cms.hhs.gov/medlearn/articleSNF1002.pdf

TABLE 4-6: BEERS' CRITERIA AND CLASSIFICATION OF INAPPROPRIATE DRUGS FOR OLDER ADULTS

Always Avoid	Rarely Appropriate	Sometimes Appropriate
Barbiturates	Chlordiazepoxide (Librium®)	Amitriptyline
Flurazepam		Doxepin
Meprobamate	Diazepam	Indomethacin
Chlorpropamide	Propoxyphene (Darvon®)	Dipyridamole
Meperidine		Ticlopidine
Pentazocine	Carisoprodol	Methyldopa
Trimethobenzamide	Chlorzoxazone	Reserpine
Belladonna alkaloids	Cyclobenzaprine	Disopyramide
Dicyclomine	Metaxalone	Cyproheptadine
Hyoscyamine	Methocarbamol	Diphenhydramine
Propantheline		Hydroxyzine
		Promethazine

Note. From Beers, M., et al. (1991). Explicit criteria for determining medication use in nursing home residents. *Archives of Internal Medicine, 151*(9), 1825-1832.

among older persons who receive psychoactive drugs (Dellasega, Klinefelter, & Halas, 2000). Even the short-acting half-life agents are associated with a significant increase in the risk of falling in this population (Ray, Thapa, & Gideon, 2000). Many of these medications or medication combinations directly or indirectly affect function. For example, a medication may affect a resident's appetite, ability to eat, ability to walk safely, or result in incontinence by causing excessive sedation or confusion. A medication may also affect the resident's ability to communicate, socialize, or participate in facility functions.

Since OBRA, the number of prescriptions for antipsychotics, sedative antihistamines, and sedative-hypnotics has decreased, the number of prescriptions for anxiolytics has increased, and prescriptions for antidepressants have undergone a qualitative shift in long-term care facilities. However, the incidence of polypharmacy has not changed (Dellasega, Klinefelter, & Halas, 2000).

Research studies have found that despite OBRA, up to 40% of residents in ECF receive one or more inappropriate drugs based on the Beers' criteria (Dhalla, Anderson, Mamdani, Bronskill, Sykora, & Rochon, 2002; Liu & Christensen, 2002). Compounding inappropriate drug choices are physician visits that occur as rarely as once per month per patient, the tendency for the clinician to prescribe medications on an "as-needed" basis, inclination toward polypharmacy, and understaffing of nurses to implement non-pharmacological interventions (Mayo Clinic, 2003). To help prevent adverse drug reactions in LTC patients, take the time to know the patient and their medications, give PRN medications judiciously, chart reactions to medications, report suspected ADRs to the patient's physician, and elicit the help of other members of the interdisciplinary care team for non-pharmacological treatment of behaviors.

Pain Medication Management

Under-treatment of pain in the elderly is also a significant problem in long-term care facilities, with 85% of the residents reporting pain and one-third of these patients reporting constant pain. Undertreatment of pain leads to increased suffering and personal distress. It also causes problems such as immobility with accompanying complications; decreased functional ability; poor or interrupted sleep; increased anxiety and depression; decreased social activities; increased isolation; loss of appetite, which often results in malnutrition; and an increased number of falls. Some of these problems are treated with psychoactive medications when pain management is what is actually needed. Inadequate education in pain management for healthcare professionals is a major problem leading to undertreatment (Gaston-Johansson, Johansson, & Johansson, 1999).

SUMMARY

In general, medications should be used only in situations where life, function, or comfort is threatened. The medication benefits should outweigh the negatives and should improve the life of the older adult or improve their function.

CHAPTER 4

Questions 22-27

22. A physiological change of aging that affects drug distribution is

    a. increase in renal function.

    b. increase total body water.

    c. fewer plasma protein binding sites.

    d. decreased fat-to-muscle ratio.

23. Which of the following statements about adverse drug reactions (ADRs) in the elderly is most accurate?

    a. OTC drug usage is not a contributing factor to ADRs.

    b. Older adults rarely utilize herbal products.

    c. Newly approved drugs are always a cause of ADRs.

    d. Polypharmacy is a common cause of ADRs.

24. The usage of OTC, herbals, supplements, minerals, and home remedies in the older adult is

    a. a method for the older adult to take control of his or her life.

    b. not a concern as these are approved by the FDA.

    c. safe, as home remedies have been used for years.

    d. common in the older adult and can lead to adverse drug affects (ADRs).

25. When working with an older adult who is non-adherent to his/her medication regimen the nurse should first

    a. take a drug history/assessment.

    b. develop a trusting relationship.

    c. determine cognitive functioning level.

    d. determine if client is able to afford medications.

26. The older adult in an extended care facility (ECF) is at risk for the following adverse drug reactions from psychoactive medications:

    a. vomiting, sedation, or falls.

    b. increased confusion, incontinence, or falls.

    c. decreased appetite, sedation, or increased socialization.

    d. increased communication, sedation, or falls.

27. Since the inception of OBRA 87, inappropriate drug usage in ECFs is

    a. no longer an issue due to the decline in prescribing antipsychotic.

    b. still an issue with the problem lying with the physician.

    c. still an issue with multiple causes.

    d. caused by the chronic nursing shortage.

CHAPTER 5

COMMON CLINICAL PROBLEMS OF THE OLDER ADULT

CHAPTER OBJECTIVE

After studying this chapter, the reader will be able to discuss clinical problems that are prevalent in the older adult.

LEARNING OBJECTIVES

After studying this chapter the learner will be able to

1. explain iatrogenesis and its effect on the older adult.

2. describe the various types of urinary incontinence and their impact on quality of life for the older adult.

3. select nursing interventions for prevention and treatment of altered bowel elimination.

4. list strategies to prevent and treat pressure sores.

5. indicate common physical functional impairments.

6. describe the impact of falls on the older adult.

7. recognize major factors that indicate a client is at nutritional risk.

8. specify the proper procedure for administering medications to tube-fed residents.

9. indicate the importance of hydration for the older adult.

INTRODUCTION

It is common for the older adult to have any number of, or be at high risk for, various clinical problems. These problems may be a persistent health issue that lasts forever such as impaired physical functioning or incontinence. Recurrent problems such as constipation, pressure sores, falls, nutrition, or dehydration are also commonly seen in this population. An unintentional injury or condition caused by the medical treatment itself is a frequent cause of clinical concerns. These problems impact the physical and emotional lives of older adults to varying degrees. The significant aspect of these problems for the nurse is that for many older adults, these problems can be prevented or eliminated with aggressive and timely nursing interventions.

IATROGENESIS

Iatrogenesis is the unintended, harmful incidents or conditions that result from diagnostic, prophylactic, or therapeutic interventions or omissions. It occurs frequently in the older adult because of their increased exposure to the healthcare system and increased vulnerability, in general. Iatrogenic complications are distressing and costly to all. The prevention of iatrogenesis is the most effective management method. The following iatrogenic problems are the most common ones seen in this population.

Medications: (The number one cause)

Adverse drug reactions (ADRs).

Infection:

Urinary tract infections (UTIs) from catheters or poor peri-care.

Respiratory: Aspiration pneumonia.

Wound: Improper sterile technique, inadequate wound assessment.

Malnutrition:

Anorexia due to medication side effects.

Restricted diets, surgery NPO orders.

Failure to provide supplements or assistance in eating, or personal choices (Wendland, Greenwood, Weinberg, & Young, 2003).

Incontinence:

Design of healthcare setting.

Lack of staff to assist in toileting.

Restraints, catheters, medications, prolonged bed rest (Potter, 2003).

Accidents & Injuries:

Falls: Unfamiliar surroundings, climbing over side rails, lack of supervision, sedation or gait disturbance from medication, lack of understanding of call bell system, restraints, clutter, wheels not locked on wheelchair, or slippery floors.

Accidents: Doors and dressers left open, needles not disposed of properly, medical equipment not functioning properly, or skin tears (Rothschild, Bates, & Leape 2000).

Sleep Disturbance:

Untreated pain, noisy bright environment, medications, and anxiety.

Functional Decline:

Medications, prolonged bed rest, surgery, depression, therapy not provided (Chin, Sahadevan, Tan, Ho, & Choo, 2001).

Decubitus Ulcer:

Lack of proper positioning, nutrition, and preventive treatment.

Nursing Interventions

• Educate patient, family, and other staff members about risks and preventative methods.

• Proper handwashing and infection control for all.

• Use interdisciplinary team for assessment of potential or actual risks and interventions for those risks (Jacelon, 1999).

URINARY INCONTINENCE

Urinary incontinence (UI) has a significant physical, psychological, social, and economic consequence on the more than 13 million older adults with this problem (Dowling-Castronovo, 2001). The prevalence of UI increases with age, but it is not a normal aging process. It is associated with skin irritation, pressure ulcers, urinary tract infections, and falls. It may also cause embarrassment, withdrawal from social life, depression, and loss of self-esteem. Excursions outside the home, social interaction with friends and family, and sexual activity may be restricted or avoided entirely. Incontinence may be stressful for family caregivers and is the second leading risk factor for institutionalization. In nursing home residents, 54% have UI and 80% require assistance with toileting. The costs of UI is enormous, approximately $30 billion per year and growing. For patients on a special care units (SCU) approximately 46% are continent upon admission and of these 42% became incontinent within 6 months of admission. Many SCU residents have the ability to maintain or regain continence with preventative and active interventions (Specht, Lyon, & Maas, 2002).

Types of Incontinence

Transient Incontinence: Commonly caused by reversible problems such as delirium, depression, infection, fecal impaction, medications, or inflammation. If the underlying problem is not treated quickly it may result in chronic UI.

Stress Incontinence: Small amounts of urine loss during activities that increase intra-abdominal pressure such as coughing or sneezing. Cause: Weakness and laxity of pelvic floor, bladder outlet, or urethral sphincter weakness. Most common in women, and in men after prostate surgery.

Urge Incontinence (UI): Abrupt and strong desire to void with sudden loss of large amount of urine, usually on way to bathroom. Cause: Overactivity of detrusor muscle causing bladder contractions attributed to central nervous system diseases such as Alzheimer's or Parkinson's, or local bladder disorder such as stones or cancer. Most common cause of UI.

Mixed Incontinence: Combination of both stress and urge.

Overflow Incontinence: Urine loss from obstruction or over-distended bladder with frequent or constant dribbling of urine. Cause: Medications, fecal impaction, diabetes and spinal cord injury. In men with prostate disorders and urethral strictures, and in women with genital prolapse.

Functional Incontinence: Urine leakage associated with inability or unwillingness to use toilet. Cause: Pain, cognitive impairment, environmental barriers, impaired mobility, and/or unavailable caregivers.

Nursing Assessment: Approximately 30 to 50% of people with UI do not report their problem to their doctor or nurse. The following questions can help determine if the client has UI and which type:

- Do you ever leak urine when you don't want to?
- Do you lose urine when you laugh, cough or sneeze, lift something heavy, walk, or sleep?
- Do you lose your urine on the way to the bathroom or toilet?
- Do you wet the bed at night?
- Do you go to the bathroom frequently because you are afraid of wetting yourself?
- Are you using perineal pads or absorbent products to collect the urine?
- Do you dribble after voiding? (suggests overflow)
- Do you void in small quantities?
- Do you have difficulty initiating urination? (suggests overflow)
- How often are you urinating?

A "yes" answer to any of the above would warrant further assessment:

- When incontinence started. (Suspect transient if recent),
- Recent or recurrent urinary tract infection (UTI) or fecal impaction.
- Medications that adversely affect the bladder (anticholinergics, diuretics, anti-Parkinsonism, or narcotics),
- Obesity, genitourinary history, or neurological diagnoses such as dementia or multiple sclerosis.
- Mobility deficits (functional).

Nursing Interventions

- Determine incontinence type.
- Determine voiding patterns using diary or other method.
- Use bladder training for urge, stress, and mixed incontinence.
- Use habit training or timed voiding for urge incontinence.
- Promoted voiding for the cognitively impaired.
- Teach Kegel (1948) exercises for urge, stress, and mixed incontinence.
- Modify environment for functional incontinence including lighting, altered clothing, or adaptive equipment.
- Provide substitution such as bedpan or urinal for functional incontinence.
- Request physical, occupational, or recreational therapy for functional incontinence.

For older adults who do not respond to these interventions, surgery, biofeedback, medications and other devices may be appropriate. Suggest a referral to a urologist for the client. In long-term care facilities make positive expectations for continence the standard. Research has found the cost of incontinence in longterm facilities to be $6,280 per year per resident (Frenchman, 2001), which should give administration the impetus to back any continence program. Include all members of the interdisciplinary care team in the planning and implementing of any interventions, particularly the nurse's aides who carry out the majority of toileting assistance needs in these settings.

ALTERED
BOWEL ELIMINATION

Constipation, fecal incontinence, and diarrhea are bowel-related problems of major concern because of the frequency of their occurrence, the distress and discomfort, costs involved, and potential for complications. Normal bowel function is dependent on physical activities, and a diet with adequate fiber and fluids. Medications, toileting habits, function, laxative and enema usage, and pathological conditions such as depression, cognitive impairment, hypothyroidism, tumors, and many others contribute to bowel-related problems. Nursing assessment includes bowel function and pattern, medication usage, current diagnoses, laxative usage, dietary patterns, activity pattern, patient expectation and emotional state.

Constipation was mentioned more than 2,500 years ago when Hippocrates noted that "the intestines tend to become sluggish with age." (Schaefer, Cheskin, 1998). The definition of constipation is highly subjective, but among older adults the most frequent descriptors are long periods between bowel movements, pain, and/or difficulty passing stool. It is a problem that affects as many as 26% of men and 34% of women over 65 years

of age. Constipation is more than an annoying problem. Persons with chronic constipation have been shown to have a diminished perception of quality of life. Fecal impaction, incontinence, colonic dilatation, and even perforation can complicate constipation.

Nursing Interventions for Constipation

- Abdominal assessment for fecal impaction (May present with liquid stool flowing around impaction, increase in confusion and agitation in those with dementia. Saline enemas and manual disimpaction to treat).

- Educate about normal bowel habits.

- Arrange an individualized regular toileting schedule (Kennedy, 2002).

- Increase fluids and fiber: High fiber enlarges and softens the stool, distends the rectum, and elicits the defecation urge.

- Increased exercise and/or activity.

- Educate client, family, and/or staff on privacy and timing issues of constipation management.

- Educate community clients on laxative types (see Table 5-1).

- For acute constipation use a saline enema.

Fecal Incontinence can be devastating. Persons with loss of bowel control may feel ashamed, embarrassed, or humiliated. Many don't want to leave the house out of fear they might have an accident in public, withdrawing from friends and family. Fecal incontinence is the loss of normal control of the bowels. This leads to stool leaking from the rectum at unexpected times. Bowel function is controlled by three things: anal sphincter pressure, rectal storage capacity, and rectal sensation. The anal sphincter is a muscle that contracts to prevent stool leakage and is critical in maintaining continence (Muller-Lissner, 2002). The rectum can stretch and hold stool for some time after a person becomes aware that the stool is there. This is the rectal storage capacity. Rectal sensation tells a

TABLE 5-1: LAXATIVE TYPES

Bulk type: (Metamucil®, Citrucel®) Onset 12-24 hours. Absorbs water to stimulate the intestine. Can harden stool and cause obstruction. Mix with 240cc fluid; follow with addition 240cc fluids.

Stool softener: (Colace®, Diocto-K®): Onset 24-72 hours. Permits water to penetrate stool. May enhance absorption of other medications.

Lubricant: (Mineral Oil) Onset 6-8 hours. Lubricates fecal matter, retards water absorption in intestine. Avoid routine regular usage to prevent dependency.

Saline: (Milk of Magnesium) Onset 1-3 hours. May cause electrolyte imbalance and dehydration.

Hyperosmotic: (Sorbitol). Onset 24-48 hours. Draws water into feces. May cause gaseous distention and flatulence.

Irritant or stimulant: (Senna, Aloe, Decholin, Dulcolax®, or Castor Oil) These alter fluid and electrolytes transport resulting in fluid accumulation. Some simulate peristalsis. Onset of action 6-10 hours. May cause dehydration, diarrhea, electrolyte imbalance, and laxative dependency. Some may cause discoloration of urine.

Enema: Use saline only. Soapsuds irritate and tap water causes electrolyte imbalance.

person that stool is in the rectum. A person also must be alert, cognizant, and mobile enough to notice the rectal sensation and do something about it. Fecal incontinence is prevalent in up to 47% of long-term care residents and contributes to the admission decision. Complications of fecal incontinence include anal pain and irritation, skin breakdown, depression, isolation, and other emotional complications. Treatment depends on the cause and severity of fecal incontinence; it may include dietary changes, medication, bowel training, or surgery. More than one treatment may be necessary for successful control, since continence involves a complicated chain of events. Start bowel training and scheduled toileting by first doing a bowel diary for a week to determine when bowel movements occur. For clients with a bowel pattern, toilet one half hour before normal bowel movement time. For clients with no bowel pattern, try training by toileting after every meal until pattern is established. In both cases allow time and privacy for bowel movements to occur.

Dietary Changes to Aid in Fecal Continence

- Eat foods that add bulk to stool (bananas, rice, tapioca, bread, potatoes, applesauce, cheese, smooth peanut butter, yogurt, pasta, or oatmeal).

- Avoid foods that contribute to the problem: Anything with caffeine, which relaxes the internal anal sphincter muscle. Foods that cause diarrhea: spicy foods, alcohol, dairy products, fatty and greasy foods, or artificial sweeteners

- Eat smaller meals more frequently. Large meals cause bowel contractions, leading to diarrhea.

- Eat and drink at different times. Liquid helps move food through the digestive system. To slow things down, drink one half before or after meals, but not with the meals.

- Eat more fiber. Fiber makes stool soft, formed, and easier to control. Fiber is found in fruits, vegetables, and grains. Add fiber to the diet slowly so your body can adjust.

Diarrhea is an increase in daily stool weight, occurring more frequently, with an increase in fluid content, and is often accompanied by urgency and pain. Acute diarrhea can be a serious health problem for older adults as they are susceptible to infections by diarrhea-causing bacterial pathogens like C. difficile and Shigella for several reasons (Simor, 2002; Slotwiner-Nie & Brandt, 2002). These include low gastric acidity which increases the viability of potential pathogens in the gastrointestinal tract; frequent use of antibiotics, laxatives and other medicines that may disrupt healthy bowel flora; and weaker immune defenses, including lower T-cell counts, impaired mucosa, and altered gut flora. Clinical features are dehydration, fever, nausea, vomiting, and watery or bloody diarrhea. Always assess the patient for fecal impaction when diarrhea occurs. If the diarrhea does not subside within 12 hours, the healthcare provider should be notified. The treatment of diarrhea is:

1. Correction of fluids and electrolytes: During hydration observe for signs of overhydration and cardiac overload such as lung base rales and jugular vein distention.

2. Symptomatic therapy: Dietary measures to reduce stool volume such as apples, bananas, yogurt, cheese, rice, and avoidance of fatty foods.

3. Specific treatment: Remove caustic agent such as medications or specific foods.

SKIN BREAKDOWN

Pressure ulcers are serious problems for older adults in the community, in hospitals, and in long-term care settings, where the incidence is as high as 24% (Ayello, 1999). Pressure ulcers in the older adult may lead to sepsis and death. The aging process changes the skin making it susceptible to breakdown. It is important to identify which clients are at risk, focus on preventing breakdown, and detect ulcers early in the development process.

Pressure sores are costly, painful, and considered a quality of life indicator by regulators. A pressure sore is necrosis and disruption of the skin and deeper tissues secondary to inadequate oxygenation and physical disruption of skin barrier. Multiple factors are involved in the development of decubitus ulcers, including trauma (e.g., friction, bruises, or multiple same-site injections); immobility; moisture from any source, but especially incontinence; and poor hydration, nutrition, circulatory, or mental status. Infection, anemia, decreased sensory perception, long-term steroid use, and edema increase the risk of skin breakdown. Mechanical factors that contribute to development include: pressure, which reduces blood flow; shear, which is the movement of one tissue plane over another, most common when sliding down a bed or chair; and friction which is the moving of skin against objects, leading to abrasions. Decubitus ulcers may cause pain, infection, protein loss, multiplication of lesions, and increased workload for caregivers. Like so many other problems of the older adult, it is best to prevent decubitus ulcers. The most common sites for pressure ulcers are the heels, ankle, ischium, sacrum, and greater trochanter.

Nursing Interventions to Prevent Pressure Sores

• Determine the client's risk by using the Braden Scale for Predicting Pressure Sore Risk. (See Figure 5-1.) It is the most widely used tool on older adults, with and without cognitive impairment in all settings. The Minimum Data Set (MDS) may also be used but research has shown that it over-predicts pressure sore development at a ratio of 2:1. Therefore, researchers recommend using both scales together (Vap & Dunaye, 2000).

• For immobile and high-risk patients who are turned and positioned at least every two hours, use preventive devices, such as pads between knees or sheepskin pads shaped to fit over heels. Keep heels off of bed.

FIGURE 5-1: BRADEN SCALE FOR PREDICTING PRESSURE ULCER SORE RISK

BRADEN SCALE—For Predicting Pressure Sore Risk

HIGH RISK: Total Score ≤ 12 **MODERATE RISK:** Total score 13 - 14
LOW RISK: Total score 15 - 16 if under 75 years old **OR** 15 - 18 if over 75 years old.

DATE OF ASSESS. →

RISK FACTOR	SCORE/DESCRIPTION				1	2	3	4
SENSORY PERCEPTION Ability to respond meaningfully to pressure-related discomfort	**1. COMPLETELY LIMITED—** Unresponsive (does not moan, flinch, or grasp) to painful stimuli, due to diminished level of consciousness or sedation, **OR** limited ability to feel pain over most of body surface.	**2. VERY LIMITED—** Responds only to painful stimuli. Cannot communicate discomfort except by moaning or restlessness, **OR** has a sensory impairment which limits the ability to feel pain or discomfort over ½ of body.	**3. SLIGHTLY LIMITED—** Responds to verbal commands but cannot always communicate discomfort or need to be turned, **OR** has some sensory impairment which limits ability to feel pain or discomfort in 1 or 2 extremities.	**4. NO IMPAIRMENT—** Responds to verbal commands. Has no sensory deficit which would limit ability to feel or voice pain or discomfort.				
MOISTURE Degree to which skin is exposed to moisture	**1. CONSTANTLY MOIST—** Skin is kept moist almost constantly by perspiration, urine, etc. Dampness is detected every time patient is moved or turned.	**2. OFTEN MOIST—** Skin is often but not always moist. Linen must be changed at least once a shift.	**3. OCCASIONALLY MOIST—** Skin is occasionally moist, requiring an extra linen change approximately once a day.	**4. RARELY MOIST—** Skin is usually dry; linen only requires changing at routine intervals.				
ACTIVITY Degree of physical activity	**1. BEDFAST—** Confined to bed.	**2. CHAIRFAST—** Ability to walk severely limited or nonexistent. Cannot bear own weight and/or must be assisted into chair or wheelchair.	**3. WALKS OCCASIONALLY—** Walks occasionally during day but for very short distances, with or without assistance. Spends majority of each shift in bed or chair.	**4. WALKS FREQUENTLY—** Walks outside the room at least twice a day and inside room at least once every 2 hours during waking hours.				
MOBILITY Ability to change and control body position	**1. COMPLETELY IMMOBILE—** Does not make even slight changes in body or extremity position without assistance.	**2. VERY LIMITED—** Makes occasional slight changes in body or extremity position but unable to make frequent or significant changes independently.	**3. SLIGHTLY LIMITED—** Makes frequent though slight changes in body or extremity position independently.	**4. NO LIMITATIONS—** Makes major and frequent changes in position without assistance.				
NUTRITION Usual food intake pattern ¹NPO: Nothing by mouth. ²IV: Intravenously. ³TPN: Total parenteral nutrition.	**1. VERY POOR—** Never eats a complete meal. Rarely eats more than 1/3 of any food offered. Eats 2 servings or less of protein (meat or dairy products) per day. Takes fluids poorly. Does not take a liquid dietary supplement, **OR** is NPO¹ and/or maintained on clear liquids or IV² for more than 5 days.	**2. PROBABLY INADEQUATE—** Rarely eats a complete meal and generally eats only about ½ of any food offered. Protein intake includes only 3 servings of meat or dairy products per day. Occasionally will take a dietary supplement, **OR** receives less than optimum amount of liquid diet or tube feeding.	**3. ADEQUATE—** Eats over half of most meals. Eats a total of 4 servings of protein (meat, dairy products) each day. Occasionally will refuse a meal, but will usually take a supplement if offered, **OR** is on a tube feeding or TPN³ regimen, which probably meets most of nutritional needs.	**4. EXCELLENT—** Eats most of every meal. Never refuses a meal. Usually eats a total of 4 or more servings of meat and dairy products. Occasionally eats between meals. Does not require supplementation.				
FRICTION AND SHEAR	**1. PROBLEM—** Requires moderate to maximum assistance in moving. Complete lifting without sliding against sheets is impossible. Frequently slides down in bed or chair, requiring frequent repositioning with maximum assistance. Spasticity, contractures, or agitation leads to almost constant friction.	**2. POTENTIAL PROBLEM—** Moves feebly or requires minimum assistance. During a move, skin probably slides to some extent against sheets, chair, restraints, or other devices. Maintains relatively good position in chair or bed most of the time but occasionally slides down.	**3. NO APPARENT PROBLEM—** Moves in bed and in chair independently and has sufficient muscle strength to lift up completely during move. Maintains good position in bed or chair at all times.					
TOTAL SCORE	Total score of 12 or less represents HIGH RISK							

ASSESS.	DATE	EVALUATOR SIGNATURE/TITLE	ASSESS.	DATE	EVALUATOR SIGNATURE/TITLE
1	/ /		3	/ /	
2	/ /		4	/ /	

NAME—Last, First, Middle   ATTENDING PHYSICIAN   ID NUMBER

BRIGGS, Des Moines, IA 50306 (800) 247-2343 PRINTED IN U.S.A.
Form 3166P

BRADEN SCALE

Note. From Barbara Braden and Nanc Bergstrom. © 1988. Reprinted with permission.

- Use sheepskin or egg crate foam to avoid compression of tissue and skin breakdown. Many products are available to reduce pressure on bony prominences, such as alternating pressure mattresses, waterbeds, silicone gel beds, or air flotation mattresses. These are not a substitute for frequent turning.

- Clients in wheelchairs should be transferred to

everyday furniture whenever possible. Assist high risk clients to shift weight every 15 minutes. Use padding if sitting in a wheelchair for greater than a half-hour.

- Encourage mobility. Perform range of motion (ROM) if tolerated to keep muscles pliant.

- Skin should be kept clean, dry, and free from urine, stool, drainage, or perspiration. Gently apply protectant ointment or film, or hydrocolloid to areas of bony prominences if needed. Do not massage area. Do not use powders.

- Use mechanical devices or a draw sheet to transfer or reposition immobile clients.

- Keep head of bed at a 45-degree angle or less, if patient can tolerate, for meals, and 30 degrees at other times.

- Use under-pads and diapers that wick away moisture. Cloth diapers, donut devices, and highly alkaline soaps such as Dial®, Ivory®, or Basis® should be avoided.

- Protein deficiency and dehydration are linked to skin breakdown, hence hydration and nutrition should be maintained. Consult or request evaluation with dietitian for clients at risk.

- Underweight patients lack body fat to provide cushioning. A generalized approach to weight gain for those who are under their optimal weight is appropriate.

- Overweight patients are at risk as the additional weight adds pressure to vulnerable parts of the body. Overweight patients also place an added burden on the nursing staff in that repositioning requires additional effort. Infrequent repositioning contributes to the pressure areas. If obesity is a concern, provide adequate calories for skin healing while avoiding excessive weight gain.

- Adequate calories must be present for the protein ingested by the body to be used in tissue restoration.

- Check serum albumin level — the body's first indicator of malnutrition.

- Family and patient teaching will help continue the preventative process.

There is much variability in how pressure sores are treated as new products and research emerge. Basic recommendations for treatment of pressure sores are to use moist wound healing and debride any necrotic tissue. Epithelium grows faster in a moist environment; keeping the wound moist promotes growth, whereas drying is harmful. Do not use wet to dry, antiseptics, or topical antimicrobial. If a wound is infected, oral antibiotics may be prescribed.

IMPAIRED FUNCTION

Maintaining optimal function, with the older adult doing as much as possible, as independently as possible, is the overriding objective of care to this population. Function means the ability to perform tasks associated with independent living and is divided into two categories:

- *Activities of Daily Living (ADLs):* Basic body self-care actions including bathing, dressing, toileting, mobility, continence, and eating.

- *Instrumental Activities of Daily Living (IADLs):* Higher, more complex activities to manage needs of independent life such as cooking, housework, transportation, shopping, financial management, medication management, or using a telephone.

Maintaining function is of utmost importance as it is the key to independent living and quality of life. More than 83% of nursing home residents receive help with three or more ADLs (Agency for Health Care Policy and Research, 1997) and for community-dwelling elders that number is as high as 20%. For those living in the community, help is most frequently provided by family and friends. The loss of function places a tremendous burden on healthcare personnel and financing. For many older

FIGURE 5-2: ACTIVITIES OF DAILY LIVING (ADL) SCALE

EVALUATION FORM

Name_____Day of Evaluation_____

For each area of functioning listed below, check description that applies. (The word "assistance" means supervision, direction, or personal assistance.)

BATHING: either sponge bath, tub bath, or shower.
☐ Receives no assistance *(gets in and out of tub by self, if tub is usual means of bathing).*
☐ Receives assistance in bathing only one part of the body (such as back or a leg).
☐ Receives assistance in bathing more than one part of the body (or not bathed).

DRESSING: gets clothes from closets and drawers, including underclothes, outer garments, and using fasteners *(including braces, if worn).*
☐ Gets clothes and gets completely dressed without assistance.
☐ Gets clothes and gets dressed without assistance, except for assistance in tying shoes.
☐ Receives assistance in getting clothes or in getting dressed, or stays partly or completely undressed.

TOILETING: going to the "toilet room" for bowel and urine elimination; cleaning self after elimination and arranging clothes.
☐ Goes to "toilet room," cleans self and arranges clothes without assistance *(may use object for support such as cane, walker, or wheelchair and may manage night bedpan or commode, emptying same in morning).*
☐ Receives assistance in going to "toilet room," cleansing self, arranging clothes after elimination, or in use of night bedpan or commode.
☐ Doesn't go to room termed "toilet" for the elimination process.

TRANSFER
☐ Moves in and out of bed as well as in and out of chair without assistance *(may be using object for support, such as cane or walker).*
☐ Moves in and out of bed or chair with assistance.
☐ Doesn't get out of bed.

CONTINENCE
☐ Controls urination and bowel movements completely by self.
☐ Has occasional "accidents".
☐ Supervision helps keep urine or bowel control; catheter is used or person is incontinent.

FEEDING
☐ Feeds self without assistance.
☐ Feeds self except for getting assistance in cutting meat or buttering bread.
☐ Receives assistance in feeding or is fed partly or completely by using tubes or intravenous fluids.

Adapted from: Katz, S., et al. (1963). Studies of illness in the aged. The index of ADL: A standard measure of biological and psychosocial function. *Journal of the American Medical Association,* 185, 914-919.

adults even the slightest decline in function may mean the difference between living independently and institutionalization. It may also result in depression, social isolation, loss of appetite, risk of injury, infection, pressure ulcers, falling, and a multitude of other damaging outcomes. Assessment of functional status is critical and should be performed initially at baseline, when reassessing, and whenever a client's status changes. See Figure 5-2 for ADL Scale and Figure 5-3 for IADL Scale. These assessments have multiple purposes:

• Identifies strengths and weaknesses.

FIGURE 5-3: INSTRUMENTAL ACTIVITIES OR DAILY LIVING (IADL) SCALE

Self-Rated Version Extracted from the Multilevel Assessment Instrument (MAL)

1. Can you use the telephone:
   without help,   3
   with some help, or   2
   are you completely unable to use the telephone?   1

2. Can you get to places out of walking distance:
   without help,   3
   with some help, or   2
   are you completely unable to travel unless special arrangements are made?   1

3. Can you go shopping for groceries:
   without help,   3
   with some help, or   2
   are you completely unable to do any shopping?   1

4. Can you prepare your own meals:
   without help,   3
   with some help, or   2
   are you completely unable to prepare any meals?   1

5. Can you do your own housework:
   without help,   3
   with some help, or   2
   are you completely unable to do any housework?   1

6. Can you do your own handyman work:
   without help,   3
   with some help, or   2
   are you completely unable to do any handyman work?   1

7. Can you do your own laundry:
   without help,   3
   with some help, or   2
   are you completely unable to do any laundry at all?   1

8a. Do you take medicines or use any medications?
   (If yes, answer Question 8b) Yes   1
   (If no, answer Question 8c) No   2

8b. Do you take your own medicine:
   without help (in the right doses at the right time),   3
   with some help (take medicine if someone prepares it for you and/or reminds you to take it), or   2
   (are you/would you be) completely unable to take your own medicine?   1

8c. If you had to take medicine, can you do it:
   without help (in the right doses at the right time),   3
   with some help (take medicine if someone prepares it for you and/or reminds you to take it), or   2
   (are you/would you be) completely unable to take your own medicine?   1

9. Can you manage your own money:
   without help,   3
   with some help, or   2
   you completely unable to handle money?   1

Note. From Lawton, M.P., & Brody, E.M. (1969). Assessment of older people: Self-maintaining and instrumental activities of daily living. *The Gerontologist, 9,* 179-186.

- Assists in determining needed services, both from formal and informal caregivers.

- Establishes baseline data and aids in setting realistic goals.

- Measure changes over time, evaluating response to interventions.

- Identifies manifestation or exacerbation of a disease (often the first sign is change in ADL).

- Deciding factor in placement decisions such as level of care needed and reimbursement.

Nursing Interventions to Maintain/Regain Function

- Teach nurses aides, family members, and friends the importance of maintaining function by allowing the patient to do as much as possible for themselves even if they can no longer do it perfectly or become messy during the process.

- Discuss with patient what goals (functions) are most important. Together develop a plan to maintain or regain these goals.

- Set up the task if necessary and provide enough time to perform.

- Use at least 2 less intrusive prompts before giving physical assistance (verbal and gestural prompts and modeling).

- Give the least amount of physical assistance required. (This may be as simple as starting the movement such as guiding a client's hand as they hold the toothbrush until they start the brushing process.)

- Praise performance and appearance.

- After an acute illness, performing past skills as soon as possible is vital for preventing further losses.

FALLS

Approximately 11 million older adults fall each year, one-third of all community-dwelling and one-half to two-thirds of all long-term care residents (Farmer, 2000). Falls are associated with mortality, morbidity, functional decline, and premature nursing home placement. Unintentional injuries are the 5th leading cause of death in older adults. Over 300,000 hip fractures occur annually due to falls. Treatment of injuries and complications from falls costs more than $20.2 billion annually (Swanson, 2001). Falls can occur anytime, any place, and to anyone while doing everyday activities such as climbing stairs or getting out of the bathtub. Older adults' number one anxiety is fear of falling. Research has shown that concerns about falling and losing function are managed by older adults by avoidance of activities (Yardley & Smith, 2002). This often leads to feelings of loss, depression, isolation, and loss of function.

There are two types of factors involved in falls: 1. intrinsic, or personal factors such as health, vision, alcohol usage, medications, and 2. fall history and extrinsic or environmental factors such as footwear, flooring, and house plan. Although some risk factors for falls, such as heredity and age, cannot be changed, several risk factors can be eliminated or reduced. Research shows that simple safety modifications at home, where 60% of seniors' falls occur, can substantially cut the risk of falling (Swanson, 2001). A study found that wearing bifocals increased fall risk (Day, Fildes, Gordon, Fitzharris, Flamer, & Lord, 2002). Other risks include wandering, gait disorders, depression, cognitive status, age, and unsafe environment (Cesari, Landi, Torre, Onder, Lattanzio, & Bernabei, 2002).

Teaching Points for Fall Prevention for Community-Dwelling Older Adults

- Get an annual eye and physical examination including evaluation of cardiac and blood pressure.

- Have medications reviewed at each physician visit.

- Maintain a diet with adequate dietary calcium and vitamin D.

- Maintain assistive devices in good working order.

- Wear non-skid, sturdy, proper-fitting shoes

- Participate in an exercise program for agility, strength, balance, and coordination.

- Eliminate tripping hazards at home, such as electric cords and clutter.

- Install grab bars, handrails, shower mats, and other safety devices.

- Remove scatter rugs and use nightlights at night.

- Keep stairs clutter free, lighted, and with sturdy handrail.

- Replace slippers that have stretched out of shape and are too loose.

- Avoid excessive alcohol intake.

- Request physical therapy (PT) for specific mobility therapy and occupational therapy (OT) for home safety evaluation.

Falls Prevention in Long-Term Care

In long-term care facilities physical restraints have not proven to reduce the number of falls and can cause serious injury. The number one predictor of a fall is past history of falls. (American Geriatric Society/British Geriatric Society, 2001). Fall prevention in long-term care facilities starts with a risk assessment to identify residents at highest risk, as falls are preventable. (See Figure 5-4.) Once a specific resident is identified, he or she should be referred to a Falls Prevention Program. This is not merely placing some symbol over the bed or door of the resident to identify them at high risk. The following are elements that should be considered for a prevention program:

- Program should consist of a team composed of all disciplines including housekeeping, maintenance, dietary, social work, recreational, occupational and physical therapies, and nursing.

- Team should meet on regular basis, preferably daily.

- Team should be responsible for training all staff members on falls prevention.

- Residents enter program based on risk or on having had a fall.

- Develop a strategy to reduce risk of falling using interventions specific to either the program participant or his/her environment.

Possible interventions and discipline responsible:

- Audit of resident room or bathroom for safety. Include housekeeping factors such as time when floors are wet. May need rearranging, grips installed, different type of bed. (OT, Maintenance, Housekeeping)

- Assess footwear, clothing for alteration needs. (Nursing, Laundry)

- Assess assistive devices. (OT, PT)

- Seating assessment for participants who fall from chair or wheelchairs. (OT)

- Assess medications, eliminating any that contribute. (Medical Director, Nursing)

- For wandering behavior provide therapeutic activities and periods of rest. (RT, nursing)

- Exercise programs, morning walking programs, Tai Chi and others. (RT, OT, PT, Nursing)

- Toileting program. (Nursing)

- Hip protectors and other protective clothing. (Nursing, Laundry)

- Alarms for bed or chair to alert staff. (Nursing, PT, OT, Maintenance)

- For residents awake at night, provide activities with supervision until ready for sleep.

FIGURE 5-4: FALL RISK ASSESSMENT TOOL

INSTRUCTIONS: Circle the score that corresponds with the risk factor listed on the lefthand side of the instrument. The tool should be administered on admission to the facility or agency and again at specified intervals and when warranted by changes in health status.

CLIENT FACTOR	Date	Initial Score	Date	Reassessed Score
History of falls		15		15
Confusion		5		5
Age (over 65)		5		5
Impaired judgment		5		5
Sensory deficit		5		5
Unable to ambulate independently		5		5
Decreased level of cooperation		5		5
Increased anxiety/emotional liability		5		5
Incontinence/Urgency		5		5
Cardiovascular/respiratory disease affecting perfusion and oxygenation		5		5
Medications affecting blood pressure or level of consciousness		5		5
Postural hypotension with dizziness		5		5
Environmental Factors				
First week on unit (facility, services, etc.)		5		5
Attached equipment (e.g., IV pokes, chest tubes, appliances, oxygen, tubing, etc.)		5		5

TOTAL POINTS: _____

Implement fall precautions for a score of 15 or greater

Note. From Funk, S.G., Tornquist, E.M., Champagne, M.T., & Wiese, R.A. (Eds.). (1992). Key Aspects of Elder Care: Managing Falls, Incontinence, and Cognitive Impairment. In L. Hollinger & R. Patterson, *A Fall Prevention Program for the Acute Care Setting*. New York, NY: Springer Publishing Company. Reprinted with permission.

• Have nourishments, such as finger foods, available 24 hours per day. (Dietary, Nursing)

NUTRITION

Between 8 and 16% of older adults do not have regular access to a nutritionally adequate, culturally compatible diet. The U. S. Department of Health and Human Services (2000) states that between 2.5 and 4.9 million older adults suffer from hunger but federal programs reach only one third of those in need. Changes in physiology and function, health, and psychosocial factors associated with the aging process have the potential to impact diet and nutritional status. Approximately 85% of older adults have one or more nutrition-related chronic conditions, and up to 15% of older adults are believed to have malnutrition. Factors contributing to risk include:

- Decrease in energy expenditure: (Decline in basal metabolic rate, decrease in physical activity). In response, caloric requirements decrease.

- Change in body composition: (Loss of lean muscle, increase in body fat. Fat requires fewer calories to be maintained than muscle). Implication is loss of strength, endurance, and range-of-motion; may impair ability to purchase and/or prepare meals. (Zembrzuski, 2000)

- Decline in oral health: (Lack of or poor fitting dentures, untreated periodontal disease or decayed teeth, or decrease in saliva). Difficulty chewing and swallowing may limit food choices, loss of taste or pleasure in food, or poor oral hygiene (may cause embarrassment over eating with others).

- Sensory Deficits: (Decreased vision, hearing, sensation of thirst, taste, and smell). Socialized eating may be difficult with vision and hearing impairments. It also affects the ability to purchase and prepare foods. Decline in taste and smell affects appetite. Dehydration risk with decreased thirst sensation.

- Constipation: (Decreased peristalsis, medication side effect, or decrease in physical activity). Leads to laxative usage and abuse, which may interfere with absorption of nutrients and dehydration.

- Urinary Incontinence (Loss of sphincter control or other causes). Older adult may voluntarily restrict fluids to help manage incontinence, risking dehydration.

- Gall Bladder (Increased incidence of stones and calculi). May cause difficulty in digesting and absorbing fats.

- Cardiovascular (Decreased volume of blood pumped, loss of vessel elasticity, fat deposits on artery walls). May cause inadequate circulation of nutrients and oxygen.

- Physical Function [May be impaired due to

tremors, stoke, multiple sclerosis (MS), arthritis, pain, cardiovascular problems, and others]. Lessen ability to obtain and prepare foods.

- Cognitive Function (Such as decreased ability to remember to eat, to state hunger or thirst, to prepare foods, or to know what a balanced diet is).

- Other Factors: (Medications, alcohol, supplements, or home remedies) Side effects may alter appetite, interfere with absorption, decrease taste, cause dry mouth, confusion, excess sedation, and others. Pain, both chronic and acute, may affect appetite.

- Psychosocial factors: Eating alone, loneliness, and depression affect appetite or motivation to eat. Transportation, income, and knowledge of social programs may affect ability to purchase or afford foods. Cultural practices often determine types of foods consumed. Smoking may decrease ability to taste foods, thereby affecting appetite.

An effort by several professional organizations targeting the nutritional health of older Americans has been distributed. This effort, which combined resources of the American Academy of Family Physicians, The American Dietetic Association, and the National Council on the Aging, Inc., is called the Nutrition Screening Initiative. The organizations have formulated several assessment tools and interventions for detecting and correcting nutritional problems in this population. Basic questions can be used in screening. Table 5-2 can be used to assess the warning signs of poor nutritional health that are often overlooked (White, Posner, & Lipschitz, 1992). It is usually self-administered. Table 5-3 describes a more detailed screening and includes measurement of anthropometric and laboratory values. Anthropometrics (measurement of body size, weight, and proportion) should always be done (NSI, 1992). Patients assessed to be at risk should be referred to a dietitian to continue with the more detailed screening.

TABLE 5-2: NUTRITION COUNSELING CHECKLIST

	YES
I have an illness that the doctor has told me needs a special diet.	2
I am supposed to be on a special diet, but I am having trouble following it.	2
I have gained or lost 10 lb. or more without trying in the past 6 months.*	2
I have one or more of these problems: insulin-dependent or adult-onset diabetes, high blood pressure, high blood cholesterol, stroke, gastrointestinal problems, constipation, diarrhea or other bowel problems, osteoporosis, osteomalacia, kidney disease, alcoholism, anemia, or metabolic problems.	**1 point for each problem**
My appetite is poor, and food doesn't taste good to me.	1
I have trouble chewing and swallowing.	1
I have oral health problems.	1
I have medication use problems.	1
I treat my illnesses with vitamin and mineral supplements I have chosen myself.	1
I have many questions about nutrition or need advice about what to eat.	1
I spend less than $30 a week on food.	1
I usually need help shopping for food or cooking.	1
	TOTAL

*Contact a physician if you have lost 10 lb. or more unexpectedly.

If you have a score of 4 or more, contact a dietitian by asking your doctor for a referral or by calling your local hospital, health department, or the American Dietetic Association (1-800-366-1655), or look in the yellow pages, under "Registered Dietitians."

Note. From The Nutrition Screening Initiative, (1992). *Nutrition interventions manual for professionals caring for older Americans.* Executive Summary. Washington, DC: Greer, Margolio, Mitchell, Grunwald, & Associates, Inc.

Three types of protein-calorie malnutrition (PCM) are prevalent in hospitalized patients and skilled nursing facility residents: marasmus (calorie deficiency), hypoalbuminemia (kwashiorkor or protein deficiency), and a mixture of both. The prevalence of PCM is 20% in hospitalized patients and 37% in nursing home residents (Guigoz, Lauque, & Vellas, 2002). PCM may develop as a result of chronic disease, isolation, poverty, diminished physical or mental function, poor oral health, and polypharmacy. Marasmus results from an inadequate supply of calories. In this type of starvation, skeletal muscle, fat, and glycogen are mobilized for sources of energy; levels of visceral protein remain

TABLE 5-3: NUTRITION SUPPORT SCREENING ALERTS

If an older person indicates that the following questions of level I and II screens are descriptive of his or her condition or life situation, nutritional counseling and support interventions may help solve nutritional problems and improve nutritional status.

DETERMINE Your Nutritional Health Checklist Alerts

I have an illness or condition that made me change the kind and/or amount of food I eat.

Without wanting to, I have lost or gained 10 lbs. in the last 6 months.

I am not always physically able to shop, cook, and/or feed myself.

Level I Screen Alerts

Lost or gained 10 lb or more in the past 6 months

$$\text{Body Mass Index (BMI)} = \frac{\text{weight in pounds}}{\text{(Ht in inches)} \times \text{(Ht in inches)}} \times 703$$

Body mass index less than 22

Body mass index greater than 27

On a special diet

Difficulty chewing or swallowing

Pain in mouth, teeth, or gums

Usually or always needs assistance with preparing food, shopping for food

Level II Screen Alerts

Lost or gained 10 or more lbs. in the past 6 months

$$\text{Body Mass Index (BMI)} = \frac{\text{weight in pounds}}{\text{(Ht in inches)} \times \text{(Ht in inches)}} \times 703$$

Body mass index less than 22

Body mass index greater than 27

On a special diet

Difficulty chewing or swallowing

Usually or always needs assistance with preparing food, shopping for food

Pain in mouth, teeth, or gums

Mid-arm muscle circumference less than 10th percentile

Triceps skinfold less than 10th percentile

Triceps skinfold greater than 95th percentile

Serum albumin less than 3.5 g/dl

Serum cholesterol less than 160 mg/dl

Clinical evidence of mental or cognitive impairment

Clinical evidence of depressive illness

Clinical evidence of insulin-dependent diabetics, adult-onset diabetics, heart disease, high blood pressure, stroke, gastrointestinal disease, kidney disease, chronic lung disease, liver disease, osteoporosis, or osteomalacia

Note. From Nutrition Screening Initiative. (1992). *Nutrition interventions manual for professionals caring for older Americans.* Washington, DC: Greer, Margolio, Mitchell, Grunwald, & Associates, Inc.

normal. Immune function usually is not affected by calorie malnutrition. Marasmus or calorie malnutrition may be indicated by weight loss and decreased weight for height.

Hypoalbuminemia is indicated by a decrease in the serum level of albumin, reflecting the depletion of stores of visceral protein. Additionally, the immune response at the cellular level is decreased. In this type of malnutrition, muscle mass and weight may be normal or even above normal as a result of obesity or edema. For this reason, malnutrition usually is not suspected. Preliminary signs and symptoms of protein-calorie malnutrition are vague and often overlooked or attributed to other chronic diseases. Signs and symptoms include anorexia, lassitude, irritability, and anxiety. Dehydration as well as protein-calorie malnutrition can cause confusion. Protein-calorie malnutrition is frequently not recognized until hospitalization, and if not treated would lead to worsening of malnutrition during hospitalization (Thomas, et al., 2002). A combination of marasmus and hypoalbuminemia is called a mixed marasmic state. Changes in body composition, weight loss, laboratory indexes, and anthropometrics can be used to assess moderate and severe PCM. All three malnourished states require an aggressive approach to resolve the condition.

Assessment of weight status is more meaningful if the person's previous weight is known. The change in weight over time expressed as a percentage is a more accurate indicator of nutritional risk than values given in the traditional height-for-weight tables. The change in weight can be calculated as follows:

$$\text{percentage weight change} = \frac{\text{usual weight} - \text{current weight}}{\text{usual weight}} \times 100$$

By using Table 5-3, the severity of nutritional deficit can be estimated on the basis of weight loss in a specified period.

Nursing Considerations for Community-Dwelling Older Adults

• Do a nutritional screening, including current height and weight and past weight history.

• Family caregivers are a vital resource in the nutrition assessment but often lack adequate knowledge to meet nutritional needs of the frail older adult (Biggs & Freed, 2000).

• Checking inside the refrigerator will give a good indication of ability to afford food items and what types of food they normally eat.

• Unintended weight loss of 1–2% in 1 week, 5% in 1 month, 7.5% in 3 months, or 10% in 6 months requires physician attention.

• Check medical diagnoses and current medications.

• Assess educational needs for special diets such as no added salt (NAS), nutritional concerns, or food safety issues.

• If the patient is having economic difficulties affording food or functional difficulties preparing obtaining and preparing meals, contact the appropriate local agency for possible options which may include food stamps, delivered meals, or congregate meals. Call Eldercare Locator, a national toll-free directory assistance provided by U.S. Administration on Aging that helps people locate aging services in every community throughout the United States. (1-800-677-1116)

• Recommend eating 4 to 6 smaller meals, as they may be easier to digest.

• Appetite loss is often the result of depression; screen for depression if suspected.

• If possible, encourage increasing physical activity levels to increase appetite.

• Certain foods may pose a significant health hazard because of the level of bacteria present in the product's raw or uncooked state. Educate the clients to avoid:

- Raw finfish and shellfish, including oysters, clams, mussels, and scallops.

- Raw or unpasteurized milk or cheese.

- Soft cheeses such as feta, brie, camembert, blue-veined, and Mexican-style cheese. (Hard cheeses, processed cheeses, cream cheese, cottage cheese, or yogurt need not be avoided.)

- Raw or lightly cooked egg or egg products included in salad dressings, cookie or cake batter, sauces, and beverages such as egg nog.

- Raw meat or poultry or raw alfalfa sprouts.

- Unpasteurized or untreated fruit or vegetable juice. When fruits and vegetables are made into fresh-squeezed juice, harmful bacteria that may be present can become part of the finished product. Unpasteurized or untreated juices, are required by the FDA to have a warning label.

Nutritional Issues in Long-Term Care Facilities (LTC)

Preventing weight loss in residents of LTC is an everyday challenge that requires well thought out interdisciplinary programs and policies (Crutchfield, 2002b). Residents with dementia are at particular risk for weight loss as a consequence of the disease. Some residents burn more calories due to the increased energy requirement of wandering and restlessness. Some lose their appetite due to side effects of medications and others to passivity. Often older adults with dementia are not capable of expressing hunger. Eight years after onset most persons with dementia will have lost all or some of the ability to self-feed. Eventually 25% will have increased food intake, 75% decreased food intake; 33% prefer sweet or spicy foods, 25% will exhibit pica activity, and an undetermined number will lose sense of taste/smell and have difficulty swallowing.

Tip to Prevent Weight Loss for Older Adults with Dementia

- Make dining environment calm and pleasant.

- Make certain toilet needs are taken care of ahead of time.

- Resident's hands and face should be washed prior and after eating.

- Glasses, hearing aides, and dentures should be worn.

- Transfer to dining room chair or assist clients to walk from wheelchair to dining chair.

- If decreased peripheral or central vision, place food within resident's visual field.

- If one-sided neglect, turn residents plate after one side is consumed.

- Encourage family members to visit/assist or eat with their loved ones at mealtime.

- Provide adequate number of staff members to assist, depending upon resident's needs.

- Individualize meal times as much as possible.

- Provide choices in foods.

- Make mealtime a social event, seating residents near friends.

- Allow residents to feed themselves whenever possible. Provide finger foods if necessary.

- For constant wanderers, provide cart to push with meals or finger foods on it.

- For restless clients involve them in recreational therapy programs such as cooking groups, dining room set-up, and pre-meal handwashing programs.

- For residents with agnosia and/or pica, remove non-edibles: straws, napkins, styrofoam cups, and plastic utensils.

- For residents with difficulty coordinating movements, use special utensils, give verbal cues, guide hand to start, request OT or recreational therapy (RT) to involve in fine motor exercise for self-feeding.

- For residents with difficulty swallowing: Always provide the right consistency and correct position. Give reminders for swallowing if they pocket foods in the mouth or are drooling.

- Behavior: Throwing foods or dishes: Give one item at a time and use non-breakables.

- Eating from others' plates: Give enough foods or if food obsessed, provide activity after meal is finished.

- Medications: Avoid passing medications during mealtime or "hiding" medication in foods; this alters the taste and promotes suspicious behavior.

- Loss of appetite in a resident who normally eats well may be caused by undetected infection, oral cavities or abscess, or medication toxicity, digoxin in particular.

- Staff consideration: Behavior of staff members can make a difference in the dining atmosphere and it is often the nurses' responsibility to supervise the dining room and the staff members. If music is used in the dining room, it should be soft background music from the residents' generation, NOT music based on staff's preference. Televisions should not be an option in the dining room. They serve one purpose only: to distract the staff from the residents. Staff members assisting residents should sit alongside the resident and converse with the residents they are helping, rather than each other. Never stand over the residents to help feed. Facility staff members not involved in the meal should not "hang out" in the dining room during mealtime socializing with staff. Staff should avoid making negative comments about the foods provided.

- Unit Considerations: Unit nourishment room should always be stocked. Provide food for the night owls, who frequently sleep through daytime meals. Have a nourishment cart stocked with snacks and fluids to be passed every 2 hours between meals. Assistance should be provided for residents who are unable to feed self.

Enteral and Parenteral Support in Long-Term Care

When a person has an intact gastrointestinal tract but is unable to ingest food, tube feeding provides a practical alternative for oral nutrition. Enteral feeding relies on the normal physiological actions of digestion and absorption. It is safe and avoids complications that are common in total parenteral nutrition. Enteral therapy is convenient and requires clean technique instead of sterile technique. With the advent of closed systems, problems of infection control are nearly eliminated. In the long-term care setting, tube feedings continue to be a method of supplying nutrients. Several considerations affect the tolerance of enteral feeding and its success. Some of these include the following: the patient's ability or lack of ability to ingest food normally, the patient's digestive capacities, and other physical and mental problems. Persons who recently have had head or neck surgery or who have cancer or neurological disorders such as a cerebrovascular accident are examples of those who are appropriate candidates for enteral feeding by tube. In some cases, tube feeding is used as an adjunct to oral feeding. In that situation, the team members work closely to ensure that nutrient needs are met and to establish a timeframe for oral feeding to be achieved. So-called weaning programs are an essential component of any rehabilitation-oriented facility.

Contraindications for the use of enteral feedings include intractable vomiting, intestinal obstruction, severe intractable diarrhea, and hemorrhaging in the upper part of the gastrointestinal tract. Persons who are at a high risk for respiratory aspiration are not good candidates for enteral therapy. The route for tube feeding depends on three factors: the length of time the tube feeding will be needed, the condition of the gastrointestinal tract, and the potential for aspiration. A nasogastric tube is preferred when feeding will be short-term and an oral diet will resume. When feeding is anticipated to be long-term, a gastrostomy can be placed surgically or a percutaneous endoscopic (PE) placement of a gastrostomy (PEG tube) can be performed that requires minimal sedation. These tubes provide increased comfort and are the best alternative for alert, ambulatory residents needing long-term enteral nutrition support. When gastric feeding is contraindicated or the individual is at increased risk for aspiration, a percutaneous endoscopic jejunostomy (PEJ) tube can be placed directly into the jejunum or through an existing gastrostomy.

Mechanical, metabolic, and gastrointestinal complications can evolve as a result of tube feeding therapy. Mechanical problems are associated with the type of tube used and the position of the tube. Examples of mechanical complications include obstruction or dislocation of a nasogastric tube, reflux of gastric contents that can lead to aspiration pneumonia, and leakage of a gastrostomy or jejunostomy tube that can lead to skin irritation or erosion. Tubes with small lumen are now used almost exclusively because of the greater comfort they provide the individual. These also can be more prone to clogging. Adequate water must be used frequently to flush the tube as well as before and after medications. When the tube becomes obstructed, it usually requires removal of the tube and reinsertion of a new one. Frequent replacement of the tube can cause irritation and breakdown of the nasal mucosa. Gastrointestinal complications may include delayed gastric emptying, nausea, vomiting, abdominal pain, malabsorption, diarrhea, and constipation. These problems are usually related to the rate and/or the concentration of the enteral formula being administered.

Aspiration pneumonia occurs frequently in the institutionalized elderly and is one of the most frequent reasons for transfer to an acute care facility. The elderly have a high risk for aspiration because of a reduced gastric-emptying rate. Foodstuffs stay in the stomach longer before digestion. The lower esophageal sphincter may also be weak and allow gastric contents to reflux into the esophagus. If feedings are given as a bolus, then the amount remaining in the stomach should be measured before the scheduled feeding is administered. If the amount is more than 100ml, the feeding should be held for 1 hour and the residual amount rechecked. If feedings are being given continuously, the residual amounts are not measured. In this case, it is important to observe the patient for abdominal distensions and monitor for complaints of "fullness." To avoid reflux of gastric contents, elevate the head of the bed to greater than a 45° angle and feed for a duration of 1 hour.

Fluid and electrolyte disturbances are particularly dangerous to older adults. Dehydration can result from serious diarrhea, excessive protein intake, or osmotic diuresis. Dehydration, hypernatremia, hyperchloremia, and azotemia-tube-feeding syndrome may result from excessive protein intake, accompanied by inadequate fluid intake. Signs include confusion and decreasing levels of consciousness. Some electrolyte disturbances that may occur include hypernatremia, hyponatremia, hyperkalemia, hypokalemia, and hypophosphatemia. Hypernatremia is usually indicative of dehydration.

Accurate recording of intake and output is essential for monitoring fluid balance. Fluid intake consists of fluid taken by mouth, intravenous fluids, and the tube feeding formula and water given via the tube. Output consists of the fluid lost through the urine and feces and the insensible loss from perspiration and water evaporation from the lungs. Additional water losses may occur through draining wounds or fistulas. Fluid intake should be approximately equal to fluid output. Fluid balance is essential for normal bodily functioning because water is a vital component of every body cell. Inadequate fluid intake is often the cause of constipation associated with tube feeding. Fluid requirements usually are estimated by assuming that the patient needs 30ml of water for each kilogram of body weight. This may be adjusted upward in the case of fever, pressure ulcers, or a history of dehydration. The total water given may be restricted in the presence of cardiac insufficiency, pulmonary disease, or decline in renal function. Nursing monitoring for signs and symptoms of edema or dehydration is an important part of tube feeding therapy.

Medications administered through the feeding tube may cause intolerance to the feeding or the feeding may interfere with the effectiveness of the drug. Certain medications can change the osmolality or pH of the feeding and may cause gastrointestinal intolerance or curdling, with resultant tube clogging. In addition, many drugs are known gastrointestinal irritants. Guidelines regarding suitability of certain medications for enteral administration are obtainable from any pharmacy. In general, it is wise to use the liquid form of a drug whenever available. Certain solid oral dosage forms can be thoroughly crushed, dissolved in a suitable diluent, and administered via the feeding tube with a water flush before and after administration. Enteric-coated, slow-release, and sublingual forms of drugs should never be given via the tube.

Special care should be taken to satisfy the psychological and social needs of individuals receiving enteral feeding. This is especially important for patients in a hospital or residents in a skilled nursing facility who require long-term tube feeding. These residents are denied the pleasures of eating and socializing with others. Although the nutrition needs of the resident may be met, the "food" no longer looks, tastes, or smells familiar. Reassessment should be done periodically to determine if the resident is a candidate for weaning to oral feeding.

Many factors must be considered if a weaning program is to be successful. Members of the healthcare team who should be involved include speech or occupational therapists, the dietitian, rehabilitation nurses, and the nursing assistants.

Nutritional needs of the patient or resident must be met during a trial-feeding program.

Total parenteral nutrition (TPN) is the alternative method of feeding for those patients who can neither accept nor absorb nutrients taken enterally. Examples of such patients include those with impaired digestive function (e.g., bowel inflammation, bowel obstruction, or Crohn's disease) and those with malnutrition associated with chemotherapy, cancer, stress, or trauma.

To provide adequately for residents who are receiving TPN, the long-term care facility should have 24-hour staffing with registered nurses, established policies and written procedures for TPN therapy, and an ongoing staff education program. Adequate refrigerated storage facilities for solutions are an additional requirement. Two routes are used for TPN: peripheral and central vein. The first route is used short-term for patients with mild-to-moderate nutritional deficiencies and for those at risk for such deficiencies. The central route is used for those who require therapy for longer than 5 to 7 days. More than 2400 calories/day can be given via this route. The hypercaloric solutions are delivered through a silicone catheter directly into the subclavian vein running into the superior vena cava and into the right atrium. The potential for infection is great, and meticulous infection control procedures must be followed. When patients begin taking food by mouth or tube, TPN can be stopped gradually. However, as with the enteral weaning program, provisions must be made to meet nutritional needs during this tapering process. TPN is associated with many complications, and strict protocols for their prevention are required. Pneumothorax may occur during placement of the central line; air embolism is a constant risk if the line is interrupted or accidentally disconnected. Strict aseptic technique is essential to prevent infections. Due to risks of hyperglycemia, blood glucose levels need to be monitored frequently. Metabolic problems similar to those associated with enteral therapy may occur, particularly in nutritionally depleted geriatric patients.

HYDRATION

Fluid intake is frequently overlooked in the diets of the older adult. Water is the medium in which all the body's various metabolic activities take place, and is an essential structural component of every cell. Digestion, absorption of nutrients, circulation (blood is 80% water), and excretion (urine is 97% water) all rely on the body's water component. Water is essential in the regulation of body temperature and in the lubrication of joints and abdominal viscera. The decreases in body water in the older adult makes them more susceptible to dehydration (Suhayda & Walton, 2002). Dehydration may refer to any one of three conditions where fluid intake does not equal fluid output:

- Hypernatremic dehydration:

body water losses > sodium losses, such as with a high fever.

- Isotonic dehydration:

body water losses = sodium losses, such as in extreme diarrhea or vomiting.

- Hypotonic dehydration:

body sodium losses > water losses, such as when using diuretics and/or sodium restricted diets.

Many older adults become dehydrated for a combination of reasons:

- Decreased thirst sensation: Hypothalamus function declines with age.

- Intentional reduction in fluid intake due to incontinence.

- Fever, internal bleeding, uncontrolled diabetes, or enteral feedings

- Physical Function: May not be able to obtain fluids or drink by self. Facility may not have a hydration program or provide hands on assistance.

- Cognitive Function: May not recognize thirst or be capable of asking for a drink.

- Communication: May not be able to express thirst.

- Swallowing: May self-restrict due to swallowing difficulty and fear of choking.

- Alcohol and many therapeutic agents, such as diuretic medications and cardiac glycosides, can increase the rate of loss of body water.

- Overexertion as a result of activity or exercise can increase fluid losses.

- Exposure to extreme heat or cold.

Signs of Dehydration, Based on Strength of Sign (++++ strong) to (+ some) (- none) (Mentes, 2000)

++++ Upper body weakness (The most accurate sign.)

+++   Speech difficulties, dry tongue with longitudinal furrows, dry pale oral mucosa with decreased saliva, acute decreased weight

++   Rapid pulse, sunken eyes, acute onset of confusion

+   Decreased axillary sweating, orthostatic hypotension

-     Decreased skin turgor

Hydration Management

- Calculate daily fluid goal, example given with 70kg patient:

  Patients weight (kg) = 70

  Subtract 20 = 50

  Multiply by 15 = 750

  Add 1500 = 2250

  Multiply by .75 = 1668 (ml fluid goal)

- Do accurate fluid intake and output for at least three days.

- Compare goal with actual intake.

- Provide fluids consistently throughout the day

with assistance when needed.

- Offer a variety of fluids and avoid caffeinated beverages.

- Offer high fluid snack such as fruits, ice pops, ice cream, and yogurt.

- Get patient involved in cooking programs to stimulate appetite.

- Involve in socialization programs such as "Wine and Cheese," "Afternoon Tea."

SUMMARY

The common clinical problems discussed in this chapter are things that nurses will commonly encounter with this population. They are quality of life issues that mean much more than a medical diagnosis does. Using all your nursing skills and an individualized approach are the methods to use for prevention and management.

EXAM QUESTIONS

CHAPTER 5

Questions 28-36

28. The number one most common cause of iatrogenesis is

    a. infection.
    b. accidents.
    c. impaction.
    d. medications.

29. Your home care patient, Mrs. Smith, has a urinary tract infection and she is concerned as she has suddenly become incontinent. You educate Mrs. Smith by telling her she has

    a. urge incontinence.
    b. transient incontinence.
    c. stress incontinence.
    d. functional incontinence.

30. Normal bowel functioning is dependent upon

    a. adequate fiber, fluids, and physical activities.
    b. physical activities, fluids, and occasional laxatives.
    c. mobility, education, and a low-fat diet.
    d. adequate fluids, activities, and laxatives.

31. The incidence of pressure ulcers in nursing home residents is

    a. 24%.
    b. 30%.
    c. 10%.
    d. 17%.

32. An example of an instrumental activities of daily living is

    a. getting dressed to go to church.
    b. balancing a checkbook.
    c. taking a shower independently.
    d. needing assistance eating a meal.

33. Safety modification for community-dwelling older adults can

    a. only be considered for intrinsic factors.
    b. only be considered for extrinsic factors.
    c. substantially reduce the risk of falling.
    d. marginally reduce the risk of falling.

34. A risk factor for inadequate nutrition is

    a. dining with a group of neighbors.
    b. eating 6 small meals per day.
    c. lacking finances to purchase food.
    d. getting daily physical activity.

35. A medication that can be crushed and administered through an enteral feeding is a

    a. compressed tablet.
    b. enteric-coated tablets.
    c. slow-release compound.
    d. sublingual tablet.

36. According to Mentes (2000), the most accurate sign of dehydration is

    a. decreased skin turgor and sunken eyes.

    b. rapid pulse and decreased sweating.

    c. upper body weakness and speech difficulties.

    d. orthostatic hypotension and confusion.

CHAPTER 6

COGNITIVE IMPAIRMENT

CHAPTER OBJECTIVE

After studying this chapter, the reader will be able to discuss clinical problems that are related to cognitive changes and dementia as a part of the aging process.

LEARNING OBJECTIVES

After studying this chapter, the learner will be able to

1. describe normal aging memory changes.

2. list medical diagnoses, medications, and other factors that may affect cognition.

3. specify the various types of dementia, their symptoms, and how they are diagnosed.

4. discuss various methods to assist the older adult with dementia and their families in dealing with a diagnosis of dementia.

5. describe therapeutic methods of interacting with clients with dementia.

6. specify strategies for management of disturbing behaviors of dementia.

7. recognize the risks factors associated with disturbing behaviors.

8. discuss implications of psychotropic medication and their side effects on the older adult.

9. detail common problems associated with older adults with dementia.

INTRODUCTION

It is currently estimated that over four million Americans have some form of dementia, and that number will grow to 14 million by 2050 unless a cure or prevention is found. Each year, in the United States, more than 1 million adults are newly diagnosed with a chronic brain disease or disorder, most of which affects cognition and behaviors (Family Caregiver Alliance, 2001). Currently 10% of persons over 65 and nearly half of those over 85 have dementia. More than 70% of people with dementia live at home with almost 75% of the care and costs provided by family and friends with very little training in dementia care. The cost of dementia caregiving to society is placed at $61 billion dollars per year (Alzheimer's Association, 2002). The need for effective treatments, especially those that assist the family caregivers are dramatic. Older adults and others often assume if a person has changes in memory that they have dementia. This is not necessarily true. Therefore an understanding of normal aging memory changes is the first step in understanding cognitive impairments.

NORMAL AGING MEMORY CHANGES

Understanding the basics of how the brain functions helps in comprehension of how memory works. The brain is made up of billions of cells called neurons that communicate with each other through small gaps called synapses with the help of neurotransmitters. Millions of signals travel back and forth across the synapse in a fraction of a second at any given time. Different areas of the brain perform different functions, but the neurons responsible for memory are generally widely spread throughout the brain. Memory is dependent on healthy neurons. However, neurons die and reduce in numbers during a natural life course. Memory peaks between the ages of 20–30 followed by a subtle decline until after age 60 when memory difficulties become more pronounced. The brain has a highly complex system of memory storage and retrieval and consists of the following:

- Short-term memory: Lasts 7–10 seconds and can only hold 4–7 items at once.

- Intermediate memory: Lasts 24-48 hours.

- Long-term memory: What happened beyond 48 hours.

Successful memory relies on all three. To recall intermediate or long-term memories this information must be brought into short-term memory. Many people assume that as people age their memories will fail. There are some memory changes that are associated with normal aging; however, the ability to learn new things does not decline.

Normal age-related memory changes:

Slower Thinking: All body systems become less efficient with age, including thinking and problem-solving abilities. The speed of learning and recall decreases, so it may require more time to learn new things and/or retrieve information. Memory doesn't necessarily fade with age; it just takes longer for the neurons to communicate with each other.

Difficulty in Paying Attention: Many memory problems are due to problems of attention, not retention. Reduction in the ability to concentrate as a person ages makes it harder to remember. Distractions are more difficult to ignore and interruptions may cause forgetfulness. Slower stimulus identification and registration are normal aging changes.

More Memory Cues Required for Recall: As people age, more memory aids or cues are needed, more often, to retrieve information from memory. A cue can be a word, picture, smell, rhyme, or anything associated with information or events to be remembered.

Physical Changes of the Brain that Occur Through Aging that Affects Memory:

1. Enlargement of the ventricular system: The volume of the ventricles (the spaces in the brain that contain cerebrospinal fluid) increases. It is thought that this enlargement occurs because cells surrounding the ventricles are lost.

2. Widening of sulci (the grooves) on the surface of the brain.

3. Reduced brain weight and brain volume: These changes are probably caused by the loss of neurons.

Other Factors that Interfere with Basic Memory:

1. **Visual changes:** If something is not seen correctly it is harder to remember.

2. **Hearing changes:** If something is not heard correctly it is harder to remember it.

3. **Sleep:** Decrease in REM sleep often results in inadequate sleep which affects cognitive ability, especially patients with existing cognitive impairments (Beullens, 2002).

4. **Pain:** When a person is in pain, it is more difficult to use the brain effectively (Demirci & Savas, 2002).

5. **Medication:** Many medications contribute to confusion and difficulty focusing on a topic.

6. **Depression and other mood disorders:** Strong correlation between depression and difficulty with memory (Kim, Stewart, Shin, Choi, & Toon, 2003).

The Five Patterns of Memory Loss

There are 5 different patterns, or stages, of memory loss that the older adult may progress through. It is only when the older adult enters stage five that a diagnosis of dementia is appropriate. See Table 6-1 for 10 warning signs of dementia.

1. **No Loss of Memory Capacity or Retrieval:** Some persons never experience any change in memory function. These people are in the extreme minority.

2. **Normal Aging:** No loss of memory capacity but a delay in recall. Memory can still be retrieved but takes longer to do so.

3. **Age Associated Memory Loss:** More pronounced memory difficulties. Forgetting items, forgetting someone's name. These develop

TABLE 6-1: TEN WARNING SIGNS OF ALZHEIMER'S DISEASE

1. **Memory loss.** One of the most common early signs of dementia is forgetting recently learned information. While it's normal to forget appointments, names, or telephone numbers, those with dementia will forget such things more often and not remember them later.

2. **Difficulty performing familiar tasks.** People with dementia often find it hard to complete everyday tasks that are so familiar we usually do not think about how to do them. A person with Alzheimer's may not know the steps for preparing a meal, using or participating in a lifelong hobby.

3. **Problems with language.** Everyone has trouble finding the right word sometimes, but a person with Alzheimer's disease often forgets simple words or substitutes unusual words, making his or her speech or writing hard to understand. If a person with Alzheimer's is unable to find his or her toothbrush, for example, the individual may ask for "that thing for my mouth."

4. **Disorientation to time and place.** It's normal to forget the day of the week or where you're going. But people with Alzheimer's disease can become lost on their own street, forget where they are and how they got there, and not know how to get back home.

5. **Poor or decreased judgment.** No one has perfect judgment all of the time. Those with Alzheimer's may dress without regard to the weather, wearing several shirts or blouses on a warm day or very little clothing in cold weather. Individuals with dementia often show poor judgment about money, giving away large amounts of money to telemarketers or paying for home repairs or products they don't need.

6. **Problems with abstract thinking.** Balancing a checkbook may be hard when the task is more complicated than usual. Someone with Alzheimer's disease could forget completely what the numbers are and what needs to be done with them.

7. **Misplacing things.** Anyone can temporarily misplace a wallet or key. A person with Alzheimer's disease may put things in unusual places: an iron in the freezer or a wristwatch in the sugar bowl.

8. **Changes in mood or behavior.** Everyone can become sad or moody from time to time. Someone with Alzheimer's disease can show rapid mood swings, from calm to tears to anger, for no apparent reason.

9. **Changes in personality.** People's personalities ordinarily change somewhat with age. But a person with Alzheimer's disease can change a lot, becoming extremely confused, suspicious, fearful, or dependent on a family member.

10. **Loss of initiative.** It's normal to tire of housework, business activities, or social obligations at times. The person with Alzheimer's disease may become very passive, sitting in front of the television for hours, sleeping more than usual, or not wanting to do usual activities.

Note. From Alzheimer's Association. (n.d.). *Ten warning signs of Alzheimer's Disease.* Retrieved December 10, 2003 from http://www.alz.org/AboutAD/10Signs.htm. Reprinted with permission.

slowly over a long period of time and gradually worsen.

4. **Mild Cognitive Impairment (MCI):** More consistent and persistent memory problems. Significant decline in short term memory, difficulty learning new materials. Problems are noticed by friends, family and co-workers. Does not affect everyday living to any great extent. Of those with MCI, 15% will develop Alzheimer's disease in 1 year, 40% in 3 years. Some people with MCI never develop Alzheimer's disease (Petersen, et al., 1999).

5. **Dementia:** For a diagnosis there must be two domains of function that are impaired; one is memory, and the other must be one of the following: aphasia, apraxia, agnosia, or executive functioning such as problems with planning, organizing, using judgment, and reasoning. Examples are difficulty paying bills or following a recipe. The impairment must be severe enough to interfere with everyday functioning.

Some examples of normal versus abnormal memory changes are

Normal: Forgetting the name of someone you were just introduced to.
Problem: Forgetting the name of your neighbor who you lived next to for the past 10 years.

Normal: Going into the living room and forgetting why you were going there.
Problem: Forget or becoming confused over how to get to the living room.

Normal: Forgetting where you left your car keys.
Problem: Finding that you put your keys in the freezer.

Normal: Taking longer to learn a new job task.
Problem: Forgetting how to tie your shoe.

Normal: Forgetting the name of the movie you saw last week.
Problem: Forgetting that you went to the movies last week.

TYPES OF DEMENTIA

Although loss of recent memory is the outstanding feature, the term dementia implies global impairment of mental functions. The signs and symptoms can include: 1. impairment in abstract thinking; 2. impaired judgment; and 3. disturbances of higher cortical function, such as aphasia (disorder of language) and apraxia (inability to carry out familiar motor activities despite intact comprehension and motor function, that is, difficulty in using objects correctly, such as brushing one's hair or dressing); agnosia, loss of perception powers (visual, auditory, and tactile), may occur with failure to recognize or identify objects despite intact sensory function. Personality changes may also occur with loss of social skills. The clinical picture is sometimes complicated by the presence of significant depressive features or delusions.

Dementia is different from mental retardation because it indicates a loss of previous abilities. Dementia differs from delirium because delirium is associated with diminished attention or temporary confusion. Delirium implies a transient loss of mental abilities. In dementia, the person is alert and the signs and symptoms are relatively stable. However, delirium and dementia may coexist.

Dementia can occur from over 70 different causes and can be diagnosed with a high degree of accuracy with a comprehensive work-up. Of the over 70 different causes of dementia, the types that are most common occur in approximately this order: Alzheimer's, which comprises approximately half of all cases, followed by vascular and dementia with Lewy bodies (DLB), frontal lobe or Picks disease, Parkinson's disease, and alcohol dementia. Determining the type of dementia is not an easy task and many clients may be given vague, inaccurate diagnoses, or merely a single diagnosis when they actually have more than one type of dementia. It is important to get a thorough history to preclude a patient's being labeled with dementia when in fact the patient may have something that is treatable or reversible. See Table 6-2 for differential diagnoses of dementia.

Alzheimer's Disease

The German physician Alois Alzheimer described the first case of Alzheimer's disease (AD) in 1906, when a 55-year-old woman with progressive dementia was found at autopsy to have senile plaques and neurofibrillary tangles (Graeber, & Mehraein, 1999). These physical changes in the brain are now recognized as the hallmark of Alzheimer's disease. On electron microscopy, the neurofibrillary tangles consist of double helical twisted tubes; the senile plaques consist of a degen-

erated amyloid center and surrounding neurofibrillary tangles. There is also a reduction of choline acetyltransferase in the brain by 50–90% and in some a 50% decrease in somatostatin. These are neurotransmitters that act as messengers between neurons, and their loss appears to be a consequence rather than a cause of the disease. Deficits in norepinephrine, dopamine, and serotonin have also been discovered in AD patients. Pharmacological treatment has been aimed at increasing the availability of acetylcholine in the brain. (See Figures 6-1 through 6-6 for brain photographs.)

Some of the risk factors for AD include increased age, female gender, head trauma, family

TABLE 6-2: DIFFERENTIAL DIAGNOSIS OF DEMENTIA

Alzheimer's Disease	Insidious onset, gradual progression. Short-term memory loss, disoriented, difficulty with familiar tasks, change in mood.
Vascular Dementia	Sudden onset, stepwise progression. Abnormal computerized tomogram (CT) or magnetic resonance imaging (MRI).
Dementia with Lewy Body	Fluctuations in cognition, hallucinations, or unexplained falls. Similar to AD in cognitive deficits.
Parkinson's Disease	History or signs and symptoms of Parkinson's disease.
Normal Pressure Hydrocephalus	Triad of gait disturbance, urinary incontinence, dementia. excessively enlarged ventricles seen on CT.
Alcohol/ Wernicke-Korsakoff	History of heavy alcohol intake, presence of cerebellar ataxia. Agnosia uncommon.
AIDS Dementia	Rapid onset and progression. Early motor difficulties.
Huntington's Disease	Family history, early onset age, choreiform movements first symptom.
Pick's Disease	Extreme personality changes, poor hygiene, preserved memory, loss of inhibition.
Creutzfeldt-Jakob Disease	Myoclonic jerks and fasciculations, ataxia, somnolence, rapid progression. Electroencephalogram (EEG) findings.
Progressive Supranuclear	Rigidity of torso with erect posture, extension of neck. Palsy of upward and downward eye movements.
Other causes:	Downs syndrome, amyotrophic lateral sclerosis, Binswanger's disease, subarachnoid hemorrhage, chronic subdural hematoma B12 deficiency, folate deficiency, multiple sclerosis, chronic fatigue syndrome,immunoglobulin deficiencies, infections, meningitis, chronic encephalitis, neurosyphilis, liver, kidney and lung disease, diabetes, Wilson's disease, head trauma dementia (Pugilistica or Boxer's syndrome), brain tumors, metastatic tumors, obstructive or non-communicating hydrocephalus, non-obstructive or communicating hydrocephalus, epilepsy, leukodystrophies

FIGURE 6-1: NORMAL HUMAN BRAIN

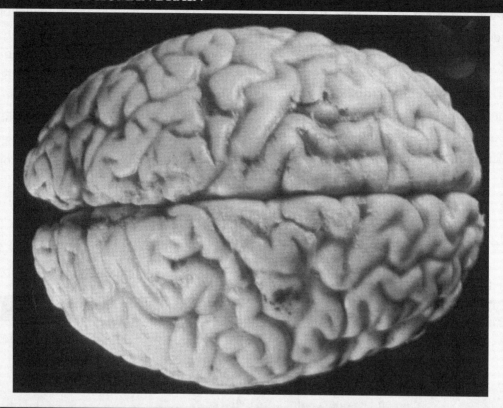

FIGURE 6-2: BRAIN OF PATIENT WITH ALZHEIMER'S DISEASE. NOTE ATROPHIC SURFACE AREA LOST BY DECREASE IN GYRI AND DEEPER, WIDER SULCI

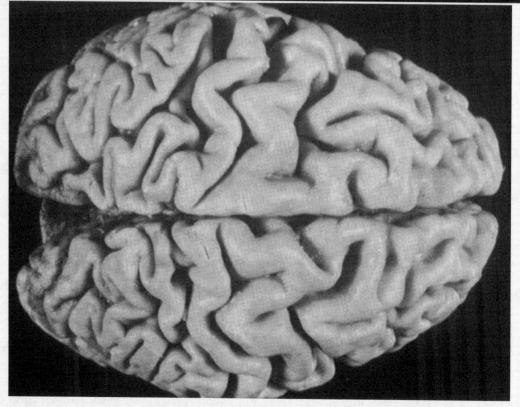

Slides courtesy of Duke University Medical Center, Durham, NC.

FIGURE 6-3: NORMAL HUMAN BRAIN SECTION

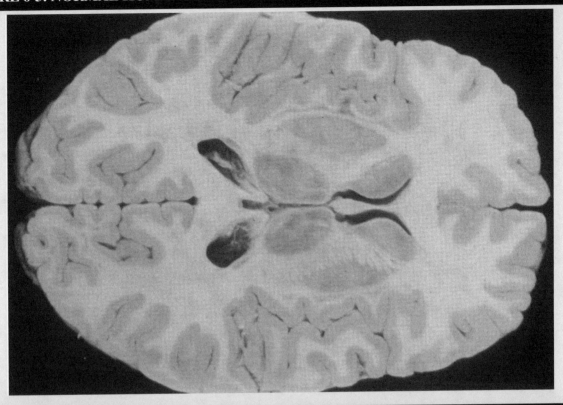

FIGURE 6-4: BRAIN SECTION OF PATIENT WITH ALZHEIMER'S DISEASE SHOWING ENLARGED VENTRICLES

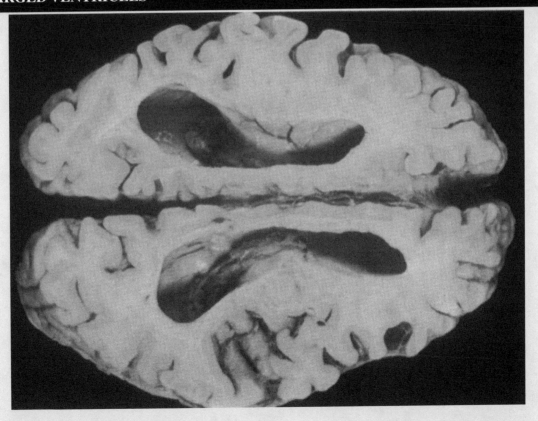

Slides courtesy of Duke University Medical Center, Durham, NC.

FIGURE 6-5: NORMAL NEURONS

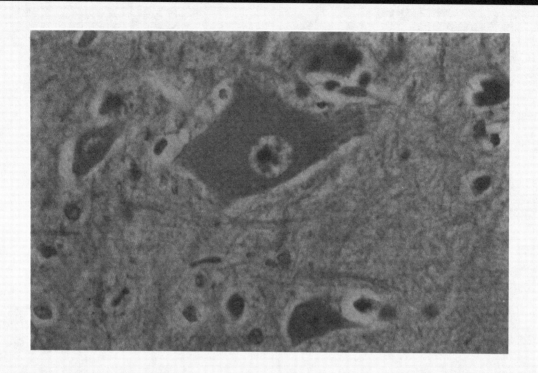

FIGURE 6-6: ABNORMAL NEURONS. INSIDE ARE NEUROFIBERS IN PAIRED HELIXES.

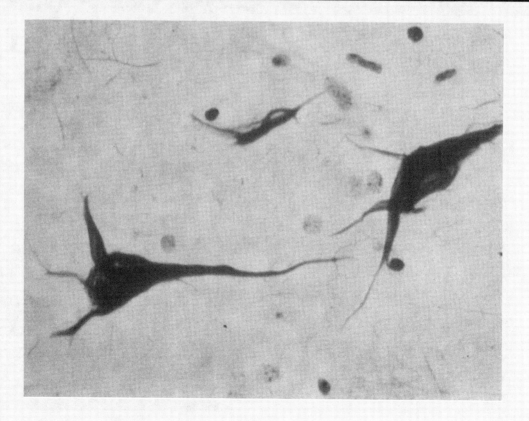

Slides courtesy of Duke University Medical Center, Durham, NC.

history, and Downs syndrome (APA, 1994). Alzheimer's disease may have several fundamental causes. An autosomal gene called apolipoprotein (APOE-4) on chromosome 19 may predispose an individual to the late onset, over age 65, form of AD. Early onset of familial Alzheimer's disease has been linked with genes on chromosomes 21, 14, and 1 (APA, 1994).

THE STAGES OF ALZHEIMER'S DISEASE

The onset of AD is insidious and there is a gradual progressive decline. It is difficult to place a specific patient with AD in stages, although symptoms often progress in a recognizable pattern. These stages provide a framework for understanding the needs of the patient. Each patient is unique and different and often stages will overlap.

First Stage: Lasting approximately 2 to 4 years leading up to and including diagnosis. First symptom is short-term memory losses (amnesia) that affect job, social, or household performance. There is often confusion about places or getting lost. Spontaneity is lost, mood changes occur frequently with anxiety, apathy, and/or depression. There are generally personality changes, mood swings, and an inability to retain new information. Visuospatial skills are often impaired, and there is difficulty orienting the individual in an unfamiliar environment. Hostility and agitation may occur, due to frustration over the losses that are occurring. Apathy has been noted as being not only the first symptom to appear but is also the most prevalent (Deruouesne, et al., 2001, 2002; Thomas, et al., 2001; Ready, Ott, Grace, & Cahn-Weiner, 2003). The presence of apathy is linked to alterations in the frontal lobe functions (McPherson, Fairbanks, Tiken, Cummings, & Back-Mudruga, 2002) and is considered a personality change.

Second Stage: 2 to 10 years after diagnosis (longest stage). Symptoms include increasing memory loss and confusion, shorter attention span, problems recognizing friends, family, or familiar objects (agnosia). Repetitive statements and/or movements, restlessness, perceptual-motor problems, language problems (aphasia), difficulty reading and writing, suspicion, paranoia, loss of impulse control, social graces, and inhibition. Additional symptoms may include resistance to personal care, difficulty with performing self-ADLs, hallucinations, wandering, physical and verbal agitation, and weight changes. The patient often has restlessness, which results in wandering, pacing, and repetitive motor movements, and they may become more physically aggressive. Motor skills are affected, making it necessary to require assistance with ADLs (bathing, eating, dressing, and toileting). The person may get lost in his or her own environment and there is a higher risk for falls.

Terminal Stage: 1 to 3 years. Symptoms include severe deterioration of intellectual and physical functioning with complete loss of language, loss of bladder and bowel control, and inability to walk or perform ADLs. The person eventually may be unable to eat or swallow and is at risk of malnutrition and aspiration pneumonia. Inability to communicate or recognize self, pica activity, and seizures, may also occur. The total time for the disease is up to 20 years.

Treatment options

At the present time, tacrine (Cognex®), donnepezil (Aricept®), galantamine (Reminyl®), and rivastigmine (Excelon®) remain the only acetylcholinesterase inhibitors approved for individuals with mild to moderate dementia. In several small studies, antiinflammatory drugs such as ibuprofen have been shown to decrease the risk of AD (Moore, 1998; APA, 1994). A relationship between AD and increased levels of the amino acid homocysteine has encouraged studies looking at increases in folic acids and vitamins B6 and B12, all which reduce homocysteine levels (Seshadri, et al., 2003). It is not known yet if this reduces the risk of AD.

Numerous studies have suggested the use of vitamin E and hormone replacement therapy, but their role is yet to be scientifically supported. As much research funding is being allocated to prevention, slowing, and cure for AD worldwide, treatment should be based on the latest recommendations.

Vascular Dementia (VD) is caused by cerebrovascular disease that results from insufficient blood flow to the brain, called cerebral insufficiency. Depending on the cause of VD, the onset may be abrupt, insidious, static, remitting, or progressive (Reichman, 1994; Roman, Tatemichi, & Erkinjuntti, 1993). Typically, there is a history of transient ischemic attacks (TIAs) with brief impairment of consciousness, fleeting pareses, or visual loss. The dementia may also follow a succession of acute cerebrovascular accidents or, less commonly, a single major stroke. If a single major stroke occurs, there are abrupt cognitive changes and one-sided function loss. VD that is not associated with a major stroke has a more gradual emergence. Symptom progression occurs and develops in a stepwise manner, including confusion, problems with recent memory, wandering or getting lost in familiar places, loss of bladder or bowel control (incontinence), emotional problems such as laughing or crying inappropriately, and difficulty following instructions. Risk factors for multi-infarct dementia include cardiac arrhythmias, hypertension, cardiovascular disease, rheumatic heart disease, stroke, and TIAs. Treatment for this type of dementia focuses on the underlying cause to prevent future decline. Many forms of VD might be preventable, especially with good control of vascular risk factors in middle age (Erkinjuntti & Rockwood, 2003).

Dementia with Lewy Bodies (DLB) requires early detection and differentiation from other conditions for determination of treatment options and to provide caregivers and clients with information and resources to help manage behaviors associated with DLB. DLB tends to affect males more than females and the age of onset typically falls between age 50 and 80, with duration of illness of about 6 years. It is considered to have a more rapid progression than pure AD. The clinical features that distinguish LBD from AD are as follows:

- Fluctuation in cognitive functioning with varying levels of alertness and attention.

- Hallucinations may occur at any time but are often worse during the times of acute confusion. The most common hallucinations are visual and involve animate objects. Most often the hallucinations are of people and usually in the same place, for example, a child always sitting in the same place.

- Spontaneous motor features of Parkinsonism with mild gait impairment including bradykinesia, characterized by slow movements, rigidity, stooped posture, shuffling gait, and difficulty initiating movement. Unexplained frequent falls occur in DLB (Walker & Stevens, 2002).

Clients with DLB are often abnormally sensitive to neuroleptic therapy, developing Parkinsonism, which is often prolonged, profound, and may even be fatal. Therefore, it is important for clients to be properly diagnosed. The occurrence of hallucination may cause a neuroleptic medication to be prescribed without consideration to a DLB diagnoses. This should be done with extreme caution and only when the benefits of the medications will outweigh the risks.

HOW DEMENTIA IS DIAGNOSED

A diagnosis of dementia is never made based on memory loss alone. Preferably a work-up should be performed at a memory clinic or by a geriatrician. The examination will attempt to rule out any physical, emotional, or psychosocial cause for the cognitive impairment. (See Chapter 9 for more on delirium.)

History: An accurate history including the patient's current mental or physical conditions, medication usage, and family history of health problems is essential in making a diagnosis of dementia. The history should be obtained from family or caregiver if possible, without the patient present, so the informant will be free to express the patient's deficits and behavior without embarrassment to the patient. The history of onset and symptoms is of utmost importance.

A mental status evaluation: The Six-Item Orientation Memory Concentration Test is short and will give an indication of the level of impairment (Katzman & Terry, 1983) (see Table 6-3). Another commonly used cognitive scale is the Mini-Mental State Examination (MMSE) (Folstein, Folstein, & McHugh, 1975). This is a 30-point cognitive screening tool that includes testing of orientation, attention, memory, visual construction, and language. This is a commonly used screening tool that takes 10 minutes to administer. The maximum score on the MMSE is 30; a score of 24–30 is considered normal, depending on age,

education, and complaints: 20–23 mild cognitive impairment; 10–19 moderate impairment; 1–9 severe impairment; and 0 profound impairment. The MMSE possesses high reliability in assessment of clinically stable patients over time. This scale is not available for reproduction but may be obtained at cost at [http://www.minimental.com].

Physical examination: Includes a through examination including nutritional status.

Neurological examination: The nervous system is tested for evidence of other neurological disorders, such as stroke, Parkinson's disease, brain tumor, or hydrocephalus.

Laboratory tests: Blood and urine tests are used to check for anemia, infections, diabetes, kidney and liver disorders, nutritional deficiencies, and abnormally high or low levels of thyroid hormone. Vitamin B12 and folate tests are ordered to rule out pernicious anemia and folate deficiency. Serological tests are done for syphilis. Brain imaging techniques, such as a CT scan or MRI, may be

TABLE 6-3: SIX ITEM ORIENTATION MEMORY CONCENTRATION TEST

	Error	Score	Weighted Score
1. What year is it now?	1	×4	_____
2. What month is it now?	1	×3	_____
Give memory phrase: "Repeat this phrase after me: John Brown, 42 Market St., Chicago." (Repeat twice)			
3. About what time is it? (within an hour)	1	×3	_____
4 Count backward 20 to 1.	2	×2	_____
5. Say the months in reverse order.	2	×2	_____
6. Repeat the memory phrase.	5	×2	_____

Score 1 for each incorrect response. Maximum weighted score: 28.
Scoring: 0–10 indicates mild impairment.
        10–20 indicates moderate impairment.
        20–-28 indicates severe impairment.

Note. From "Validation of a short Orientation-Memory-Concentration Test of cognitive impairment," by Katzman et al., 1983, *Am J Psychiatry, 140*;734-739. Reprinted with permission.

ordered to rule out the presence of tumors, stroke, blood clots, or other factors.

Psychiatric, psychological, and other evaluations: Designed to rule out the presence of other illnesses such as depression, bi-polar disorders, anxiety, and other disorders which might be causing the symptoms. These evaluations test memory, reasoning and writing, vision-motor coordination, the ability to express ideas, and provide more in-depth information than the mental status evaluation alone. The importance of a comprehensive work-up early in the course of the disease cannot be overemphasized. Once an older adult has been diagnosed with dementia, they may never again be re-evaluated.

TABLE 6-4: TIPS FOR OLDER ADULTS WITH ALZHEIMER'S DISEASE AND OTHER DEMENTIAS

1. **Recognize that you are going through a roller coaster of emotions.**
   - You may respond to your diagnosis and to your memory changes with a variety of emotions.
   - You might feel angry, embarrassed, frustrated, afraid, or sad. These emotions are very normal and may come and go. Let those close to you know how you are feeling.
   - Your family will also be experiencing the same type of emotional roller coaster.
   - Often people with Alzheimer's disease get depressed. If your feelings are overwhelming and won't go away, talk to your doctor.

2. **Tell people.**
   - Let the people closest to you know that you are living with Alzheimer's disease.
   - Explain how it is affecting you. This will help them to understand your difficulties.
   - Knowing this will also allow you to tell them how they might be able to support you.
   - Find people you are comfortable with to share your feelings and emotions.
   - Some people also find writing their thoughts, feelings and experiences in a journal helpful.

3. **Learn as much as you feel you can.**
   - Write down your questions and bring these with you to your next doctor visit.
   - Contact the Alzheimer's Association (1-800-272-3900) for information about the disease, treatment options, and resources. They can tell you what services are available.

4. **Recognize that you have a disease that affects your abilities.**
   - Focus on what you can do, not what you can't do.
   - Find ways that might help you cope with these changes. For example, writing down important things in a memory book, labeling cupboards, or marking a calendar.
   - People who have the disease say you need to simplify your life, follow a routine. Learn to be patient and try not to be hard on yourself.

5. **Plan for the future.**
   - If you are working, it is important to prepare for your retirement.
   - If you own a business or a home you need to plan now for when you can no longer do things on your own.
   - If there are decisions about your life that you have been putting off, make them now
   - Chose someone to make financial and health-care decisions for you for when you are unable.

6. **Explore treatment options.**
   - Currently there is no cure for Alzheimer's disease or the other types of dementia.
   - Medications are available that can help some people with some of the symptoms.
   - Discuss their risks and benefits of available treatments with your doctor and family.
   - Ask you doctor about any research study that you might participate in.

7. **Live each day.**
   - Live one day at a time, some days will be better than others.
   - You will continue to have abilities…focus on them.
   - Do the things you enjoy and that bring you meaning and fulfillment.
   - Maintain your physical health, exercise and eat a healthy diet.

Note. From Fitzsimmons, S., & Buettner, L. (2002). *Health promotions for the body, mind & spirit. A college course for persons with Alzheimer's disease.* Fort Myers, FL: Florida Gulf Coast. Reprinted with permission.

Helping the Patient and Family Deal with the Diagnosis

A diagnosis of AD can be stressful, frightening, and overwhelming to an older adult and his/her family. The older adult may have questions that may be difficult to formulate, refuse to believe the diagnosis, fearful of the future, or the family may hide the diagnosis from the client. If the patient wishes to talk about his/her diagnoses, by all means do so. See Table 6-4 for how to help discuss the diagnoses with the patient.

Family Caregiver

Assist the family caregiver to find a support group to share their feelings and concerns. Members of support groups often have helpful ideas or know of useful resources based on their own experiences. Not every caregiver wants to, or is capable of, participating in a support group, and for them an online support group may be offered as an option. Encourage the caregiver to study their day and develop a routine that makes things go more smoothly. If there are times of day when the patient is less confused or more cooperative, plan the routine to make the most of those moments. Caregivers should also be flexible and adapt their routine as needed. To prevent excessive stress, consider using adult day care or respite services. Families should plan for the future. This may include getting financial and legal documents in order and investigating long-term care options. See Table 6-5 for interaction tips.

Family caregivers often find socializing with neighbors, friends, and family members to be strained. Oftentimes, social invitations stop and friends drift away. Family members, friends, neighbors, and persons working in the community may be unsure of how to treat their old acquaintances, now that they have dementia. The person with dementia and their caregiver often become isolated, lonely, and depressed. Table 6-6 shows tips on how to treat a neighbor, friend, or relative who has

dementia. Provide family members with several copies of this to hand out to friends, neighbors, and others they want to share this with.

INTERACTING WITH CLIENTS WITH DEMENTIA

"If you know one person with dementia, you know one person with dementia."

Although persons with dementia share similar characteristics and cognitive deficits, each patient is uniquely different with different wants and needs. Information provided here are suggestions that work with some, but not all, patients. Keep in mind that even interventions with evidenced-based research rarely works for everybody. For the nurse working with older adults with dementia, keep in mind that approaches and interventions that are individualized to each specific patient usually work the best.

How to interact with persons with dementia is important for both professional and family caregivers. Positive interactions can prevent behavior problems, prevent frustration for all parties, and help in understanding and meeting the needs of the patient. The following are basic techniques to use to enhance interaction and prevent problem behaviors:

- Approach the patient from the front, establishing eye contact, speaking slowly, and using short sentences and simple words.

- Ask yes/no questions. An open-ended question is difficult to answer for a cognitively impaired patient. Provide a communication board if needed.

- Repeat, restate, and paraphrase, as needed, to help the patient understand.

- Speak literally in concrete terms. Abstract thought is difficult for a patient with dementia to interpret.

- Break down directions or tasks into simple steps, and cue the patient as needed at each step.

TABLE 6-5: INTERACTION TIPS

Tip One: Approaching the person with dementia
1. Approach slowly and calmly; speak slowly, clearly, and distinctly. Introduce yourself each time and state what you are doing.
2. Use a friendly tone and facial expression that is pleasant.
3. Make eye contact and call the person's name.
4. Do not touch the person from behind or the side, or without his or her permission.

Tip Two: Instructing the person with dementia to complete tasks
1. Use one step instructions.
2. Use gestures and demonstrations to supplement words.
3. Be patient and repeat instructions the same way.
4. When possible tell the patient what to do, not what not to do.

Tip Three: Getting dressed
1. Allow the person to do as much as possible for himself or herself.
2. Make a pile of clothing to put on in the order in which one would dress.
3. Get easy to put on clothes and limit the choices.
4. Use a consistent method each day.
5. Simplify closets and dressers and add written cues.

Tip Four: Bathing
1. Try to set up a bath time routine. Bathe the same time of day.
2. Set up the bath area with everything within reach before you start. Make sure area is warm.
3. Talk reassuringly during the bath.
4. Provide privacy and the opportunity to do as much as possible for self.
5. Use soothing music, laminated photos, and snacks as distractions.
6. Bath mitts are often useful to keep the individual involved in self care.

Tip Five: Eating – food preparation is a great activity for the person with dementia.
1. Make sure the person is sitting upright and is comfortable at meal time.
2. Simplify the table and the environment. (e.g. turn off TV, radio, etc.) Avoid crowding.
3. Serve small amount of food at a time, do not clutter the area with distractions.
4. Assess ability to use silverware and provide finger foods as needed.
5. Assess ability to sit for required amount of time, provide mobile foods & fluids.
6. Give preferred foods. Continue to reassure the individual about safety of foods.
7. Observe and assess for swallowing problems.

Tip Six: Wandering and mobility
1. Allow the individual to have as much freedom as possible. "Use it or lose it" philosophy.
2. Safe proof dangerous areas, put up stop signs, make sure the bathroom is marked with a visible sign or a different colored door.
3. Provide lots of activities and things to do throughout the home.
4. No medication will stop the individual from wandering. Sensorimotor activity is a basic need.

Tip Seven: Aggressive or hostile behavior
1. First make sure the person is safe and will not cause harm to others. A quiet homelike area may prove useful. Try a calming diversion, a rocking chair, or a relaxation program.
2. There is a reason for every behavior. Ask yourself the following:
   Is there a basic need such as thirst, tired, hunger, pain, toilet need, lonely, or bored.
   Is this a new behavior? Does it occur with a specific other person, time or place?
   Is the person medically ill?
   Is there something new in the environment? Too much stimulus? Not enough?
   Has there been any change in medication?
   What triggered the behavior? How could this be prevented in the future?

Tip Eight: Rummaging and hoarding and repeated verbalization
1. Try redirecting the individual by giving something to do such as a game, magazines or books, puzzles, a newspaper to read, music to listen to.
2. Create a rummaging dresser in an area the individual frequents.
3. Provide walking and exercise on a daily basis.
4. Provide with sensory activities in a variety of locations.
5. Provide with structured daily activities and programs to meet needs for stimulation.
6. Who is a problem for? Is the behavior harmless but irritating to staff or family? Can the behavior be ignored? Answer repeated questions calmly each time.

Tip Nine: The environment
1. People with dementia need a quiet, orderly environment.
2. For safety, maintain uncluttered rooms and hallways.
3. Doors of different colors may help the individual find the bathroom, signs are helpful.
4. Avoid high gloss, slick floors and table tops.
5. Avoid using scatter rugs, especially dark colored rugs.
6. Create activity areas throughout the home with interesting things to do.

Tip Ten: Take care of yourself
1. Remember the person you care for has a serious brain disease. Do not take the behaviors personally, they are part of the illness.
2. Eat right, exercise and get regular check-ups.
3. Ask for help when you need it, don't wait till you can no longer cope.

Note. From Buettner, L. (1997). *The art of dementia care.* Bingham, NY: Bingham University. Reprinted with permission.

- Refrain from arguing with the patient or attempting to use logic. If the patient says something that is untrue, use distraction and redirection instead.

- Reduce environmental stimulus (television, radio) and avoid having more than one person directing the patient at one time.

- Allow the patient the time to do as much as he/she can do for him/herself.

BEHAVIORAL PROBLEMS

Dementia has two sets of symptoms that all caregivers need to be aware of: cognitive symptoms and behavioral symptoms. Cognitive symptoms are the difficulty in word finding, remembering, understanding, and other tasks that rely on cognition. Behavioral symptoms are often the most problematic for both family and professional caregivers. The types of behavioral symptoms that have been identified as disturbing are shown in Table 6-7.

TABLE 6-6: TIPS ON HOW TO TREAT YOUR NEIGHBOR, FRIEND, OR RELATIVE WHO HAS DEMENTIA

- Dementia is not contagious
- Treat them as you always did. They are still adults.
- Include them in social events, especially ones that get them out of the house. Isolation from friends can easily lead to depression.
- Talk to them about the "Good Old Days" as these memories remain intact the longest.
- Don't talk about them in their presence. Don't laugh or stare.
- When greeting them state your name. "Hi, Mary, its me your neighbor Bob".
- Don't ask if they can remember you.
- Offer your assistance: Provide transportation, offer respite.
- Be honest and don't pity them.
- Ask if they can help you.
- Don't ask questions that rely on direct memory.
- Give simple choices. Don't make every choice for them. Ask yes/no questions.
- Be upbeat and cheerful, humor works great. Depression is a contagious condition.
- Don't give complex instructions.
- Realize that they would rather drive, shop, do bills, by themselves.
- If they have trouble finding the right word, help them.
- Don't announce to a group that they have dementia. This, like any other disease, is something personal, and their feelings will get hurt.
- Remember that they have a disease that affects the brain and they can not help the way they act. Thinking that they do things intentionally or that they could stop their behavior if they try really hard is like expecting a person with a cardiac condition to have good cardiac function if they tried really hard.
- If you're having difficulty understanding what they want, respond to their emotion.
- They may not always be able to verbalize their needs, remember to ask occasionally if they need a drink, use the toilet, have pain, are hungry or tired.
- Realize that they will be more confused in unfamiliar places or in a noisy, crowded environment.
- If they are doing somthing they should not do, don't say stop, instead tell them what they should do and help them start it.
- Keeping them active in meaningful activities is the best way to prevent depression, behavior problems and loss of function. Activities that they one loved in the past can be modified for their current ability. Going for a walk together is an excellent activity.
- Keep in mind, that if you make it to 85, you have a 50% chance of having dementia. Treat others as you would like to be treated.

Note. From Fitzsimmons, S., & Buettner, L. (2002). *Health promotions for the body, mind & spirit. A college course for persons with Alzheimer's disease.* Fort Myers, FL: Florida Gulf Coast. Reprinted with permission.

A ten-year, population-based longitudinal study found that 80% of the participants with AD had exhibited behavioral symptoms (Lyketsos, et al, 2000). The most prevalent symptoms, in this study, were apathy (36%), depression (32%), and agitation (30%). Tractenberg, Weiner, and Thal (2002) found 67.5% of community-dwelling elders with dementia have agitation. In an acute-care hospital setting, 95% of clients with dementia were reported to have at least one agitated behavior (Sourial, McCusker, Cole, & Abrahamowicz, 2001). This shows that the majority of persons diagnosed with dementia, in any given setting, will have behavioral problems at some point in time.

TABLE 6-7: DISTURBING BEHAVIORS OF DEMENTIA

- Apathy: Passive, lack of interest or motivation, withdrawal, and social isolation.
- Psychiatric: Depression, anxiety, psychosis: paranoia, delusions, and hallucinations.
- Physical non-aggressive: Motor-restlessness, repetitive movements, wandering, rummaging, hording, hiding things, intrusive, spitting, pacing, picking, and rubbing.
- Physical aggressive: Spitting, hitting, biting, kicking, pushing, destroying things, and self-injurious.
- Verbal: Non-aggressive: vocalizing, repetitive questioning, complaining, screaming, weepy, crying, and moaning.
- Verbal: Aggressive: arguing, yelling, threatening, irritability, cursing, and angry outburst.
- Other: Refusing care, medications, foods or liquids, socially inappropriate (disrobing, urinating), gluttony, pica, sleep-wake disturbance, sun-downing, sexually inappropriate, and disinhibition (Neugroschl, 2002; Gurvich & Cunningham, 2000; LoBuono, 2001; Allen, 1999).

The occurrence of behavioral manifestations in older adults with AD develop due to many factors including degenerative changes that are occurring in the brain. Clinical and research findings have identified the following risk factors for disturbing behaviors:

- Individuals with cognitive impairments (Algase et al., 1996)
- Impaired communication (Talerico, Evans, & Strumpf, 2002)
- Females (Burgio, et al., 2000)
- Fatigue or loss of reserve (Algase, et al., 1996)
- Change of environment, caregiver, or routine (Hall & Buckwalter, 1987)
- Pain or infection (Algase, et al., 1996)
- Overwhelming influx of external stimuli (sensory bombardment) (Ragneskog, Gerdner, Josefsson, & Kihlgren, 1998)
- Deprivation of environmental stimuli or activity (Aubert, et al., 2001)
- Individuals receiving personal care (Burgio, et al., 2000)
- Impaired physical function (Rapoport, et al., 2001)
- Individuals with dementia and depression (Menon, et al., 2001)
- Physical restraints (Talerico, Evans, & Strumpf, 2002)
- 3-month prior pattern of antipsychotic drug usage (Talerico, Evans, & Strumpf, 2002)

THE NEEDS-DRIVEN DEMENTIA-COMPROMISED BEHAVIOR MODEL

The Needs-Driven Dementia-Compromised Behavior Model (NDB) offered a view that behaviors are expressions of unmet needs (Kolanowski, 1999; Algase, et al., 1996). The NDB

Model focuses on the interaction of relatively stable individual characteristics (background factors) and current situational variables (proximal factors) to produce disruptive behaviors. A long-term care unit, with its proximal factors or triggers (physical and social environment) may lead to anxiety, confusion, boredom, or fear. This interplay of factors produces need-driven dementia compromised behavior, which is the most integrated and meaningful response a person with cognitive impairment can make (Figure 6-7). The NDB Model asserts that disruptive behaviors arise because of an unmet need. The individual

---

FIGURE 6-7: NEED-DRIVEN DEMENTIA-COMPROMISED BEHAVIOR MODEL

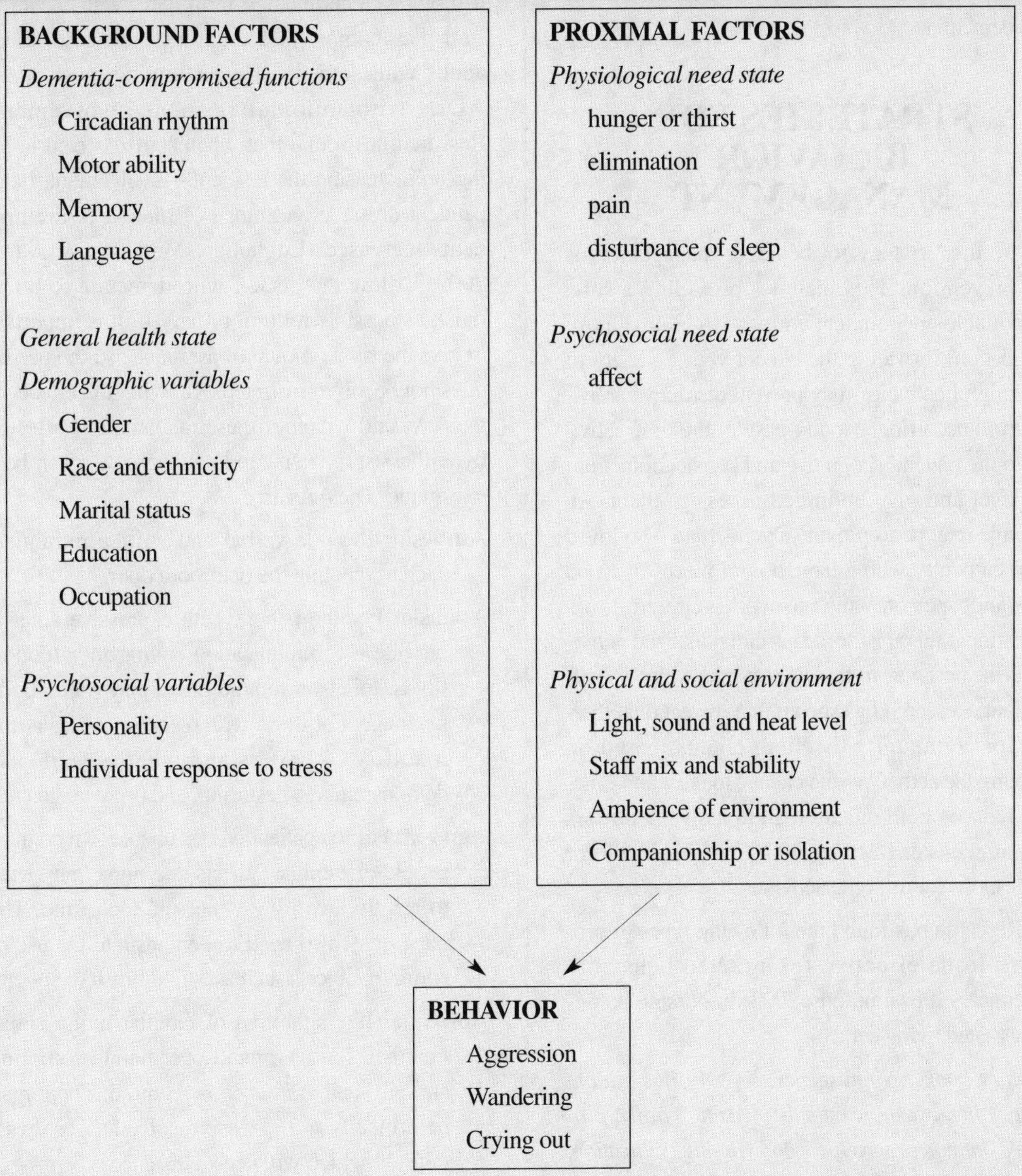

BACKGROUND FACTORS

Dementia-compromised functions

    Circadian rhythm

    Motor ability

    Memory

    Language

General health state

Demographic variables

    Gender

    Race and ethnicity

    Marital status

    Education

    Occupation

Psychosocial variables

    Personality

    Individual response to stress

PROXIMAL FACTORS

Physiological need state

    hunger or thirst

    elimination

    pain

    disturbance of sleep

Psychosocial need state

    affect

Physical and social environment

    Light, sound and heat level

    Staff mix and stability

    Ambience of environment

    Companionship or isolation

BEHAVIOR

    Aggression

    Wandering

    Crying out

Adapted from Kolanowski, A. (1999). An overview of the Need-Driven Dementia-Compromised Model. *Journal of Gerontological Nursing, 25*(9), 7–9.

with dementia is pursuing a goal and (or) trying to express this need. Interventions for NDB are developed by isolating proximal factors (physical and social environment) and manipulating them in a way to prevent, reduce, or eliminate the behaviors. The implication is that all behavior has meaning and is driven by a need. Research is ongoing as to how this model can enhance the quality of life for individuals with dementia.

STRATEGIES FOR BEHAVIOR MANAGEMENT

The first strategy for behavior management is prevention. This includes providing a safe, comfortable environment with the right amount of stimulation. Providing the patient with a variety of meaningful activities may prevent disruptive activities from occurring. Modify past leisure time activities to the patient's cognitive and physical functioning level and give unlimited access to them. An example may be to provide a gentleman who loved to do carpentry with a large box of pieces of wood and sandpaper on which to work. A referral to a recreational therapist to adapt individualized activities is the best way to find what works with a specific client. Research has shown that recreational therapy for community-dwelling clients, based on adapting the activity to the clients' interest and function reduces both agitation and passive behaviors (Fitzsimmons & Buettner, 2002). See Table 6-8 for suggestions for in-home activities.

Research has found the following types of programs to be effective for agitated behaviors (Buettner & Fitzsimmons, 2003) in nursing homes and assisted living centers:

Memory books, reminiscence, sensory integration, sensory handwashing, simple pleasure garden programs, humor programs, woodworking, relaxation, airmat therapy, animal-assisted therapy, nurturing dolls, intergenerational programs, social dancing, exercise for function, walking groups, newsletter programs, cognitive games, or music

Providing the right amount of assistance is also important. Oftentimes caregivers do too much for the patient with dementia, as the task is completed faster and perhaps neater when the caregiver does it. For residents in long-term care, well-meaning staff may compromise the independence of older adults with dementia by performing most of the ADLs with minimal resident involvement. Research has found that when staff received training on increasing the resident's involvement, independent dressing and range of motion of the residents increased (Engleman, Mathews, & Altus, 2002). Allow the person with dementia to do as much as possible for him or herself. It is important to give the right amount of assistance so the person does not become frustrated. Knowing the effects of the 4 As and which of these the patient is affected by will assist the nurse in knowing how much help to provide. The 4 As are:

Amnesia: Provide verbal and written reminders such as labeling the bathroom door.

Aphasia: For the patient with expressive aphasia provide a communication board, offer food or fluids, toilet on routine basis, and watch body language. For those with receptive aphasia (the inability to understand what is said) use demonstrations, gesturing, and body language.

Agnosia: For the patient who is unable to recognize people or familiar objects, the nurse may need to reintroduce him or herself each time. The nurse may also need to demonstrate the use of common objects such as a toothbrush or spoon.

Apraxia: This is the loss of familiar motor skills. For these clients, hand-over-hand prompting and physical assistance is required. There may be difficulty in tasks such as feeding or dressing self, which will need assistance.

TABLE 6-8: SUGGESTIONS FOR IN-HOME ACTIVITIES

1. Make your loved one an activity box, brief case, or luggage case. Place interesting and meaningful things from the past in the box. Fill it with magazines, photographs, cards, letters, things to tinker with. Put some small jewelry boxes in the case that say "open here" on each of them. Each small box can be filled with trinkets and objects the person might enjoy. Take care that the items are not small enough to be swallowed or mistaken as edible.

2. Make an apron or table cloth with lots of pockets. Using elastic or velcro and string attach a variety of interesting objects to each pocket. Some suggestions include: a small music box, a ball of socks with an object inside, small photo albums, old jewelry items, a calculator, a watch, a wooden spoon, ribbons. Be sure all items are removable for washing. Elastic and velcro work well.

3. Dominoes or cards are good to fill time before meals. Matching skills are often intact until later in the disease. The person does not necessarily have to play a game by the rules, but simply sorting or manipulating the items is often fun.

4. For individuals who like to sew make simple sewing cards. Use any size poster board, decorate with beautiful fabrics or pictures, punch holes around the edges. Take a ball of yarn and dip the end in school glue to harden into a needle. The individual can sew the cards together or sew them separately. Make seasonal decorations and door decorations.

5. Scrapbooks and photo albums are interesting and stimulate cognitive functioning in people with cognitive impairments. It is a good idea to label the pictures for the individual who can read.

6. Take an old dresser and fill the drawers with interesting items to rummage through. The individual may enjoy finding items, sorting, or folding. Fill one drawer with towels and socks. Fill another will old toys. Old food boxes from pop tarts, cereal, etc can be cleaned and placed in another drawer. Watches, jewelry and personal items can fill another drawer.

7. Develop a place for the individual's leisure time stuff. The idea is the individual should learn where to look for stimulation or activity. Use familiar things owned in the past. For example, safe proof fishing gear or art supplies. Music should be available if the individual chooses to listen to it.

8. Expressive arts are valuable for the individual with dementia. Some suggestions include: homemade nontoxic clay, chalk and black paper, colored pens and pencils. Make your own holiday cards or gift wrap with stencils and stamps. Use items from nature walks in your projects: dried leaves, flowers, rocks, etc.

Note. From Buettner, L. (1997). *The art of dementia care.* Bingham, NY: Bingham University. Reprinted with permission.

When disturbing behaviors do occur, the first step is to rule out any underlying basic need such as thirst, toilet need, pain, cold, boredom, or sleepiness. Keep in mind that a common symptom of delirium is a change in behavior, for the better or worse. Therefore, a patient with a new behavior may have an underlying medical cause. An example is a patient who suddenly becomes physically aggressive when attempting to toilet or change their clothing. This patient may have a urinary tract infection or be constipated. Make certain to describe the behavior accurately: What happens? Who's involved? When does it occur? How often? What precedes the behavior? What consequences result for patient, caregivers? From this a pattern may be detected such as a patient who gets agitated around only one particular caregiver or a particular time of day or a particular place. Education for that particular caregiver may be all that is needed.

Distraction and redirection are effective techniques to use in working with cognitively impaired patients. One of the benefits of a short-term memory deficit is that as a patient becomes upset or agitated over a particular situation, the caregiver can often distract the patient from that situation and redirect focus to a less upsetting subject.

Reality Orientation

It is appropriate to say a word here about reality orientation. This refers to a technique designed to decrease confusion and disorientation in a confused person. It consists of reorienting the patient to basic information on a consistent basis such as time, place, and person. Reality orientation is an appropriate process for a patient temporarily confused because of an acute confusional state or a patient with mild cognitive impairment who is seeking information to help orient himself or herself. (Spector, Orrell, Davies, & Woods, 2001). For patients with moderate to severe impairment, it is not an appropriate technique and may cause agitation. For these individuals a structured environment is an effective method of assisting a confused patient to meet their means. The goal of reality orientation is to correct the patient's misperception of the environment. Because of the physiological changes in the brain, patients with dementia have lost the ability to think in the abstract, reason, and correctly interpret stimuli; therefore, they have a different perception of reality. If a nurse continues to force reality on a patient who is too impaired to understand, a catastrophic reaction will likely ensue. Validation is a better technique for these individuals. In validation therapy, the caregiver enters the demented person's reality, avoids confronting delusions or hallucinations, uses reminiscence, listens carefully for meaning, and provides reassurance of safety (Feil, 1992, 1994).

Passive Behaviors

Professional and informal caregivers often overlook passivity as a problem. Passivity or apathy is a lack of motivation that is not attributable to diminished level of consciousness, cognitive impairment, or emotional distress. Apathy has several components: lack of initiation and persever-

ance, lack of emotional expression, and lack of goals. The apathy spectrum includes decreases in interest, motivation, spontaneity, affection, enthusiasm and emotion (Marin, 1991; Levy, et al., 1998). Most patients with agitated behaviors also have passive behaviors, with the agitated behaviors increasing as the day goes on (Fitzsimmons & Buettner, 2002). These patients should be engaged in meaningful activities during the time of day that they are passive, to prevent boredom and restlessness that leads to agitation

Passive behaviors place the patient at risk for a decline in both cognitive and physical functioning. They are also susceptible to malnutrition, skin breakdown, incontinence, constipation, infection, and a host of other problems brought on by lack of movement. The patient does less and less for his or herself. Quality of life becomes severely impaired and caregiver burden increases. Passive behaviors may also accompany depression but may occur without depressed mood. Older adults with passive behaviors should be encouraged to participate in activities based on past and current leisure interests and current cognitive and physical functioning. There is a large amount of research data supporting the use of psychosocial, music, physical, and art programs for passivity by increasing social interactions, communication, and engagement (Buettner & Fitzsimmons, 2003). A referral to a recreational therapist can provide activities that are adapted to a specific client.

PHARMACOLOGICAL TREATMENT

It is the nurse who attempts to structure the environment to prevent problem behaviors, attempts nonpharmacological management of the behaviors when they occur, and both assesses the patient and reports the behavior to the physician when pharmacological treatment is being considered. Frequently the behavior occurs when a nurse's aide provides care such as dressing and bathing. If this is the case, it is wise for the nurse to observe and critique the aide's approach. Assisting and modeling proper interaction techniques may eliminate the behavior and thus the need for psychotropic medications. It is therefore vital that nurses understand how to adequately assess the need for psychotropic medications. To understand what pharmacological agent is appropriate for use in a cognitively impaired patient, the first step is to determine the target sign or symptom one is trying to extinguish. This not only helps prevent the inappropriate use and overuse of psychotropic medications, but also provides a standard from which to assess the effectiveness of the treatment. Medications are not effective for all behaviors. Behaviors that do not respond well to medications are personality symptoms, screaming, wandering and verbal nonaggressive behaviors. Verbal non-aggressive behaviors are the ones that are typically harmless but annoying to staff such as repetitive questions. Caregivers should be instructed to be patient over behaviors that are annoying but harmless. When an attempt is made to halt these behaviors with medications it often results in excessive medication usage. Enough medication will stop most behaviors by sedating the patient and placing them at risk for a multitude of side-effects and losses of function. Medications should be used when all other methods of management have failed and the benefits outweigh the risks. (See Table 6-9.) Benefits would include increased quality of life and increased or maintained cognitive and physical functioning. Used appropriately in judicious amounts, psychotropic medications can make a remarkable difference in the quality of life for both the patients and the patients' caregivers; however, used without a good initial assessment and frequent evaluation, these agents can cause a significant amount of morbidity in and of themselves. See Chapter 5 for more on appropriate usage of medications for behaviors.

The usage of as-needed (PRN) psychotropic medications is discouraged and if used more than twice in a seven-day period, should be re-evaluated by the prescribing physician. When PRN medications are used the nurse should be detailed in the documentation of its usage. *"Resident agitated, prn Ativan given with good results"* provides little information for others. Use objective charting methods instead such as *"Resident pacing back and forth in front of nursing station yelling at other residents. Resident refused to attempt a relaxation program. Denied hunger, thirst, pain, or toilet needs. Ativan given at 1400. At 1500 resident noted to be smiling while participating in music group with recreation therapy."* The second example provides much more detailed information.

As older adults with dementia lose the ability to orient themselves, reason, correctly interpret their surroundings, and think logically, psychotic signs and symptoms can develop. Those usually associated with Alzheimer's disease include wandering, restlessness, agitation, paranoia, hallucinations, delusions, belligerence, and unprovoked outbursts of rage. The patient may require a neuroleptic medication at some point to help control psychotic symptoms (Stolley & Buckwalter, 1992). When a psychotic or delusional behavior does occur, the nurse must assess the patient to determine if there is any truth behind them. An example is an older adult living by herself who is accusing her family of stealing money from her. She tells everyone that she "has seen someone walk out of her bedroom" while she awoke while napping on the couch in the early evening. Her family members states that she is hallucinating about seeing people in her house and requests she is placed on antipsychotic medications. Eventually an investigation by adult protection discovered that her grandson had stolen a total of over $8,000 from her in the past 6 months. Always investigate any hallucinations, paranoia, and delusion prior to requesting medication. Hallucinations that are not disturbing

TABLE 6-9: HANDLING BEHAVIORAL SYMPTOMS OF DEMENTIA

VERBAL

Repetitive questioning: Due to loss of short-term memory. *Give consistent answers, distract, and provide activities. Write answer on pad for patient to keep.*

Complaining: Generally caused by unmet need that can't be verbalized. *Listen for feelings in addition to content. Observe body language for clue as to pain, fatigue etc.*

Asking for the impossible: (such as a deceased relative): Long-term memory intact, short-term impaired. *First talk to them about person they are asking for, look at photos of the person, they miss them, do not tell them the person is deceased, then attempt to distract.*

Screaming: Over/under-stimulated, unmet need, underlying untreated physical/ emotional condition. *Depression is a frequent cause of screaming. Provide comfort items.*

Manipulative: Frustration, confusion. *Provide simple tasks, focus on feelings not facts.*

Anxiety: Confusion, fatigue, or over-stimulated. *Assess needs, reassure, and provide comfort and outlets.*

Paranoid/Suspicious: Common in middle stages, often caused by forgetting where items are. *Do not argue or try to reason. Investigate the suspicion, it may be based on fact. Offer simple answers. If forgetting whereabouts of belongings have multiples of items if possible, learn hiding places. Do not take personally.*

Withdrawn/Isolated/Weepy/Apathy: *Assess for depression.*

Cranky: *Check for unmet need, pain, or fatigue. Remove from over-stimulating environment.*

PERSONAL CARE DIFFICULTIES

Refusing to bathe, brush teeth , not wanting to change clothing, dressing inappropriate to temperature: *Establish daily routine. Be patient, set up task, and assist in starting. Inform what you are doing and give one step commands. Provide simple choices, lay out clothes in order that they go on, provide privacy, and allow ample time for self-care. Provide comfortable easy to put on clothing. Praise appearance. If grabbing items give something to hold.*

INAPPROPRIATE BEHAVIORS

Hallucinations/Delusions: Hearing or seeing things that are not there or unfound beliefs. *Investigate if it is in fact a hallucination. Check for visual or hearing impairment, increase lighting, remove clutter. Check for sensory depravation. Check medication side effects.*

Socially Inappropriate Behavior/No longer remembers social graces. *Avoid situations that precipitates inappropriateness. Don't scold, distract by giving simple tasks.*

Impulsive Sexual Behavior: *Remain calm and reply consistently. If self-stimulating, provide privacy. Increase opportunity for touch and warmth. Offer soothing objects. Don't argue or reason, change subject. Ignore that which is harmless.*

Undressing: *Provide comfortable clothes, praise appearance, check for skin irritation, urinary tract infections, and bathroom needs. If persistent, provide clothing with fasteners in back, provide activity to keep hands busy.*

Urinating in public/inappropriate places: *Place signs on bathroom door. Provide bedside commode. Toilet before leaving home and check for need every half hour. Establish toileting schedule. If persistent get assessment for urinary tract infection or prostate problem.*

Spitting: *Check for swallowing difficulties, dental exam for oral pain, and provide tissues or cup.*

AGGRESSIVENESS

Verbal: Under- or over-stimulating environment, frustration, pain, constipation, fatigue. *Only one person should address the patient, having many people talking at once will add to the aggression and confusion. Use soft voice, don't argue or attempt to reason, try distracting by changing the subject or engage in an activity. When all else fails ignore the outburst and give time for both of you to cool down. Quiet the environment. Check basic needs especially pain or fatigue.*

Physical: Under- or over-stimulating environment, frustration, pain: *Stay calm, protect yourself, remove dangerous items from environment, give personal space, do not confront or accuse, offer reassurance that you will keep them safe. If holding onto you tight, keep relaxed, attempting to pull away will cause increased grabbing. Calmly state that this hurts. Take to quiet controlled environment. Determine what triggered reaction and prevent situation from reoccurring.*

RESTLESS

Pacing, picking: *Substitute an activity for the behavior. Allow freedom to move safely, find outlets for energy. Walk, exercise, dancing, craft activity.*

Rummaging/Hoarding: *Provide dresser or space for rummaging, and provide activities. Ignore behavior that causes no harm.*

REFUSING

Medications: Inability to understand the need, difficulty with swallowing. *Give only essential medications. Tell that the MD, or other influential person wants them to have it. Make simple medication chart and post to give control to the patient.*

Foods: *Give one food at a time, give small servings, provide many small meals throughout the day, provide calm environment, eat with others, allow to feed self even if messy, provide finger foods, oral assessment. Check medication side effects.*

Fluids: *Offer fluids on a regular basis. Check for oral pain. Give high fluid content foods such as popcicles, pudding, or fruit.*

OTHER

Overeating: Forgotten that they have eaten. *Provide low cal snacks such as crackers, involve in cooking and other activities, allow her to plan menus and post them.*

Pica behavior: Inability to recognize an item as being inedible, eating non-edible items: *Remove harmful items such as plants, Styrofoam, paper products. Provide finger foods, gum, or crackers. Involve in activities to keep hands busy.*

Note. From Buettner, L., & Fitzsimmons, S. (2003). Dementia problem guidelines for recreational therapies: Treatment of disturbing behaviors. Alexandria, VA: American Therapeutic Recreation Association. Reprinted with permission.

to the patient should not be treated with medications, as the benefits would not outweigh the risk of the side effects.

These medications should be used as a last resort after all other interventions have failed. There is little evidence that neuroleptics control behavioral symptoms of AD. These medications have some significant, irreversible side effects; therefore, they should be used only to manage specific symptoms for which other interventions are not effective. The side effects of concern with the neuroleptics include level of sedation, anticholinergic effects, potential for orthostatic hypotension, and extrapyramidal syndromes.

The prescribing physician generally chooses a particular psychotropic medication based on target behavior and by determining the side-effect profile the patient would best be able to tolerate. It is up to nursing to assess for side effects and the patient's need for that particular medication at that particular dose. AD is not a static disease. The patient shows a gradual but continually declining course and may no longer need a medication for behavior management. Trial medication reductions are encouraged every 6 months.

GENERAL SIDE EFFECTS OF PSYCHOTROPIC MEDICATIONS

There are 4 general areas of side effects with psychotropic medications:

1. Anticholinergic effects

2. Orthostatic hypotension

3. Level of sedation

4. Extrapyramidal symptoms

Anticholinergic effects: Patients with AD lose a significant number of the cholinergic cells in their brain; additionally, there is diminished activity of choline acetyltransferase. These changes give the patient with Alzheimer's disease an increased sensitivity to the anticholinergic side effects of many of the psychotropic medications (Ray, Taylor, Meador, & Gideau, 1993). Anticholinergic delirium, which is a frequent cause of increased confusion in elderly demented patients, can result. The peripheral anticholinergic side effects are dry mouth, constipation, urinary retention, blurred vision, tachycardia, and dry skin and mucous membranes. Anticholinergic effects on the central nervous system can cause delirium, with symptoms including agitation, anxiety, disorientation, restlessness, assaultiveness, hallucinations, and paranoia. A patient with AD suffering from an anticholinergic delirium will appear to have worsening behavior. It is possible that the care providers may mistakenly increase the patient's dose of psychotropic medication to extinguish the behavior, when the patient actually needs a reduction in the number of medications with anticholinergic side effects. Pharmacological agents with significant anticholinergic effects therefore are used cautiously in patients with AD.

Orthostatic hypotension is defined as a drop of 20mm Hg or more in the patient's blood pressure when the patient stands up. Orthostatic hypotension can be dangerous for the elderly, because it can lead to falls and associated injuries. Nursing actions appropriate for patients with orthostatic hypotension include evaluating for symptoms of dizziness or falls, especially when a new medication or dose increase occurs. Nurses should teach the following safety precautions both to the patient and the patient's caregiver: Make changes in position slowly. Arise slowly from bed in several stages. From a lying position, sit at the side of the bed with the legs dangling over the side for a few moments to allow the blood pressure to stabilize before standing up.

Sedation: The degree of sedation an agent causes is also considered in choosing a psychotropic drug. If the patient needs energy and already has psychomotor retardation, then a less sedating agent would be appropriate. For highly anxious and hypervigilant patients, a more sedating agent might be a better choice. The patient should be assessed for excessive sedation with the addition of any new medication or dosage increase. This would include increased and excessive sleeping, increased confusion, and declines in abilities to communicate, feed self, ambulate, and perform other ADLs.

Extrapyramidal symptoms are side effects of neuroleptic treatment. The 3 extrapyramidal symptoms that are most common in the elderly are: Parkinsonism, akathisia, and tardive dyskinesia.

- Parkinsonism consists of bradykinesia, muscular rigidity, stooped posture, shuffling gait, masked facies, tremor, and drooling. These parkinsonian side effects occur during the first few months of treatment and then usually resolve over several months as tolerance develops (Ray et al., 1993).

- Akathisia is an extrapyramidal symptom that consists of motor restlessness and pacing. The patient has a subjective feeling of anxiety with an inability to sit still and a pressured need to move. Because akathisia can make it seem that the patient's psychotic symptoms are worsening, it can be mistakenly treated by increasing the dose of neuroleptics. This is wrong, however; when akathisia occurs, the dosage of the antipsychotic medication should be reduced.

- Tardive dyskinesia is an involuntary, primarily oral-facial movement disorder. It consists of sudden movements of the tongue known as the "fly-catcher syndrome," lip smacking, lip puckering, and facial grimacing. It may be accompanied by rolling chorea movements of the arms and trunk (Perry, Alexander, & Liskow, 1991). This frequently irreversible side effect of the neuroleptics is not only disfiguring but can also significantly interfere with the patient's ability to eat and drink. The elderly

seem to be more sensitive to this effect; it develops more frequently and at smaller doses than in the young. Tardive dyskinesia may be reversible if detected early; therefore nurses working with patients under treatment for psychotic symptoms need to assess frequently for its early signs. These include rhythmic, wave-like movements of the tongue or trunk; mild, choreiform movements of the fingers or toes; and facial tics or frequent eye blinking (Perry et al., 1991).

If any of these develops, consideration should be given to reduction of the dose or discontinuation of the neuroleptic. The list of neuroleptic medications is quite extensive with newer atypical medications being developed and marketed. The nurse should learn the side-effect profile on all of the specific medication prescribed for his or her patients. In the days of Thorazine® and Haldol®, the prescription of psychoactive medications came with the understanding of the great risks for side effects. Since the advent of newer, "safer" atypical antipsychotics, nursing may feel more comfortable with these medications. This is validated by research that shows over 50% of long-term care patients with dementia are on one or more psychoactive medication (Gibbs-Brown, 1997). Medications always carry the risk of an adverse event and are correlated with falls, loss of function, hip fractures, decreased cognition, and premature institutionalizations (Dellasega, Klinefelter, & Halas, 2000). A recent warning from the FDA and Janssen Pharmaceutica "Risperdal® has not been shown to be safe or effective in the treatment of patients with dementia-related psychoses" resulted from four separate research studies linking its usage to cerebral vascular accidents (Janssen Pharmaceutica, 2003). It makes one wonder what will be discovered next about other "safe" commonly prescribed medications. This makes the use of non-pharmacological intervention an avenue to pursue vigorously.

OTHER COMMON PROBLEMS

Sleep disturbances can be stressful and cause exhaustion in caregivers. Encourage physical activity in the afternoon and limit daytime napping and caffeine. Create a quiet, peaceful tone in the evening to encourage sleep. Keep the lights dim, eliminate loud noises, and play soothing music if the person seems to enjoy it. Developing a bedtime routine may help. Use night-lights in the bedroom, hall, and bathroom if the darkness is frightening or disorienting. See Chapter 9 for additional information.

Wandering

Five different types of wandering may be seen in older adults with dementia:

1. Tactile wandering occurs in the end of the ambulatory dementia phase and individuals use their hands to explore their environment, remain calm, and appear to feel their way through the facility.

2. Environmentally cued wanderers follow cues in their environment; if the individual sees a window, she looks out. A chair may cue him or her to sit. These individuals are usually in the middle of the ambulatory phase.

3. Reminiscent walking stems from the individual's delusions from the past (e.g., seeing parents, going to school, or doing chores). These individuals are calm and in the ambulatory phase.

4. Recreational wandering may be in the older adult who had an active lifestyle in the past. May serve a need for exercise. The individual is calm unless stopped.

5. Agitated purposeful wandering is seen in individuals who are upset or exhibit stress-related behaviors like angry outbursts. They are preoccupied with leaving, and may pack suitcases to take with them (Hall, et al., 1995).

Keeping the person safe is one of the most important aspects of caregiving. For a patient that wanders, make certain he/she has sturdy non-skid footwear that fits correctly and a safe place to wander. For a constant wanderer, provide extra nourishment and fluids to prevent dehydration and malnutrition. Encourage sitting to rest every hour by providing a favorite activity or relaxation method such as calm music. Research has shown that relaxation, exercise, doll therapy, music, outdoor gardens, and cognitive programs all have a positive effect on wandering (Buettner & Fitzsimmons, 2003). Providing community outings is another intervention for patients who wander. Riding in a car may provide needed rest while still enjoying a moving scenery that occurs while wandering.

Make sure that the person carries some kind of identification or wears a medical bracelet. If he or she gets lost and is unable to communicate adequately, this will alert others to his or her identity and medical condition. Keep a recent photograph or videotape of the person with AD to assist police if the person becomes lost. Keep doors locked. Consider a keyed dead-bolt or an additional lock up high or down low on the door. If the person can open a lock because it is familiar, a new latch or lock may help.

Nutrition/Hydration

Patients with AD commonly lose weight. This weight loss is felt to be multifactoral; that is, the patient forgets to eat, cannot complete the task of eating without someone cueing at each step, has apathy towards eating, has become much more active with increased movement, difficulty swallowing, or feeding apraxia. Weight loss and inadequate protein intake places the patient at risk for skin breakdown, particularly in combination with urinary incontinence. Adequate nutrition may become a problem both for family and professional caregiver. High-protein supplements can be bought commercially or made at home. Making sure the patient actually drinks the supplement is vital. In some patients, an occasional sweet will stimulate the appetite.

Cognitively impaired patients are also at risk for dehydration. The older adult with dementia has a diminished thirst sensation and may not correctly interpret the thirst signal when it does occur. Additionally, he or she may not understand environmental cues that remind a person to drink, that is, water pitchers or glasses or where to find a drink. Dehydration can lead to delirium and puts patients at high risk for stool impaction, respiratory and urinary infections, and medication side effects. Caregivers need to offer patients with Alzheimer's disease fluids on a regular basis (see Chapter 5 for further discussion of hydration and nutritional information). A simple reminder to drink is not adequate. A patient with dementia may agree that he or she should be drinking fluids but may not be able to initiate the activity or perform the necessary sequencing to actually drink the fluids. The nurse must pour the water, hand the glass to the patient, and cue the patient at each step until swallowing is completed. Because of the high risk for dehydration, fluid restriction should not be used as a technique for managing incontinence. Ice pops, gelatin, ice cream and high water fruits should be encouraged for those that resist fluids.

The nutrition and hydration management issues for the patient with AD requires creativity and flexibility on the caregiver's part. Early in the disease, the patient needs easy-to-eat finger foods, if apraxia is affecting the ability to use utensils. Eating alone, or in a small group, is better than eating in the chaos of a large dining room, which may precipitate a catastrophic reaction in some patients. If a patient coughs while eating, aspiration may be developing. Aspiration begins in patients with AD, as the disease progresses. A speech or occupational therapist can teach the patient's family feeding techniques to prevent aspiration, including swallowing twice, checking for food pocketing, using

thickened liquids, and using different textures and temperatures of food. A feeding syringe should never be used to feed a patient at risk for aspiration. Frequent evaluation of the weight of all patients will allow the caregiver to detect any weight loss early. The nurse must keep a high index of suspicion regarding a developing depression when weight loss occurs early in the disease.

Home Safety

Caregivers of people with AD often have to look at their homes through new eyes to identify and correct safety risks. Creating a safe environment can prevent many stressful and dangerous situations. The following should be considered for community-dwelling patients.

- Install secure locks on all outside windows and doors, especially if the person is prone to wandering.

- Place STOP, DO NOT ENTER, or CLOSED signs in strategic areas of doors. Secure the yard with a locked fence. Obtain devices that alarm when a door is opened.

- Remove the locks on bathroom doors to prevent the person from accidentally locking in himself or herself.

- Use childproof latches on kitchen cabinets and any place where cleaning supplies or other chemicals are kept.

- Label medications and keep them locked up. Also make sure knives, lighters and matches, and guns are secured and out of reach.

- Keep the house free from clutter. Remove scatter rugs and anything else that might contribute to a fall. Make sure lighting is good both inside and out.

- Consider installing an automatic shut-off switch on the stove to prevent burns or fire. Install smoke detectors and keep refrigerator free of spoiled foods.

Medical Visits

It is important that the person with AD receive regular medical care including routine dental examination and treatment. Planning these trips in advance can help the trip go more smoothly.

- Try to schedule the appointment for the person's best time of day and when the office is least crowded.

- Notify the office staff in advance that the patient has dementia. If there is something they could do to make the visit go more smoothly, ask.

- Inform the patient about the appointment the day of the visit or even shortly before it is time to go. Be positive and matter-of-fact.

- Bring along something to eat and drink and any activity that he or she may enjoy.

- Have a friend or another family member go with you on the trip, so that one of you can be with the person while the other speaks with the doctor.

SUMMARY

The nurse caring for older adults with dementia will undoubtedly need continual education to keep informed of the latest research and approaches to care. Educating the patient's family and friends, the nurse's assistants, and other staff members should be considered an ongoing process. As this is perhaps the most vulnerable population to be working with, nurses should remain alert to their patients' needs and actively advocate for them. Providing care to this group is challenging and stressful yet enlightening, rewarding and heartwarming. Consider the following exchange:

While working on a special care unit I spotted Gladys, a constant wanderer, walking down the hall towards me. I noticed that she had her nitroglycerin patch stuck on the end of her nose.

"Gladys, what is this doing on your nose?" I asked.

"Keeps my nose warm" replied Gladys.

Assuming she had taken it off of her chest I removed it and placed it on her back, where she could not reach it, while saying to her "I think this will be better for you on your back."

Gladys turned and started down the hall, then paused, just briefly, in front of another resident.

She pointed her thumb towards me and said "Boy, is that one confused. She thinks this little thing will keep my back warm!"

EXAM QUESTIONS

CHAPTER 6
Questions 37-47

37. Normal aging is characterized by

    a. inability to learn new information.

    b. normal response time and reflexes.

    c. decreased speed of learning and recall.

    d. increased ability to concentrate.

38. A factor that often contributes to confusion and difficulty focusing on topic is

    a. medications.

    b. education level.

    c. marital status.

    d. ambulation status.

39. Your client Mrs. Jones has been complaining of fluctuating cognition and hallucination, and has reported to have fallen several times in the past month. These symptoms are most consistent with

    a. Alzheimer's disease.

    b. dementia with Lewy Bodies.

    c. vascular dementia.

    d. alcohol dementia.

40. A diagnosis of Alzheimer's disease can be stressful, frightening, and overwhelming to an older adult and his/her family. If your client states he/she wants to talk about the diagnosis

    a. change the topic and hope they forget.

    b. ask a family member to talk to the client.

    c. tell the client to discuss this with their doctor.

    d. by all means do so.

41. A technique that will enhance communication with patient with dementia is to

    a. ask open-ended questions.

    b. use abstract terms.

    c. repeat, restate, and paraphrase.

    d. use logical examples.

42. The percentage of older adults with Alzheimer's disease that exhibit behavioral symptoms is

    a. 50%.

    b. 25%.

    c. 80%.

    d. 40%.

43. The client on a dementia special care unit who has the most risk factors for disturbing behaviors is

    a. Mr. Thomas, 80 years old with diabetes.

    b. Mrs. Hardy, 90 years old with hypertension.

    c. Mrs. Jones, a new admission with chronic pain.

    d. Mr. Smith, a new admission with mild COPD.

44. The first strategy for behavior management in patients with dementia is

    a. prevention.

    b. medications.

    c. restraints.

    d. validation.

45. Reality orientation is a technique that should be used

    a. with patients with mild cognitive impairment who are seeking information.

    b. with all patients with dementia, routinely throughout the day.

    c. with all patients in a post-operative acute care setting.

    d. only with patients who are cognitively intact.

46. The side effects of psychotropic medications that include dry mouth, constipation, urinary retention, blurred vision, tachycardia, and dry skin and mucous membranes are considered

    a. anticholinergic effects.

    b. sedative effects.

    c. hypotension effects.

    d. extrapyramidal effects.

47. Mrs. Jones uses her hands to explore the environment and remains calm as she feels her way through the special care unit. This type of wandering behavior is considered to be

    a. environmental.

    b. recreational.

    c. tactile.

    d. reminiscent.

RESOURCES

Alzheimer's Association: On-line and print publications plus local chapter with support groups, education programs and other services. 1-800-272-3900, Web: http://www.alz.org

Alzheimer's Disease Cooperative Study: Coordinates clinical trials. 858-622-5880, Web: http://antimony.ucsd.edu/

Alzheimer's Disease Education Center (ADEAR): Publications and booklets, information on clinical trials, and information specialists for local resources. 1-800-438-4380, Web: http://www.alzheimers.org

Children of Aging Parents: Information and referrals for nursing homes, retirement communities, elderlaw, adult day-care, insurance, respite and state and county agencies. 1-800-227-7294, Web: http://www.caps4caregivers.org

Eldercare Locator: Nationwide directory to help locate local services. 1-800-677-1116, Web: http://www.eldercare.gov

Family Caregiver Alliance: Support services for caregivers. 1-415-434-3388, Web: http://www.caregiver.org

RECOMMENDED READINGS

Ballard, E.L., & Poer, C.M. (1999). *Lessons learned: shared experiences in coping.* Durham, NC: The Duke Family Support Program. Silver Spring, MD: Alzheimer's Disease Education and Referral (ADEAR) Center. Documents the experiences of people caring for loved ones with AD. Filled with short stories and advice.

Davies, H.D., & Jensen, M.P. (1998). *Alzheimer's: the answers you need.* ForestKnolls, CA: ElderBooks. This book is for people in the early stages of AD. It provides information about the nature and causes of AD, the symptoms, and how to deal with them.

Mace, N.L., & Rabins, P.V. (1999). *The 36 hour day: a family guide to caring for persons with Alzheimer's disease, related dementing illnesses and memory loss in later life* (3rd ed.). Baltimore, MD: Johns Hopkins University Press. Practical and detailed reference book provides a wealth of information for families.

Shenk, D. (2001). *The forgetting. Alzheimer's: portrait of an epidemic.* New York, NY: Random House, Inc. An eloquent and moving description of AD. Readable description of the history of AD, research and the human impact of the disease. The author, calling AD a "death by a thousand subtractions," describes AD in terms that are easy to understand.

CHAPTER 7

COMMON CHRONIC CONDITIONS

CHAPTER OBJECTIVE

After studying this chapter, the reader will be able to discuss the implications of, and strategies for, management and coping with common chronic diseases and conditions in the older adult.

LEARNING OBJECTIVES

After studying this chapter, the learner will be able to

1. describe the various cardiovascular conditions common to older adults.

2. discuss the differences between a TIA and a CVA.

3. explain the difference in left and right brain damage as it pertains to patient needs.

4. identify methods to maintain optimal mobility for patients with Parkinson's disease.

5. describe the impact of the major musculoskeletal disorders on the older adult.

6. identify the primary signs and symptoms for the most common endocrine disorders.

INTRODUCTION

Older adults experience an increased prevalence of chronic illness as they age. Approximately 79% of the aged population have at least one chronic illness, and a larger percentage have several chronic conditions (National Center for Health Statistics, 1999). The health of the older adults is a reflection of lifelong health practices, genetics, emotional strength, availability of adequate health care services, and perhaps a bit of chance. Nursing interventions are aimed at managing chronic conditions while maintaining quality of life. This chapter examines some common health problems as they apply to older adults and methods of assisting the patient to manage these problems. (The student is referred to a medical-surgical textbook for specific information on nursing care of adults for each specific health problem). This often includes psychosocial problems as well as physical problems specific to the elderly that interfere with management and adherence.

DISEASES OF THE CARDIOVASCULAR SYSTEM

The most prevalent cardiovascular disease is hypertension. Current estimates show that it effects 28 million older adults, of whom only 24% have it under control. It is especially prevalent in African Americans and elderly women (Kilker, 2000). Four major cardiovascular complications are associated with hypertension: coronary heart disease (CHD), cerebral vascular accidents (CVA) peripheral vascular disease (PVD) and heart failure (HF) (Noel, Saunters, & Smolensky, 2000).

Classification of Blood Pressure for Adults 18 and Older*

- Optimal <120/<80 mm Hg

- Normal <130/<85 mm Hg

- High-Normal 130-139/85-89 mm HG

- Hypertension** >140/90 mm Hg

- Stage 1 140-159/90-99 mm Hg

- Stage 2 160-179/100-109 mm Hg

- Stage 3 > 180/ > 110 mm Hg

* Not taking hypertensive drugs and not acutely ill. When systolic and diastolic fall into two different categories, the higher category should be selected.

** Based on the average of two or more readings taken at two or more visits after initial screening.

In developing countries, cardiovascular disease is the most common cause of death and hospitalization in the older adult, and coronary atherosclerosis is the most common underlying pathology (Samraj & Kuritzky, 2002). Coronary artery disease (CAD) increases in prevalence, complications, intensity and mortality as persons become older, and may lead to myocardial ischemia or myocardial infarction. The same factors that cause stress and strain on the younger heart cause stress in the aged and are considered to represent risk for cardiac ischemia or infarction. These factors include continuation of a diet high in animal fat (elevated serum lipid levels), salt, and calories; excessive weight or obesity; a high pack-a-day smoking history; physical inactivity; internalization of emotions; exposure to high-density air pollutants; and various existing medical conditions such as infection, anemia, pneumonia, cardiac dysrhythmia, poorly controlled hypertension, surgery, fever, diarrhea, hypoglycemia, malnutrition, avitaminosis, circulatory overload, renal disease and prostatic obstruction. Myocardial oxygen supply is affected when arteriosclerosis or occlusion causes narrowing of coronary arteries. Ischemia can result when myocardial oxygen supply through coronary arter-

ies fails to meet oxygen demand and myocardial tissue is forced to change from aerobic metabolism to anaerobic metabolism, which is less effective. Tissue anoxia and necrosis can result from a myocardial infarction (MI). Congestive heart failure (CHF) indicates a decompensation in the pumping ability of the heart, and is not an uncommon finding in older adults with arteriosclerosis. Decreased cardiac output and stroke volume compounds this condition. The term congestive generally relates to the development of edema in the lungs or in the extremities, with the end result of an increased workload on the myocardium.

Older adults should not be ruled out of active rehabilitation programs solely because of age, as they often respond well to these programs. For patients with cardiovascular disease, lifestyle modifications are not easy to implement. Physical training for older adults can produce profound improvements that affect strength and cardiac endurance, counteracts osteoporosis and results in many other positive health outcomes. Research also shows that exercise may help with depression, sleep, appetite and socialization. Contraindications to physical exercise are in Table 7-1. Encourage healthy lifestyle changes but keep in mind that many older adults are not willing to change at this point in their life and that this is their choice. Educate, in a nonjudgmental manner, on the risks versus benefits of any behavior or habit the patient is unwilling to relinquish. Nursing interventions should focus on prevention of further disease by minimizing risk factors.

Dietary Education Points

- Healthy food habits can help reduce three of the major risk factors for myocardial infarction: high blood cholesterol, high blood pressure, and excess body weight.

- Healthy food habits also help reduce the risk of stroke, as heart disease and high blood pressures are major risk factors for stroke.

TABLE 7-1: CONTRAINDICATIONS TO PHYSICAL EXERCISE

Absolute contraindications:

Severe CAD	Unstable angina	Uncontrolled arrhythmias
Decompensated CHF	Severe valvular heart disease	B/P > 200/105
Pulmonary hypotension	Infectious disease	Recent PE or DVT

Relative Contraindications (Need order /guidance from physician):

CHD, CHF	Significant valvular disease	Arrhythmias
HTN	Fixed rate pacemaker	PVD
Uncontrolled DM	Marked obesity	Anemia
Serious systemic disorder	Congenital anomalies	Severe lung disease

CAD – Coronary Artery Disease CHF – Congestive Heart Failure DVT – Deep Vein Thrombosis
DM – Diabetes Mellitus HTN – Hypertension PE – Pulmonary Embolius
PVD – Peripheral Vascular Disease

- Eat a variety of fruits and vegetables. Choose 5 or more servings per day.

- Eat a variety of grain products, including whole grains. Choose 6 or more servings per day.

- Include fat-free and low-fat milk products, fish, legumes (beans), skinless poultry and lean meats.

    Choose fats and oils with 2 grams or less of saturated fat per tablespoon, such as liquid and tub margarine, and canola and olive oil.

- Balance the number of calories you eat with the number you use each day. To determine the number of calories, multiply current weight by 15 calories if moderately active, by 13 if less active. To lose weight, do enough activity to use up more calories than you eat every day.

- Limit intake of foods high in calories or low in nutrition, including foods like soft drinks and candy that have a lot of sugars.

Cardiac Emergencies

The patient should be informed on when to seek help when experiencing chest discomfort. Most cardiac incidences involve discomfort in the center of the chest that lasts more than a few minutes, or that goes away and comes back. It can feel like uncomfortable pressure, squeezing, fullness, or pain. There may be discomfort in other areas of the upper body such as one, or both arms, the back, neck, jaw or stomach. Some may experience shortness of breath, breaking out in a cold sweat, nausea, or lightheadedness. Many older adults display atypical symptom or "silent" symptoms. If the patient has nitroglycerin for chest discomfort, make certain he/she knows the correct method of administration. Inform the patient to call 911 if experiencing any of the symptoms above or those unrelieved by nitroglycerin. Emphasize to patient not to delay in calling 911 as rapid treatment dramatically improves mortality and morbidity. Educate the patient not to drive him or herself to the hospital and not to allow a friend or relative do so. Having a myocardial infarction while driving, or as a passenger, severely delays urgent medical attention.

Nursing Intervention for Patients with Cardiovascular Disease

- Educate patient and family members on how to recognize a cardiac emergency.

- Include family members, friends and others who may influence or care for the patient.

- Review dietary recommendations with patient.

- Educate on dietary recommendations, reduced sodium, saturated fats and cholesterol intake.

- Encourage reduction and eventual stopping of

smoking.

• Assist patient in making plans and setting realistic goals for weight loss if overweight.

• Encourage limiting of alcohol to no more than 1 ounce per day.

• Limit caffeine intake.

• Determine patient's activity preferences and assist in gradually incorporating daily exercise into lifestyle.

• Teach how to take blood pressure and/or heart rate reading, set up recording method and instructions on what to do for high or low readings. Find alternative method of reading B/P if patient is unable to perform.

• Assess for dyspnea, edema, chest pain, leg pain, dizziness, changes in vision, irregular heartbeat, palpitations, confusion, syncope, fatigue, shortness of breath, and appetite.

• Assess for adherence to medication regimen. If non-adherent, determine cause and attempt to find solutions.

• For those on daily digoxin, assess patient knowledge, and usage. Educate on the signs and symptoms of digoxin toxicity: loss of appetite and seeing rings around lights.

• Assess frequency of PRN medication usage.

• Assess for depression, fatigue and life stressors.

• Teach relaxation techniques for stress reduction.

• More information is available through the American Heart Association 1-800-242-8721 or www.americanheart.org.

Transient Ischemia Attack (TIA) and Cerebral Vascular Accidents (CVA)

Cardiovascular accidents are the leading cause of disability in the country and the third leading cause of death (Bryant-McKenney, 2000). A TIA is sometimes called a little stroke but actually it is a precursor to a cerebral vascular accident for up to 35% of people with TIAs. It is characterized by transient focal neurological signs that occur suddenly, and last a short time, usually less than an hour and never longer than 24 hours. Most TIAs are caused by partial blockage of arteries in the neck. As small blood clots attempt to pass through these partially blocked carotid arteries, they may become temporarily lodged in that area, temporarily preventing blood flow to a part of the brain. As the blood flow is restored, the symptoms the patient experiences generally disappear without any permanent damage. The specific signs of a TIA vary greatly but may include blurred vision or speech, flashes of light, migraine, vertigo, facial weakness, confusion, and ataxia. A physician should see patients who experience a TIA so a disabling stroke may be prevented by medications or a carotid endarterectomy. The major role of nursing is the early identification and referral of patients suspected of having TIA's.

A cerebral vascular accident (CVA), often called a stroke, is the term used to describe neurological deficits resulting from an interruption of the blood supply to the brain. Cerebral thrombosis (most common) is the formation of a blood clot in a vessel supplying cerebral tissue. The term hemorrhagic stroke refers to neurological deficits that occur as a result of bleeding within the cranial cavity. This is caused by a balloon-like deformity in the wall of a blood vessel. The wall weakens as the balloon grows larger, and eventually bursts, causing a hemorrhage. The brain, which requires more than one-fifth of all cardiac output, suffers inadequate oxygenation and tissue death occurs. The severity of neurological deficits depends on the extent of brain damage. The specific signs and symptoms are determined by the precise location of the cerebrovascular involvement and the extent of brain damage. Instruct patients to seek immediate hospital care if experiencing signs and symptoms of a cerebral vascular accident as early treatment with thrombolytics can minimize neurological deficits if the cause is a clot.

There are two stages associated with recovery from a CVA: the acute stage and the rehabilitative stage. Cerebral edema occurs initially and is the leading cause of death during the first week post stroke; however, patient outcome is greatest if in a neurological intensive care unit (Marik, 1997). The focus in nursing care during the acute stage is the prevention of complications such as pressure sores, contractors, malnutrition, and pneumonia.

The rehabilitation stage may take days or months, depending upon the amount of brain damage that has occurred. Usually a plateau is reached in 3 to 6 months after the event. The focus during this stage is to regain function, prevent further strokes, and prevent complications. These patients require an interdisciplinary team, which may include speech, recreational, physical, and occupational therapists. The nursing needs are complex and varied and often depend upon the side of the brain affected. More information may be obtained from the American Stroke Association 1-888-478-7653 or www.strokeassociation.org.

Left Brain Damage (right side paralyzed)

Behavior: Slow, cautious, disorganized, anxious, or underestimates abilities.

Cognition: Memory deficits, short attention span, or lack of awareness of effects of the stroke.

Communication: Expressive and receptive aphasia. Cannot name objects but understands how to use them. Repeats a word or phrase over and over (perseveration).

Movement: Paralysis or weakness on the right side of the body, poor balance, loss of ability to plan how to move (apraxia), too much muscle tone (spasticity), or too little (flaccidity).

Other: May have swallowing difficulties (dysphagia).

Suggestions for Caring:

- Do not underestimate ability to learn and communicate even if he or she can not speak.

- Try other forms of communication such as a board with words or pictures.

- Do not shout; keep the message simple.

- Divide tasks into simple steps.

- Give the patient time to think and form thoughts.

- Do give lots of feedback, encouragement and praise progress.

Right Brain Damage (left side paralyzed)

Spatial-perceptual deficits: Impaired ability to judge distance, size, position; affects self-care ability, and causes left-sided neglect.

Behavior: Quick and impulsive behavior, lack of insight, temper flare-ups. Emotional lability, apathy, or lack of motivation and initiation. May be irritable, depressed, or self-centered.

Cognition: Memory deficits, short attention span and lack of awareness of effects of the stroke.

Communication: Speaking and understanding is not usually affected. May have trouble with starting a conversation, taking turns in conversation, rambling speech, or writing and spelling.

Movement: Paralysis or weakness on the left side of the body, poor balance, loss of ability to plan how to move (apraxia), too much muscle tone (spasticity) or too little (flaccidity).

Other: May have swallowing difficulties (dysphagia).

Suggestions for Caring:

- Do not overestimate their abilities. Spacial-deficits are easy to miss.

- Approach from the left side.

- Use verbal cues.

- Break tasks into small steps.

- Watch if they can safely perform something rather than take their word.

- Minimize clutter in the environment.

- Avoid rapid movements.

- Highlight visual reference points.

PARKINSON'S DISEASE

Parkinson's disease (PD) is a progressive disorder of the central nervous system. Individuals with Parkinson's disease lack dopamine, which is important for the nervous system to control muscle activity. It is estimated that up to 10% of individuals over the age of 80 are affected by PD. The only known identified risk factor for PD is age. The cardinal features are 1. Resting tremors, usually "pill-rolling" but may also occur in the head, feet, lips, or tongue, 2. Rigidity, which is passive resistance to stretching or movements and can be felt as "cog-wheeling," and 3. Bradykinesia, which is slowness of movement and akinesia which is absence of movement such as freezing in place. Other symptoms that may be noticed are postural instability with a displaced center of gravity, stooped stance, lack of arm swing, and shuffling gait. Associated problems are depression, neurogenic bladder, perfuse perspiration, excessive secretions by sebaceous glands, loss of sexual functioning, drooling, sleep disturbances, flat affect, difficulty talking, and night terror from medication side effects. The prevalence of dementia in older adults with Parkinson's disease is 27%. The age of the patient, rather than the duration of the disease, is usually more of a risk for developing dementia. A large meta-analysis found that the older adult with Parkinson's and dementia had a mean age of 70.3 years compared to the patients without dementia at 64.3 years (Lieberman, 2002).

PD slows gastric motility. Swallowing is prolonged and the stomach takes longer to empty and for food to traverse through the intestines. For this reason, the body better utilizes food when small amounts are eaten frequently rather than 3 large meals per day. Patients on Sinemet® derive greater benefits if medication is taken on an empty stomach. Patients who experience significant motor fluctuations and take Sinemet 6 or more times per day may need to alter the amount or timing of protein intake to avoid interfering with Sinemet absorption. Medication management often requires close monitoring and frequent dose and time changes that may be difficult for the older adult to remember. Anti-Parkinson drugs also "dry out" the body. It is important to tell the patients to drink throughout the day to enhance the absorption of both nutrients and medications, and reduce the risk of dehydration. Many of these medications cause psychiatric symptoms such as hallucination and night terrors. Inform the patient's physician if these are occurring. Abnormal dreaming and increased sleep disruption may precede the development of psychotic symptoms by weeks to months and provide an important early clue to their potential occurrence. The treatment of drug-induced psychosis generally begins with reduction in the antiparkinsonian medication, beginning first with any adjunctive agents followed by lowering the levodopa dosage.

The major nursing goals for these patients is medication management, maintaining current functioning level, and the prevention of weight loss, falls, and injuries.

Tips for Working with Patients with Parkinson's Disease

- Keep environment on the cool side due to sensitivity towards heat.

- The patient may show lack of coordination, stiff muscles and joints, difficulties initiating movement, freezing, and gait disturbances, which can be addressed with various exercise programs. Exercise programs may be selected to: improve mobility and strength, maintain

TABLE 7-2: MOBILITY CONSIDERATIONS FOR CLIENTS WITH PARKINSON'S DISEASE

- Use verbal and physical cuing.

- Make sure client's legs are not crossed when rising from a chair.

- Remind client to lift up toes with every step or when they are "frozen." This helps eliminate muscle spasm.

- Encourage to lift head and eyes up when standing or walking.

- Have client walk with legs spread 10" (rather than close together) to provide wide base of support.

- For greater safety in turning, encourage small steps with feet widely separated.

- Encourage client to swing the arms freely when walking. This helps to take body weight off the legs, reduce fatigue, and loosens arms and shoulders.

- Encourage client to take as large of a step as possible, raising with the toe and striking the ground first with the heel, and keeping legs apart.

- Sitting down should be done slowly, with body bent sharply forward, until client touches the seat.

- If client has difficulty rising from seated position encourage him/her to rise fast to overcome the 'pull of gravity.'

- If the client 'lists' to one side when walking, encourage him/her to carry a weight in the other hand to decrease the bend.

- To improve balance, have client stop and "march in place" several times during ambulation.

- Try using a weighted wheelchair for balance when walking (to prevent fast forward ambulation).

range-of-motion (ROM), improve balance, increase ADL functioning, increase sleep quality, reduce stress, aid constipation, and reduce risk of falling. Examples of these types of therapy are exercise, dance, aquatics, gardening, calisthenics, airmat therapy, and ambulation.

- Encourage evening walking or physical activities to promote sleep and appetite.

- Patient may have significant fluctuations in function during the course of the day. Schedule active programs when functioning level is greatest.

- Patients may have difficulties maintaining sleep. Providing physical evening activities, outdoors, are useful.

- Assist patient in setting up medication manage-

ment reminder system if needed.

- Provide a safe environment, free of clutter; avoid horizontal lines on flooring as these may cause the patient to freeze in place.

- Educate all staff and family members on gait and ambulation techniques (Table 7-2).

- More information may be obtained from:

  - Parkinson's Disease Foundation 1-800-457-6676 www.pdf.org

  - The National Parkinson's Foundation 1-800-317-4545 www.parkinson.org

  - For support group referral: 1-800-327-4545 x2985

MUSCULOSKELETAL CONDITIONS

Musculoskeletal conditions are commonly seen in older adults. More than 100 different entities can produce joint and muscle signs and symptoms. These conditions are of great importance, for they affect a person's lifestyle as well as general feelings of health and wellness. They are generally associated with pain, stiffness and disturbances of gait, all of which can alter the functional status of older adults. Emotional factors can exacerbate the disease and contribute to increased morbidity. The gradual bone loss that occurs with aging, beginning in late midlife, causes bones to become weakened, making them more susceptible to fracture. Changes in the cervical and thoracic curves of the spine may impair balance and walking. Aging causes an atrophy of all muscles, with a consequent decline in muscle strength, tone, mass, endurance, agility, and efficiency. A decrease in elasticity of tendons and ligaments results in a generalized stiffening of the joints, particularly the knees, hips, and spine. Even with these changes, older adults remain mobile and independent unless an underlying disease process develops.

Osteoarthritis

Osteoarthritis is a noninflammatory, progressive, degenerative disorder of the movable, weight-bearing joints. It is a common rheumatology disorder. It is estimated that 40 million Americans, 70 to 90% of persons older than 75 years, are affected by osteoarthritis. Although symptoms of osteoarthritis occur earlier in women, the prevalence among men and women is equal. In addition to age, risk factors include joint injury, obesity, and mechanical stress. The diagnosis is largely clinical because radiographic findings do not always correlate with symptoms (Hinton, Moody, Davis, & Sean, 2002).

Osteoarthritis has been associated with various factors, including aging, mechanical trauma to joints, obesity, genetic predisposition, congenital abnormalities, joint infection or inflammation, immobility, normal daily wear and tear, and neuropathic, endocrine, and metabolic disorders such as diabetes mellitus. The disease process includes destruction of the articular cartilage and changes in ligaments, tendons, and synovial fluid, with pain resulting from synovitis, inflammation, and spasm. Loss of bone density and erosion usually lead to increased calcium production and the formation of osteophytes, or bony spurs, in the joints. The pain resulting from these osteophytes is caused by formation of a mechanical block, synovitis and inflammation in the articular capsule, contracture, and spasm. Osteophyte formation and cartilage deterioration are mechanical deformities that frequently lead to pain and enlarged, stiff, and immobile joints.

Signs and Symptoms

The most common signs and symptoms include the following: stiffness after a long period of immobility; morning stiffness, which usually subsides in less than 30 minutes; joint pain that occurs with activity; bony enlargement or deformity, particularly Heberden's nodes, bony enlargement's found on the distal interphalangeal joints (DIP); and Bouchard's nodes, found on the proximal interphalangeal joints (PIP); limitation of movement and crepitus; aching or nagging discomfort, usually experienced with motion, weight-bearing, or activity; and "flare-ups" of the disease that are associated with the use or abuse of the joint or trauma, and are often relieved with rest.

The major goals of treatment include preservation of function, reduction of pain, and minimization of further damage to involved joints. Because of the irreversibility of the condition, treatment is medical, with aspirin and nonsteroidal anti-inflammatory drugs (NSAIDs) as the main pharmacological agents prescribed. Treatment may also include range-of-motion, recreational and physical therapy exercises to correct muscle atrophy; cold and heat therapy; weight reduction (if needed); and support with a cane, crutches, or splints along with rest and prevention of trauma to involved joints. If the conservative approach is unsuccessful, surgical intervention may be necessary in the form of joint fusion, prostheses, or total joint replacement. The joint replacements are reserved for severe joint destruction and pain or a disability that has been refractory to conservative treatment; these are usually total hip or knee replacements.

Nursing Interventions

- Prevention of falls and injuries

- Encouragement of low-intensity exercise

- Pain management and pain medication management

- For more information: Arthritis Foundation 1-800-283-7800 www.arthritis.org

Osteoporosis

In 2002, it is estimated that over 10 million people already have osteoporosis. Approximately 80% of these people are women over the age of 50. Osteoporosis has reached epidemic proportions in this country with 25 million people affected by the disease and over 1.5 million related fractures annually (Wehren, 2002). The estimated national direct expenditures (hospitals and nursing homes) for osteoporotic and associated fractures was $17 billion in 2001 ($47 million each day) – and the cost is rising. The universal loss of bone that occurs with aging is the result of the uncoupling of the relationship between osteoclastic bone resorption and osteoblastic (new bone) formation. Osteoporosis is often called the "silent disease" because bone loss occurs without symptoms. People may not know that they have osteoporosis until their bones become so weak that a sudden strain, bump, or fall causes a fracture or a vertebra to collapse. Collapsed vertebrae may initially be felt or seen in the form of severe back pain, loss of height, or spinal deformities such as kyphosis (stooped posture).

Certain people are more likely to develop osteoporosis than others. Traditionally it has been considered a disease of elderly white women. However, this view has recently changed as more women of various racial and ethnic heritage and more men are being diagnosed. For men, mortality after hip fracture is disproportionately high as they are twice as likely to die than women are (Wehren, 2002). The risk factors that have been identified:

- Female gender.

- Thin and/or small frame.

- Advanced age (greater than 65).

- A family history of osteoporosis.

- Postmenopause, including early or surgically induced menopause (Women can lose up to 20% of their bone mass in the 5–7 years following menopause).

- Abnormal absence of menstrual periods (amenorrhea).

- Anorexia nervosa.

- Diets low in calcium.

- Use of certain medications, such as corticosteroids, and anticonvulsants.

- Low testosterone levels in men.

- An inactive lifestyle.

- Cigarette smoking.

- Excessive use of alcohol.

- Being Caucasian or Asian, although African Americans, and Hispanic Americans are at significant risk as well.

- For more information: National Osteoporosis Foundation (202) 223.2226 www.nof.org

Osteoporosis is a silent disease that does not become apparent until midlife when a fracture occurs, although loss of height and back pain may signal the onset of this condition long before then.

Fractures occur during normal activities such as lifting, bending, stepping off a curb, or coughing or with minimal trauma such as an aggressive hug or bumping a bedside table. Specialized tests called bone density tests can measure bone density in various sites of the body. A bone mineral density (BMD) test can detect osteoporosis before a fracture occurs, predict the chances of fracturing in the future, determine the rate of bone loss and/or monitor the effects of treatment if the test is conducted at intervals of a year or more. For postmenopausal women the BMD is interpreted as normal, osteopenia (low bone mass), osteoporosis, or severe osteoporosis. Various medications that reduce reabsorption of bone are effective in increasing bone density and decreasing fractures. Response to these medications cannot be expected in less than one year, with repeat BMD testing measurements taken after two years being more dependable. The ultimate measurement for effectiveness is the incidence or lack of fractures (Andrews, 2002). Hormone replacement therapy (HRT) was once thought to be a safe method of not only helping to slow the rate of bone loss but also offering cardiovascular protection. Research now shows that HRT increases the risk of ovarian and breast cancers and that it does not have the cardiovascular benefits that were once believed. Studies have concluded that the use of HRT in some women actually increases the risk of heart attacks, strokes and thromboembolic events. The National Institutes of Health (NIH) terminated the Women's Health Initiative (WHI) study prematurely because the adverse effects of estrogen/progesterone replacement therapy outweighed the benefits (Rossouw et al., 2002). As more research is performed on HRT, better guidelines for its usage will be developed. Patients currently on HRT should be evaluated by their physician to determine if it is safe to continue its usage.

Nursing Interventions

- If patient is being treated with medications assess adherence to regimen, particularly drugs

with specific instructions for administration such as Fosamax.

- Assess and teach intrinsic and environmental safety issues for falls prevention.

- Encourage a balanced diet rich in calcium and vitamin D. Good sources of calcium are milk, cheese, yogurt, broccoli, green leafy vegetables, kidney beans, and ice cream. The best source of vitamin D is 15–30 minutes of sun exposure per day.

- Encourage weight-bearing exercise, starting slow and mild on alternate days, increasing as tolerated.

- Encourage a healthy lifestyle with no smoking or excessive alcohol intake.

ENDOCRINOLOGIC PROBLEMS OF OLDER ADULTS

Diabetes

Diabetes is a growing health problem that affects 20.1% of older adults, or 7 million people. It was the sixth leading cause of death listed in the United States in 1999. Diabetes mellitus (DM) is a group of diseases characterized by high levels of blood glucose resulting from defects in insulin production, insulin action, or both. There are two types of diabetes. Type 1 diabetes was previously called insulin-dependent diabetes mellitus (IDDM) or juvenile-onset diabetes. Type 1 diabetes develops when the body's immune system destroys pancreatic beta cells, the only cells in the body that make the hormone insulin that regulates blood glucose. This form of diabetes usually strikes children and young adults, who need several insulin injections a day or an insulin pump to survive. Type 1 diabetes may account for 5% to 10% of all diagnosed cases of diabetes. Risk factors for Type 1 diabetes include autoimmune, genetic, and environmental factors. Type 2 diabetes was previously called non-insulin-dependent diabetes mellitus (NIDDM) or adult-onset diabetes. Type 2 diabetes accounts for up to 95% of all diagnosed cases of diabetes. It usually begins as insulin resistance, a disorder in which the cells do not use insulin properly. As the need for insulin rises, the pancreas gradually loses its ability to produce insulin. Type 2 diabetes is associated with older age, obesity, family history of diabetes, prior history of gestational diabetes, impaired glucose tolerance, physical inactivity, and race/ethnicity. African Americans, Hispanic/Latino Americans, American Indians, and some Asian Americans and Pacific Islanders are at particularly high risk for Type 2 diabetes. Symptoms of diabetes include increased urination, unintended weight loss, thirst, hunger, weakness and fatigue, irritability, change in vision, slow healing cuts, frequent infections, tingling in feet or hands, and skin infections.

Patients with Type 1 diabetes must have insulin delivered by a pump or injections. Patients with Type 2 diabetes may be able to control their blood glucose by following a careful diet and exercise program, losing excess weight and taking oral medication. If unsuccessful they will require insulin by pump or injection. Complications from diabetes include heart disease, stroke, high blood pressure, blindness, end-stage renal disease, nervous system damage, and amputation of lower extremities. The needs of older adults with diabetes are complex and require the skills from a variety of disciplines. Nursing goals should focus on preventing complications and reinforcing the instructions of other disciplines.

Nursing Interventions

- Many medical centers have a diabetes teaching center. Arrange for patient to take self-management courses, if available.

- Reinforce instructions on insulin or oral medication usage.

- Reinforce instructions on glucose monitoring.

- Evaluate knowledge of diabetic diet. Arrange for dietitian to work with patients who are having difficulty complying with diet.

- Encourage physical activity.

- Evaluate blood pressure (Blood pressure control can reduce cardiovascular disease by approximately 33% to 50% and can reduce microvascular disease (eye, kidney, and nerve disease) by approximately 33%.

- Control of blood lipids through medications, diet and exercise. Improved control of cholesterol and lipids (for example, HDL, LDL, and triglycerides) can reduce cardiovascular complications by 20% to 50%.

- Monitor for vision loss. Detection and treatment of diabetic eye disease with laser therapy can reduce the development of severe vision loss by an estimated 50% to 60%. Diabetic retinopathy causes from 12,000 to 24,000 new cases of blindness each year.

- Assess feet every week and teach proper foot care to patient. Arrange for podiatrist visits. Comprehensive foot care programs can reduce amputation rates by 45% to 85%.

- Detection and treatment of early diabetic kidney disease can reduce the development of kidney failure by 30% to 70%.

- American Diabetes Association 1-800-342-2383 has lots of free information. www.diabetes.org

Thyroid Disease

Thyroid disease is the second most common endocrine problem in the older adult, affecting over 10% of women (Elliott, 2000). Detection of thyroid disease becomes difficult because the symptoms of hypothyroidism and aging, overlap, and the symptoms of hyperthyroidism are often blunted. Untreated thyroid disease can lead to cardiac dysfunction with heart failure, functional decline, and dementia. Signs and symptoms of hyperthyroidism in the older adult are atypical and may include depressed affect, failure to thrive, and skin changes. Signs of hypothyroidism include fatigue, weight gain, dry skin, constipation, cold intolerance, depression, decline in cognition, coarsening of hair, weakness, and voice changes. Laboratory evaluations are performed on any patient with suspected thyroid problems and usually include those that measure TSH and FT4. Thyroid hormone replacement treatment must be individualized and should include follow-up labs.

Patient Education

- Instruct patient to take thyroid replacement hormone at the same time each day, optimally before breakfast. Take 4–5 hours apart from iron, antacids, or cholesterol-lowering agents.

- Notify healthcare provider of any symptoms of intolerance or inadequate dose: palpitations, chest pains, dyspnea, anxiety, or sudden increase in size of thyroid.

- Instruct patient not to adjust their does by themselves.

- Instruct patient that symptoms should begin to abate in 2 weeks.

- Instruct patient that thyroid replacement therapy is life-long and labs will be required at least every 6 months.

- For additional information: National Hormone Foundation 1-800-HORMONE www.hormone.org

SUMMARY

This chapter discusses many common chronic health care problems of the older adult including cardiovascular disease, cerebrovascular accidents, Parkinson's disease, diabetes, osteoarthritis, osteoporosis, and thyroid disorders. Problems that chronically ill persons face include preventing and managing medical conditions, recognizing signs and symptoms, managing health regimens, and dealing with the emotional aspects of coping with these conditions. The goal of nursing for these conditions is to optimize function and quality of life while preventing complications and physical or emotional injuries.

EXAM QUESTIONS

CHAPTER 7
Questions 48-53

48. The percentage of the 28 million older adults with hypertension under good control is

    a. 75%.

    b. 52%.

    c. 24%.

    d. 18%.

49. Your home care patient is 79-year-old Mrs. Smith. Her daughter calls you and states that her mother had a bout of confusion and slurred speech that lasted 20 minutes, but she is fine now. You tell her that her mother probably had a

    a. TIA but not to worry about it.

    b. stroke but not to worry about it.

    c. stroke and she should see her doctor.

    d. TIA and she should see her doctor.

50. Which of the following most describes a client left brain damage as a consequence of a stroke?

    a. Quick, impulsive with difficulty communicating

    b. Slow, cautious with expressive and receptive aphasia

    c. Slow, cautious with left-sided neglect

    d. Quick, impulsive with left-sided neglect

51. The best method of improving mobility in a client with Parkinson's Disease is to provide

    a. a motorized wheelchair and instructions on usage.

    b. a walker to prevent loss of balance and falls.

    c. an exercise program to increase ROM, and improve balance and strength.

    d. a chair equipped with mechanical lift.

52. The following is considered a modifiable risk factor for osteoporosis:

    a. current cigarette smoker.

    b. advanced age.

    c. family history.

    d. dementia.

53. Complaints of increased thirst, urination, weakness, and weight loss are signs of

    a. diabetes.

    b. hypothyroidism.

    c. hyperthyroidism.

    d. thyroid tumor.

CHAPTER 8

COMMON SENSORY PROBLEMS

CHAPTER OBJECTIVE

After studying this chapter, the reader will be able to discuss the implications of and strategies for management and coping with problems related to the aging sensory system.

LEARNING OBJECTIVES

After studying this chapter, the reader will be able to

1. state the problems with identifying and treating pain in older adults.

2. describe normal physiological changes that occur in aging that affect the senses.

3. select interventions to promote safety for older adults with sensory impairments.

4. identify factors associated with loss of taste and smell in older adults.

5. describe why older adults have a difficulty with thermal regulation.

INTRODUCTION

Older adults experience a multitude of sensory losses that effect not only quality of life, but how they interpret and interact with their environment. Unfortunately, the sense of pain remains intact and many live with it daily. These impairments place the older adult at high risk for injuries, decreased ability to function, depression, and feelings of loneliness and isolation. Nursing interventions are aimed at preventing or reducing these risks to maintain quality of life.

PAIN

Pain is whatever the individual says it is, existing wherever the individual says it does.

The number of older adults, in all settings, who experience chronic pain is reported to be at least 70%, with as many as 83% of nursing home residents reportedly having pain (Horgas & Dunn, 2001). The high prevalence of pain in this population is related to chronic health disorders, particularly osteoarthritis, neuralgia and osteoporosis. The effects of arthritis cause the older adult to place limitations on movements. This response leads to deconditioning, increased pain and creating a pain-movement cycle that is constant. The consequence of pain includes falls due to restricted or awkward movements, malnutrition, gait disturbances, slow rehabilitation, depression, decreased coping skills, social isolation, sleep deficit, behavioral problems, and increased healthcare utilization and costs (American Geriatric Society, 1998; Teno, et al., 2001). Pain dictates the amount of activity that can be tolerated by an individual in one day. This inactivity contributes to loss of bone, muscle, and connective tissue and decreased range of motion.

Despite the prevalence and consequence of pain, most research indicates that pain is under-detected, underreported and poorly managed. Current research shows 26% of older adults residing in long-term care facilities who reported experiencing daily pain received no analgesics (Won, et al., 1999). If untreated, pain becomes chemically ingrained in the central nervous system. Delayed treatment exacerbates chronic pain until it is difficult to manage with conventional treatments. Early aggressive treatment ultimately decreases the amount of medication needed to control the pain. Pain may be not be treated for many different reasons.

The older adult may:

- Have difficulty describing pain or its location.

- May believe it is part of aging and must be endured without complaint.

- May neglect to report pain to prevent being labeled a complainer or out of fear of diagnosis (Davis, Hiemenz, & White, 2002).

- Believe nothing can or will be done to help.

- Not report pain, as their culture is to be stoic.

- Rather endure pain than the side effects of medications.

- Be fearful of addictions.

- Not be able to afford medications.

- Use words other than "pain" such as discomfort, ache, or hurt.

Healthcare providers may:

- Lack assessment skills and not recognize the signs of pain, especially in patients with cognitive impairment (Farrell, Gibson, & Helme, 1996).

- Be fearful of addiction with opiate usage.

- Believe in myths: Pain is not harmful. The elderly always complain of pain. Older adults with dementia do not feel pain. Pain is not a serious problem in the elderly. Age-related changes reduce pain perceptions. Pain is a normal part of aging (Closs, 1996).

- Not recognize pain due to symptoms being masked by depression.

When assessing pain include past pain history and determine the current level of pain using some sort of objective pain scale. Always use the same scale each time on a patient. Examples of numerical, visual, and categorical scales are in Table 8-1. Keep accurate records of pain and pain relief methods. For some patients the nurse may need to ask questions about self-imposed limitations of function due to pain rather than actual pain rating. For patients with cognitive and/or sensory impairments there may be a lack of objective measures for gauging and measuring pain. The greater the severity of dementia, the less reporting of pain. Visual analog and numerical scales may be of no value, due to abstraction and loss of memory of previous pain. Often the nurse must look for subtle signs and symptoms that may be noticed only after the patient has been observed for some time. The Discomfort Scale for Dementia of the Alzheimer's Type has been supported as an appropriate instrument for evaluating pain in patients with cognitive impairment (Hurley, Volicer, & Hanrahan, 1992). Nonspecific signs and symptoms that suggest the presence of pain include (AMDA, 1999):

- Frowning, grimacing, fearful facial expressions, or grinding of teeth.

- Bracing, guarding, or rubbing.

- Fidgeting, increasing or recurring restlessness.

- Striking out, increasing or recurring agitation.

- Eating or sleeping poorly.

- Sighing, groaning, crying, or breathing heavily.

- Decreasing activity levels.

- Resisting certain movements during care.

- Change in gait.

TABLE 8-1: PAIN ASSESSMENT

What they tell you – subjective: (The more you listen, the more they tell)

- Do you have pain or discomfort? (Ask more than "Are you OK?")
- What does it feel like? (Sharp, burning, shocking, aching, etc.)
- Where do you feel the pain? (location and radiation)
- How severe is the pain? Select and use consistent pain scales.
- What makes the pain better? What makes it worse?
- What was the effect of the last treatment? (medication, ice, heat, position, or stretch)
- Is the pain intermittent, or is it always there? (Is there a daily pattern?)
- How does pain affect sleep, appetite, energy, mobility, relationships, or mood?
- Other symptoms: nausea, vomiting, constipation, cough, drowsiness, confusion, or new incontinence?
- Patients with memory deficits may not remember the effect of the last treatment. They must be assessed frequently.

What you see – objective:

- Facial signs: grimace, fear, sad, frown, or scowl.
- Verbal signs: grunts, grimace, groan, hushed or breathy tones, shortened sentences, monotone, repeating the same words, or yelling.
- Body signs: stiffening, guarding, limping, fidgeting, jittery, rubbing of body part, clenched fist, knees pulled up tight, wringing hand, or restlessness.
- Behavior changes: irritability, negative feelings, depression, loss of sleep, withdrawing, anxiety, disruptive behavior, agitation, aggression, vocalization, or demanding.
- Respirations: Signing, grunting, negative sound on inspiration or expiration, labored, gasping, bursts of breathing, hyperventilation, or holding one's breath.

Examples of scales to assess pain include faces, numeric, visual analog and category. Your patient may want to make up his or her own scale. Use whatever scale works best with each of your clients. It probably means using different scales on different clients. The important feature is to use that same scale on your patient every time.

Numeric Rating Scale

0	1	2	3	4	5	6	7	8	9	10
No Pain		Mild		Moderate		Severe		Very Severe		Worst Possible Pain

Visual Analog Scale

No pain   Worst pain ever

Directions: Ask the patient to indicate on the line where the pain is in relation to the two extremes. Qualification is only approximate; for example, a midpoint mark would indicate that the pain is approximately half of the worst possible pain.

Categorical Scale

None (0)   Mild (1-3)   Moderate (4-6)   Severe (7-10)

TABLE 8-2: NON-PHARMACOLOGICAL APPROACHES TO PAIN

Physical Relief Techniques

- Change position, seating, lie down for a rest, use pillows and cushions.

- Slow gentle stretching.

- Cold helps reduce pain by slowing nerve conduction. It decreases inflammation, itching and swelling and reduces muscle spasms. Cold is helpful for acute muscle strains and sprains, acute inflammation and lower back and abdominal pain. For acute injuries, ice packs can be applied for 20 to 30 minutes at least every 2 hours.

- Heat allows more oxygen and nutrients to reach the damaged area and reduces muscle spasms. Heat is helpful in chronic musculoskeletal injuries such as tendonitis and the noninflammatory stages of arthritis as well as before stretching or exercise. It should not be used in the first 48 hours after injury. The recommended temperature range for heat is 40-45°C (104 –113°F). As lamps and electric pads do not automatically turn off, they should not be used on sleeping patients. Contraindications include recently radiated skin, poor sensation, or acute inflammation and trauma.

- Massage manipulates soft tissue and can reduce edema, increase blood flow, decrease muscle spasms, break up adhesions, and relieve pain. Massage also relaxes and relieves fatigue. It can be helpful for muscle pain. Do not use with open lesions, local infections or malignancy, deep vein thrombosis, and predisposition to bleeding.

- Tub Bath: Warm water is helpful for achy joints and muscles.

- Quiet environment.

Cognitive Techniques

- Relaxation techniques are helpful when muscle tension contributes to the pain or when fear and frustration augments the pain. Cognitive techniques can alleviate pain by decreasing the patient's focus on the pain, cognitively redefining the pain and giving the patient control over his or her reaction to the pain. Physiologic changes during relaxation include decreases in blood pressure, heart or respiratory rate, and oxygen consumption. Endorphin level changes also occur, perhaps contributing to the change in blood flow and pain relief. Physiologic changes occur in five minutes, but deep relaxation may require 20 minutes. Effects may last 45 minutes. The patient must practice the techniques to obtain the most relief. These include slow rhythmic breathing, progressive muscle relaxation and guided imagery: pleasant images to replace the painful experience.

- Biofeedback, hypnosis.

Distraction Methods

- Music, dance, art, humor, prayer, exercise or activities: focuses the patient's attention, and alters the level of pain awareness.

- Humor, hugs, pets, loved ones, and love.

- Change in behavior.

- Loss of physical function.

Non-Pharmacological Treatment of Pain

There are two classes of non-pharmacological treatments for pain. The first are physical relief approaches such as massage, hot packs, and repositioning. The second class is the cognitive behavior approaches that are aimed at improving coping and altering the perception of pain. Examples of these are distraction, humor, biofeedback, relaxation techniques and hypnosis. Use of non-pharmacological approaches may, by itself, relieve mild pain, and when used in combination with analgesics, result in more effective pain management and less medication usage (Herr, 2002). See Table 8-2 for non-pharmacological approaches to pain.

Analgesic Usage

Analgesics can be used safely in older adults with careful evaluation of benefits and risks as well as careful evaluation of pain relief and side effects (Herr, 2002). Recommendations include:

- Using the least invasive medication administration route.

- For episodic pain, using short-acting agents.

- For chronic or continuous pain, using around-the-clock administration.

- Using long-acting agents or sustained-released preparations for continuous pain only.

- Always starting low and going slow.

- If not contraindicated for the patient, using acetaminophen or NSAID, for mild to moderate pain.

- Short-acting opioids: morphine, hydromorphine, oxycodone, hydrocodone, and fentanyl are choices for severe, chronic pain.

- Sustained-released opioids are appropriate for older adults with continuous pain, whose opioid dosing has been stabilized.

- Anticipating and preventing side effects such as constipation, nausea, vomiting, sedation, and possible respiratory depression.

- Drugs to be specifically avoided in older adults include Meperidine, methadone, and propoxyphene.

SENSORY DISORDERS

Alterations in the senses that occur with aging can have a profound effect on older adults' communication abilities, perceptions, behaviors, moods, and personalities. As the senses diminish, older people become more vulnerable to accidents, injuries and falls, social isolation, disorientation and cognitive decline, sometimes resulting in death.

Loss of Hearing

Hearing loss is extremely common in older adults, especially among men. Of the 28 million Americans who have a hearing loss, only 20% seek help (Olive, 2002; Van Houten, 2002). Hearing loss leads to social isolation and the older adult may appear and feel cognitively impaired. Many older adults are not aware of their impairment or are reluctant to report any problems. This causes frustration among spouses, family members, and friends. Hearing difficulties can also interfere with the delivery of health care and overall quality of life. For patients who acknowledge a hearing loss, a referral to an audiologist for complete assessment and determination of technological aide, is in order. For patients who do not admit to a loss or who refuse treatment, apply good communication skills, and insure that they understand what is told to them. The following are common symptoms of hearing loss that is untreated:

- Missing parts of conversations and continually asking people to repeat themselves.

- Loss of high and low tones, no longer able to hear birds singing.

- Turning the TV, radio, or telephone volume loud.

- Unable to distinguish speech from background noises, unable to follow dinnertime conversation while others are talking and/or music is playing.

- Straining to read lips and facial expressions.

Loss of Vision

One in 6 Americans age 65 and older are blind or severely visually impaired (Lighthouse, 2002). Although visual acuity may remain sharp for many older persons, the quality of an individual's vision generally is not what it was in younger years. Vision is altered in older adults by 4 major physiological changes: an elevation of the minimal threshold for light perception, decreased visual acuity and peripheral fields, decreased ability to adjust to changing amounts of dark and light, and a loss of accommodative power. Loss of elasticity in the lens and atrophy of the ciliary muscle decrease the ability to focus on fine details. The lens increases both in thickness and size throughout life because of the continual proliferation of new cells. This interferes with the transmission and refraction of light. The ciliary muscle, which governs the convexity of the lens, decreases in length and replaces its muscle with collagen. The collagen causes stiffness of the ciliary muscle and, together with changes in the lens compromises the focusing or accommodation of the lens. This change results in the condition called presbyopia or farsightedness. The lens becomes more opaque, resulting in a sensitivity to glare, and a decreased ability to focus on details, as the visual reflexes slow results in changes in dark adaptation. Peripheral vision and depth perception decline with age. Visual field effects the performance of tasks like driving and walking in crowded places, which require a broad perception of the environment and moving objects. Depth perception is the visual skill that is responsible for localizing objects in three-dimensional space and enables a person to use objects effectively and maneuver safely in the environment. Alterations may lead to falls and mobility problems because of miscalculations about the distance and height of objects.

Most older adults have impaired vision, the most common being *presbyopia*. Loss of accommodation and loss of elasticity in the lens capsule cause the common symptoms of not being able to see near objects clearly, headaches, and eyestrain after doing close work. Presbyopia is easily corrected by wearing glasses or contact lenses.

The major risk factor for *cataracts* is age. More than 50% of adults over 65 have a cataract (National Eye Institute, 2002). Other risk factors include diabetes, poor nutrition, cigarette smoking, long-term exposure to ultraviolet and infrared radiation, and some drugs. Any clouding or opacity occurring in the normally clear crystalline lens is a cataract and as opacification increases, visual acuity diminishes. The earliest change may be an increase in myopia progressing to disturbed distance vision and yellowing of colors. There is a susceptibility to glare and a general darkening of the world. Cataracts usually develop bilaterally and treatment is surgical removal and replacement with an intraocular lens, contact lenses, or glasses. The decision to operate is influenced by the location of the cataract, the degree of visual impairment, and the effect on quality of life and ability to carry out ADLs. For an early cataract, vision may improve by using different eyeglasses, magnifying lenses, or stronger lighting. If these measures don't help, surgery is the only effective treatment. A cataract should be removed even if it doesn't cause problems with vision it prevents examination or treatment of another eye problem, such as age-related macular degeneration or diabetic retinopathy. Laser cataract removal is one of the most common operations performed in the U.S. today; performed almost exclusively on an outpatient basis. In 2002, approximately 2.7 million Americans underwent cataract surgery, with 95% of those patients experiencing improved vision (Hardten, 2003).

The prevalence of *glaucoma* increases with age. It is characterized by increasing intraocular pressure (presumably resulting from some impairment in the outflow of aqueous humor from the eye), degeneration and cupping of the optic disc, atrophy of the optic nerve head, and loss of peripheral visual fields. Untreated it may result in visual field abnormalities and irreversible blindness. Treatment may be with eye drops, surgery, laser coagulation, or a combination of these, depending on the disease.

Macular degeneration involves degeneration of the macula due to decreased blood supply and tissue atrophy, which results in diminished sharpness of "central" vision. Although those affected cannot see straight ahead, they can see peripherally and do not become totally blind. They see a gray shadow in the center of their field of view, making impossible any "fine" or close work such as reading, watching television, or sewing. Eyeglasses are not effective, but some "low-vision aids," essentially magnifiers, help patients use their remaining vision more effectively. Treatment is aimed at arresting the process of retinal destruction by using laser photocoagulation.

Approximately 10% of cognitively intact older adults with vision-impairments experience hallucinations (Stegbauer, Mojica, & Bailey, 2000). This condition, Charles Bonnet Syndrome (CBS), causes individuals without contributory psychiatric illness or altered consciousness to experience complex visual hallucinations. This is frequently misdiagnosed as psychoses or dementia. The criteria for CBS include the presence of formed, complex, repetitive, stereotyped visual hallucinations, and full or partial retention or insight. They are usually described as one image, a child, flowers, or an animal, that moves, has different colors, and is a pleasant or neutral experience. The appearance and disappearance is associated with darkness, stress and fatigue. CBS does not respond well to anti-psychotic agents and medications usage is controversial. Further deterioration of sight, changes in lighting, and relaxation techniques have shown some response for some patients. Empathy and understanding and educating the patient that they do not have a psychiatric illness may be all the management that is required. Many older

adults, once educated on CBS, ignore, or even enjoy the hallucinations.

Some elderly experience dry eye because of diminished tear production, and alteration in the composition of the tears. Prescription and over-the-counter drugs can contribute to or cause dry eyes. Symptomatic relief can be obtained from daily use of over-the-counter artificial tears, especially if used before reading and other frequent eye movement activities.

Nursing Interventions

- Encourage eye examinations every 1 to 2 years.

- Assess eyeglasses, magnifiers, and other assistive devices.

- Arranging the home for safety and comfort.

- Educate for safe food preparation and medication management.

- Assess ability to maintain financial records and use the telephone.

- Assess ability to perform ADLs.

- Assess need for labeling clothing by color.

- Assess transportation: getting around safely indoors and outside.

- Assess social contact and physical activities.

Older Adults with Severe Visual Impairments

- Need to learn new ways to accomplish routine daily tasks. These skills enable the patient to live independent and productive lives, minimizing the need for costly in-home or nursing home care.

- Need specially trained rehabilitation teachers, orientation and mobility specialists, low-vision specialists, and vision rehabilitation therapists teach essential skills, including independent living skills — using specialized adaptive devices and techniques for personal and household management; communication skills — using large print, writing guides, and time-telling devices, and using braille for reading or labeling and making notes; mobility skills — using specific orientation and mobility techniques, long canes, and other mobility tools for safe and independent travel.

- Need low-vision services – using special low-vision optical and adaptive devices.

- For additional information:

  The American Foundation for the Blind: 1-800-232-5463. Website: www.afb.org/

  The National Association for the Visually Handicapped: 212-889-3141. Website: www.navh.org/

  Lighthouse International: 800-829-0500. Website: www.ligtouse.org/

Loss of Senses

Lost or impaired smell, taste, and touch are serious issues as they put the older adult at higher risk for safety issues such as detecting gas leaks, smoke, and rotting food. They may also reduce quality of life as they take away the enjoyment of some of life's pleasures, such as the fragrance of flowers, the taste of good food, or the soft touch of a pet. Sensory losses may cause safety risks, depression, malnutrition, and weight loss.

Some losses are due to the aging process, while others are caused by medications, medical conditions and lifestyle. Due to changes that occur during the aging process, it becomes increasingly difficult for older adults to "sense" the environment around them. The "threshold" or minimum amount of stimulation necessary for the body to sense a smell, taste, or touch, usually rises, thereby requiring a greater level of stimulation.

Loss of Touch

During the aging process there is a loss of sensitivity to light touch, small changes in joint position, and vibration. These changes are caused by a decrease in the number of receptors for most forms of sensation, structural changes in remaining functioning receptors, and proprioceptive losses. Loss of sensitivity to vibration starts at around 50 years of age and is greater in the lower limbs than in the upper. This loss is linked to imperceptible changes in the blood circulation to the legs or the spinal cord. This decreased sensitivity to touch, temperature, and vibration affects the ability to distinguish different stimuli and/or may reduce reaction time. The patient may have difficulty differentiating coins or picking up small objects. Slower reaction to stimuli may result in injuries or burns, as the stimulus is perceived slowly. Decreased reactions time to toxic products—such as paint, solvent, or high temperatures may result in serious health injury. Blood circulation to the capillaries diminishes, thus predisposing the elderly person to feeling chilly and more vulnerable to temperature changes. Ceiling rotary fans are recommended over air conditioning, as these do not bring about sudden temperature changes.

Illnesses of neurological, muscular, cutaneous, or osteo-articular origin greatly affect the sense of touch (e.g., multiple sclerosis, muscular dystrophy, arthritis, rheumatism, psoriasis, or eczema). These may result in deformations, pain, skin lesions, and marked losses of tactile sensitivity. Certain disturbances such as paraesthesia (abnormal sensations such as formication, itching, or burning) or paralysis, upset the daily living activities of an individual. These disturbances create a high risk for injuries due to deprivation of the normal defense mechanisms that touch provides. An older adult with paralysis may not feel a burn caused by a cigarette. The sense of touch is not solely affected by aging or disease. Solitude and isolation may result in great damage to all of the bio-psycho-social components of the patient including difficulties in tactile and vibratory perception. The need to touch or to be touched is necessary for human physical and mental health. Older adults, who are deprived of touch stimuli, due to prolonged isolation for example, are subject to various reactions such as anxiety, affective and perceptual disturbances, hallucinations, aggression, somatization, and disorientation. The more common problems related to touch mainly involve minor accidents such as damages to the skin, but may be serious such as bathing in water that is too hot or being burned by a heating pad. For vibration, the older adult may have difficulty keeping his/her balance on escalators and moving walkways, because the receptors transmit messages less well.

Loss of Taste and Smell

Gradual reduction, or loss, of taste is a common consequence of aging. According to estimations, almost everyone has some type of smell impairment by age 60, and half of those in their 80s are anosmic (Mann, 2002). Loss of smell can also be one of the early symptoms of Alzheimer's and Parkinson's diseases, and is common with multiple sclerosis, Bell's palsy, head injury, diabetes, liver and kidney diseases, hypertension, and zinc or niacin deficiency. Persons with AD have a reduction in saliva that carries the enzymes that break down foods, assists in taste and smell, and starts the digestive process. In many, the loss follows a viral upper respiratory tract infection and the only treatment is to reassure patients that the problem may resolve if the damaged sensory cells regenerate. Loss of smell may also be caused by mechanical obstruction such as in rhinitis, nasal polyps, or tumors.

Sensitivity to taste also decreases with aging. One-third to one-half of a person's taste buds die by age 70. As one ages, sensory receptor cells in the nose and on the tongue are not replaced as often. Although smell and taste are two separate functions, they are intertwined as flavor involves taste, smell, texture, and temperature. Reduced taste sensations may also be the result of dental problems and treatments, including oral trauma, dry mouth, periodontal disease, burning mouth syndrome, and denture-related inflammation. Common treatments associated with taste and smell losses include full or partial dentures, and over-the-counter preparations such as

toothpastes, denture adhesives, and cleansers and mouthwashes. Losses may be the result of life habits such as smoking and eating spicy foods. More than 250 drugs have been implicated in altered smell and taste sensations. These include cholesterol lowering drugs, antihistamines, antibiotics, anti-cancer agents, asthma medications, antihypertensives, muscle relaxants, antidepressants, and anticonvulsants. Maximizing quality of life and preventing injuries are goals for patients with sensory impairments.

Nursing Interventions

- Check temperature of hot water heater; should be less than 120 degrees.

- Check for smoke detectors in basement, kitchen, and by bedroom doors.

- Check for visually apparent gas-detection devices on heaters and stoves.

- Enlist family members or friends to check for spoiled food and pet wastes.

- Set up dating system for foods to be thrown out.

- Encourage use of a variety of spices for cooking.

Loss of Thermal Regulation

Aging is associated with physiological and pathological changes that make temperature regulation challenging. These changes are skin atrophy, autonomic dysfunction, inability to alter environment (poor mental and functional status), decreased ability to detect temperature changes, and presence of comorbidity such as heart failure, chronic obstructive pulmonary disease, and diabetes mellitus. Loss of subcutaneous fat and a decrease in heat production and shiver response make it harder to maintain body heat, resulting in the need to wear layers of clothing in order to feel warm. Keeping cool is also more difficult. Skin changes include reduced ability to sweat and becoming overheated quicker. Aging causes a decrease in the ability to adjust to hot and cold and to sense these temperature extremes. Nursing interventions are aimed at preventing hypo- and hyperthermia.

SUMMARY

This chapter discussed the common problems of pain and loss of hearing, touch, vision, taste, smell and thermal regulation. The older adult must adapt to these sensory losses while maintaining a healthy lifestyle. The goal of nursing for these conditions is to reduce risk of injury or functional decline, maintain quality of life and assist the patient and family members in coping with these losses.

EXAM QUESTIONS

CHAPTER 8
Questions 54-58

54. What percentage of older adults residing in nursing homes are reported as having pain?

    a. 26%
    b. 50%
    c. 70%
    d. 83%

55. The most common visual problem of older adults is

    a. cataracts.
    b. presbyopia.
    c. macular degeneration.
    d. glaucoma.

56. To live more independently older adults with severe visual impairments need

    a. nursing home placement.
    b. round the clock nurses.
    c. specialized training.
    d. live with family members.

57. Normal aging changes, nasal polyps and Alzheimer's disease may increase the loss of

    a. smell.
    b. touch.
    c. hearing.
    d. vision.

58. Loss of subcutaneous fat, decrease in heat production, and decrease in shiver response makes the older adult susceptible to

    a. diabetes.
    b. hypothermia.
    c. hypothyroidism.
    d. infections.

CHAPTER 9

MENTAL HEALTH
AND THE OLDER ADULT

CHAPTER OBJECTIVE

After studying this chapter, the reader will be able to discuss the common mental health problems and the impact these have on the older adult population.

LEARNING OBJECTIVES

After studying this chapter, the learner will be able to

1. list two examples of the mind-body connection.

2. specify two developmental tasks that occur for the majority of older people.

3. identify how older adults cope with common life events.

4. identify nursing assessment strategies for assessing mental health in older adults.

5. recognize that rapid onset of mental changes is a component of delirium and requires immediate intervention.

6. describe how the aging process affects quality of sleep.

7. specify two emotional, two cognitive, and two physical symptoms that are indicators of depression.

8. specify alternatives to drug therapy in the treatment of mental and emotional problems.

9. discuss the problem of suicide as it pertains to the older adult.

10. recognize exemplars of anxiety, phobia, personality disorder, paranoia, and psychosis.

11. select indicators that point to excessive alcohol use.

12. discuss the consequences of gambling in the older adult population.

INTRODUCTION

Older adults with mental illness may be the most complex population with which to work with. Little research has been done on the mental health and responses to treatment on the older population. Treatment modalities have vastly changed during their lifetime. Many of these adults are survivors of mental institutes where they received harsh and numerous electroconvulsive therapy (ECT) treatments, wore physical restraints for months on end, and took strong medications that resulted in the tardive dyskinesia seen in some of these patients today. This chapter begins by describing elements of mental and emotional functioning, and the interaction of mind and body. Next comes a description of aspects of interpersonal interaction that are an inevitable part of our experience as social beings. A discussion of common life events and successful and unsuccessful coping patterns follows. Then nursing assessment of mental and emotional health is discussed. Last, some specific psychological problems are covered, including delirium, depression, anxiety, abuse, personality disorders, psychosis, and addictions.

THE MIND-BODY INTERACTION

The division of mind, or psyche, and body, or soma, is an artificial one that is used to attempt to analyze and understand people better. Our thoughts are dependent on what the sensory system perceives, and can occur only if the physical mechanisms of the nervous system are working properly. In turn, thoughts can affect how we perceive the world, and how one reacts physically to that world. An area that has received much attention in the mind-body connection is depression. Although the Diagnostic and Statistical Manual of Mental Disorders, fourth edition (DSM-IV), emphasizes emotional symptoms such as sadness and anhedonia, the criteria for diagnosing depression includes physical symptoms (fatigue, sleep disturbances, or appetite changes). Research has shown that the physical symptoms associated with depression extend to other areas beyond the DSM-IV, notably pain and gastrointestinal complaints. One study of irritable bowel syndrome showed markedly higher rates in depressed patients vs. controls. Headache, back pain, or nonspecific musculoskeletal complaints commonly represent the pain associated with depression. In fact, in one study of 1146 patients with major depression, physical symptoms were the chief or exclusive complaint for 69% of those identified (Simon, vonKorff, Piccinelli, Fullerton, & Ormel, 1999). Many other studies have found these types of correlations. Persons with diabetes, who are depressed, tend to have poorer blood glucose control. Patients who had a stroke, and are also depressed, do more poorly in rehabilitation programs. Depression after an acute myocardial infarction is associated with higher

mortalities, independent of the severity of cardiovascular function. Depression appears to reduce the life expectancy of older adults. Hospitalized patients with co-morbid depression are less likely to survive life-threatening illnesses (Manning, 2002). With these examples, it is easy to see that ones mind and body is inevitably interrelated. Use of the categories of mind and body, however, do help to examine and learn about how these systems work, just as creating a division between heart and lung in order to study them, always keeping in mind that these organs are intimately interrelated.

INDIVIDUAL-SOCIAL INTERDEPENDENCE

Our minds not only interact with the internal system of our bodies, they are also in constant interaction with the outside world, perceiving, interpreting and reacting. One of the major external influences on our mental health is the social support we receive from family, friends, neighbors, and other caregivers. Social support is a subjective feeling of belonging, being loved, esteemed, valued and needed for oneself, not for what one can do for others. Individuals assess socially supportive resources and then accept or reject them based on perceived societal norms and individual needs. Social support is considered a protective mechanism of health promoting and health maintenance behaviors. Having family members and friends available to provide emotional support, instrumental help, and companionship is important for well-being and health. Social groups can create growth promoting environments, decrease stressful life events, provide feedback or confirmation of actions, and buffer the negative effects of stressful life events. The loss of social support, however, is linked to a variety of disease states and indicates that an absence of social support may increase the incidence of illness. As with people of all ages, older persons function best within a supportive social context. Selectively reducing social interaction begins early in adulthood. Emotional closeness with family, close friends and relatives increases while people who are more peripheral are phased out. By late adulthood, social networks are emotionally condensed, consisting of high emotional closeness with fewer people. The smaller number of social ties reported by older adults is partly due to the elimination of peripheral or unsatisfactory relationships. These condensed social networks may be efficient in increasing well-being, but their reduced numbers create vulnerability. Attrition can lead to the loss of intimate relationships that can never be replaced. Though it is common for people as they age to experience the loss of family members and friends, people who have had a good social support system tend to find new friends, or become close to younger members of their family.

THE DEVELOPMENTAL TASKS OF AGING

Erik Erikson (1963) described 8 developmental stages of mankind, ending with the task in later life of achieving ego integrity rather than surrendering to despair. Ego integrity is the development of a sense of wholeness and satisfaction with one's life. It can also be defined as emotional maturity. It may include promotion of intellectual vigor, redirection of energy toward new roles, acceptance of one's life and development of a point of view about death. Several lesser developmental tasks go into the achievement of emotional maturity, and different authors describe different elements, including the following:

- Flexibility in adapting to the environment, and the ability to solve problems.

- Acceptance of personal strengths and limitations with a good sense of identity.

- The ability to balance conflicting influences.

- Autonomy, independence.

- Social sensitivity, treating others as worthy of concern.

- Striving to live up to one's highest potential.

No one ever becomes perfectly "mature" in all aspects of emotional and social life. A person who functions adequately in society, maintains appropriate life roles and relationships, and evaluates his or her own life as a positive experience, is generally considered emotionally mature. The ability to reach emotional maturity, to develop ego integrity, depends on many factors. Erikson (1963) suggests that each developmental task depends upon the successful completion of previous developmental tasks. At each developmental stage, a person is dependent on the resources available, on the people who serve as role models, and on experience in coping with life. It is possible to continue to develop throughout the life span, improving one's adaptation to life and moving toward the achievement of ego integrity. Further research into the eight stages of Erik Erikson (1963) has uncovered a ninth stage of development. This was introduced by Ms. Joan Erikson, collaborator and wife of the late Erik Erikson (Hobgood, 1997). This stage describes the very old and the challenges faced by elders whose years of autonomy over their bodies and life choices are impacted by the inevitable wages of time. She outlines the critical role that hope and faith must play in the lives of 80 and 90 year olds, and questions the role of wisdom in ones final stage in favor of a role of withdrawal.

COMMON LIFE EVENTS AND COPING STRATEGIES

One universal fact of life is change. As people grow older these changes are more and more often characterized by loss. Losses can be grouped into three broad categories: loss of relationship or of people; loss of ability or roles one has held; and loss of objects, or possessions. An example of loss of ability is the development of chronic disease. In coping with this loss, a person can focus on remaining abilities and specific skills that can improve function. Or a person can focus on negative aspects, focus on the loss itself, with self-blame or wishful thinking, or avoidance, all of which tend to decrease the ability to adapt to the illness.

Coping with loss becomes a major task for older people. Losses can be obvious and large, such as the loss of a spouse or the ability to walk independently, or they can be smaller, such as the loss of a neighbor or a personal possession. The extent to which a loss is felt by an older adult can only be determined by that person and depends on the meanings the person associates with the loss. The death of a distant relative can mean little ("After all, I hardly knew her"), or it could be severe ("We were the same age, and lived through the Depression together"). A person's ability to cope with loss is a major factor in determining whether old age will be a satisfying experience or a catastrophic one.

The use of coping mechanisms tends to remain stable throughout adult life and are developed by experiencing stress, and learning useful ways to react. Unfortunately the coping skill used in the past does not always work for new problems and losses. Sometimes maladaptive coping, such as excess alcohol consumption, leads to even greater problems and losses. A model for successful aging was developed by Paul and Margaret Baltes (1998) after studying how older adults cope with losses. It involves "selective optimization with compensation." In the face of inevitable restrictions of aging, "selection" involves focusing on high priority areas of life. These are areas that give older adults a feeling of satisfaction and personal control and will be different for different people. "Optimization" is deciding to take on behavior that will enrich and enhance the abilities they still have. This helps them make the most of what they want out of life. "Compensation" involves using resources — either their own or others' — to

gain their objectives. This can involve casting aside vanity to get hearing aids or bifocal glasses. It may mean purposefully becoming dependent on others for routine needs, so they can save energy for the activities they really want to do. Even in nursing homes, clients can allow themselves to be dressed by a nurse, so they can engage in favored activities like playing the piano later.

PERSONALITY

Longitudinal studies of personality traits have found that basic personality traits remain relatively consistent throughout one's adult life (Field & Gueldner, 2001). Research has found remarkable stability in personality for periods of up to 30 years. Interviews with older adults themselves have found that individuals' own self-images seem to change relatively little as they age, leading some to believe that the self is essentially "ageless." Personality traits are important determinants of the ways in which people deal with stress. For example, extraversion is associated with forms of coping that involve humor, talking about feelings and seeking support; and agreeableness is associated with stoic and compliant attitudes in the face of stress. In summary, a person seems to become "more of the same" with increasing age, retaining and possibly strengthening many of the traits that were developed at a younger age. With this increasing development of a "unique" personality, there is at least as much variation among older people as there is among younger ones.

OLDER ADULTS AND MENTAL HEALTH SERVICES

Almost 20% of older adults experience mental disorders that are not a normal part of aging. Of these, less than half receive any treatment, and fewer than 3% receive treatment provided by a provider who specializes in mental health (O'Neil, 2002). Although there are effective treatments available for most disorders, many older adults are never screened for or diagnosed with these disorders, therefore they are never treated. The underutilization of mental health services has many causes. The older adult may view problems, such as depression, as a normal part of aging. Older adults with mental disorders tend to display physical complaints, making detection more difficult. This generation is also concerned about the stigma of being diagnosed with mental illness. When an older adult does receive care and treatment for a mental illness, it is usually in the context of a visit to their primary healthcare provider. Unfortunately many primary care physicians receive insufficient training in mental health and in geriatric assessment and care. This is quite significant when considering that older adults who commit suicide had visited their primary provider close to the time of the suicide: 20% on the same day, 40% within one week, and 70% within one month (Conwell, 1994; Andersen, Andersen, Rosholm, & Gram, 2000). Another barrier to mental health care is insurance policies. Medicare requires much higher co-payment (50%) for mental health services, than the 20% it requires for physical health services. As geriatric nurses are in a variety of different settings, and often in close relationships with their clients, they are in the optimal position to detect an untreated mental health problem in older adults.

MENTAL HEALTH ASSESSMENT

Mental health depends on a wide variety of factors. The ability to adapt to the outside world and cope with the stresses of life is a central component of mental health. Another essential component is the ability to maintain interpersonal relationships by interacting appropriately with the people in one's life. Nurses can evaluate the mental and emotional health of older people by asking questions about these two areas of life.

Questions about coping can include the following:

- How are you feeling today?

- What are the sources of stress in your life?

- What have you done in the past when you were under stress?

- What do you do in a typical day?

- What do you do to have fun?

- What do you do when you are angry? Sad?

- What are your strengths?

- What do you like about yourself?

- How did you get through the tough times in the past?

Questions about social and interpersonal interaction can include the following:

- Whom in your family do you feel close to?

- Do you have close friends?

- Can you talk about your feelings to anyone?

- Do you belong to any groups?

- Who helps you when you are in trouble?

While asking such questions, nurses can also be evaluating other aspects of a person's mental health. To evaluate speech, determine whether the speech is at a normal, fast, or slow rate. Is the tone normal? Is the amount of speech appropriate, or does the person answer with monosyllables or talk continuously? Thoughts should be expressed logically. Are thoughts expressed disjointedly, with the patient jumping from topic to topic? Are thoughts constructive? Are they self-destructive, or do they indicate an obsession with fears or delusions? Do the thoughts indicate an obsession with bodily concerns? Nonverbal behavior or "body language" can give important clues about a person's mental state. Does the person make eye contact? Is motor activity depressed or excessive? Is posture relaxed, tense, or blocking, as with crossed arms and legs? Mood or affect can also be evaluated by using observation. Does the patient seem happy, sad, angry, fearful, up, down, high, and so on? Is a range of emotions expressed? Do facial expressions and nonverbal behavior match the person's expressed mood?

Validating observations with the patient can strengthen the nurse's assessment of these aspects of mental status. This is performed by stating the observation and asking the patient if he or she is aware of the behavior and if it is normal. An example would be to observe that a person is fidgeting during the interview and ask, "You seem to be moving a lot. Is this normal for you, or do you think it's because of how you're feeling?" To a patient who speaks slowly in a low tone of voice, answers in monosyllables, and sits slumped in a chair, the nurse could say, "You seem sad to me. Are you feeling sad?" Either a yes or a no answer could then be further explored.

One factor nurses need to consider when evaluating someone's behavior is the cultural norm for that person. People of different cultures may express their mental state in very different behaviors. If unsure of a patient's ethnic background, it is appropriate to ask the patient what that background is. Another factor to consider is how distressed a person is. Perhaps you are confronted with someone who is talking incessantly in a loud, high-pitched voice, with disjointed thoughts and delusions that someone is trying to hurt him. It would obviously not be a good time to try to validate your observations; This person is simply in too much distress to hear what another person is saying.

An additional component of mental health includes cognitive function. Cognitive function is the ability to process and remember data, pay attention, reason and calculate, use judgment, be oriented, and use language and motor skills appropriately. The chapter on dementia goes into more detail on cognitive function. One example of change in cognitive function is delirium, which is a short-term, acute change and is a nursing and medical emergency.

DELIRIUM

Delirium is from the Latin, de Lira, meaning not on track. It was known during the time of Hippocrates (Huth, 1985). Clinical features have been described in the medical literature since the 16th century, and were noted to be more common after surgery and in the elderly. It is defined as an *acute* reversible organic mental disorder, manifesting as confusional state characterized by an impairment of cognitive function (thought, perception, recall) of acute (*sudden: hours or days*) onset with attendant disturbance of consciousness/attention. There is a reduced ability to maintain attention to external stimuli and disorganized thinking as manifested by rambling, or irrelevant or incoherent speech. There is also a reduced level of consciousness, sensory misperception, and disturbance of the sleep wakefulness cycle and level of psychomotor activity, disorientation to time, place or person and memory impairment. Delirious older adults will often act out and manifest psychiatric behaviors. This state is often caused by a *reversible* condition (see Table 9-1). It is a poor prognosis and is often *life threatening*. Delirium is common, preventable and often reversible, using interventions that targets the underlying etiologic factor (Foreman, Wakefield, Culp, & Milisen, 2001). The longer an older adult remains delirious, the more likely there will be serious complications. Often there is a delay in diagnosing delirium as it may be assumed the person has dementia, or a dementia that is getting worse. As an older adult may be afebrile due to a slower immune system, delirium due to infection may not be obvious. Suspect delirium if his/her cognitive status change has an acute onset, has fluctuations, has inattention, and either disorganized thinking or altered level of consciousness (Milisen, et al, 2002).

TABLE 9-1: POSSIBLE CAUSES OF DELIRIUM

Infections: Such as urinary, sepsis, oral, respiratory, or decubitus.

Medication: Toxicity, withdrawal, side effects, adverse reaction; especially sedative and hypnotics.

Central nervous system disease: CVA, TIA, seizures, trauma, or subdural hematoma.

Electrolyte abnormalities, or dehydration.

Hepatic or renal failure, decreased cardiac output, hypoxia, MI, or CHF.

Blood loss, Trauma (fractures, burns, MVA).

Fecal impaction, constipation, urinary retention, vomiting, or diarrhea.

Recent surgical procedure.

Nutritional deficit or hypo/hyperglycemia.

Pulmonary emboli, multiple sclerosis, or AIDS.

Hypo/hyperthermia or hypotension.

Thyroid, pituitary, or adrenal hormone abnormalities.

Pain, depression, alcohol usage, or anxiety.

Sensory depravation, sensory overload, isolation, or immobility.

Bereavement, unfamiliar/new environment.

Restraint usage, impaired sensory function, or sleep depravation.

The nurse, who notices that a patient is suddenly more agitated and calls a physician for an order for a tranquilizer might, be ignoring the real possibility that a delirium exists. This leads to a failure in obtaining appropriate treatment for the underlying condition. Inouye et al., (1990) proposed a simple and elegant method for detecting delirium called the confusion assessment method (CAM). To evaluate whether an abnormality of attention and cognition is a delirium, ask the following four questions:

1. Does the abnormal behavior have an acute onset and fluctuating course?

2. Is the person characterized by inattention, having difficulty concentrating or keeping track of what is being said?

3. Is the person showing disorganized thinking, with rambling or incoherent speech, irrelevant or incoherent ideas, and jumping from subject to subject?

4. Does the person demonstrate an altered level of consciousness, such as hypervigilance, lethargy, stupor, or coma?

To arrive at a diagnosis of delirium, the patient needs to demonstrate both 1 and 2 as well as either 3 or 4.

Table 9-2 is a Delirium Checklist for nurses that can help find the cause of a delirium. When assessing for delirium, obtain the oral history from someone other than the patient for accuracy. Keep in mind that a behavior change for better or worse is cardinal sign of delirium in persons with dementia.

SLEEP DISTURBANCES

Sleep disturbances affect more than 50% of older adults who live at home and over two-thirds of those in long-term care facilities (Grandjean & Gibbons, 2000). The age-related changes of sleep have a significant impact on the quality of sleep of the older adult. Stage 4 sleep, which is rapid eye movement (REM) stage, is decreased resulting in a reduction in sleep efficiency and increased awakenings. This also causes early morning awakenings and frequent daytime naps. Sleep problems may include difficulty falling to sleep, remaining asleep, and/or feeling fatigued upon awakening. The primary sleep disorders of the older adult are sleep apnea and periodic leg movement. There are also many chronic conditions that are disruptive to sleep: angi-

TABLE 9-2: DELIRIUM CHECKLIST

Vital Signs _____

Lungs _____

Sputum/cough/nasal/eyes _____

Oxygen Saturation _____

Pain _____

Skin

  Decubitus _____

  Color, temperature, edema _____

  Rash, itchiness, bruise _____

  Dehydration _____

Oral Assessment _____

Neuro Assessment _____

  TIA activity _____

  Pupils _____

  Hand grips _____

  Abnormal movements _____

Loss of Consciousness (LOC)/Hallucinations __

Bowel/Bladder/Abdomen Assessment _____

  Bladder distention _____

  Last void _____

Vaginal/penile drainage _____

Urine color/dip _____

Bowel sounds _____

Abdomen palpation/tympany _____

Last Bowel Movement _____

Occult blood _____

Appetite _____

Nausea/vomiting _____

Fingerstick _____

Swallowing difficulty _____

Motor Function Changes

  gait _____

  fine motor movements _____

Medications

  Possible toxicity _____

  New medications _____

  Refusal history/PRN usage

Medical History

  Old diagnosis _____

  Previous labs _____

Other _____

Recent Fall or injury _____

MD/NP notified   Date _____ Nurse _____

Family notified   Date _____ Nurse _____

Request orders for:

  Labs _____ Results _____

  Urinalysis _____ Results _____

  Skin Culture & Sensitivity _____ Results _____

  X-ray _____ Results _____

  Electrocardiogram (EKG) _____ Results _____

  Dental evaluation _____ Results _____

  Speech evaluation for swallow ____ Results _____

  PT evaluation for pain _____ Results _____

  Psychiatric evaluation _____ Results _____

  Other _____ Results _____

Assessment completed by _____   Date _____

Resident _____ Room _____

Note. From Fitzsimmons, S., & Buettner, L. (2003). Therapeutic recreational interventions for needs-driven dementia-compromised behaviors in community-dwelling elderly. *American Journal of Alzheimer's Disease, 17*(6), 362-381. Reprinted with permission.

na, asthma, anxiety, benign prostatic hypertrophy, pain, depression, diabetes, gastro-esophageal reflux disease (GERD), heart failure, migraines, seizures, Parkinson's Disease, Chronic Obstructive Pulmonary Disease (COPD) and dementia (Onen & Onen, 2003). Other factors that disrupt sleep are bowel and bladder incontinence, immobility, pressure sores, or pain (Zanocchi, et al., 1999), cough, contractures, poor sleeping environment, unfamiliar environment, nightmares, physical restraints, uncomfortable medical equipment, nursing care, and medications.

Treatment for sleep problems should start with non-pharmacological interventions with medications being used only as a last resort. Community-dwelling elders often self-medicate with over-the-counter agents, such as Benadryl, which is an inappropriate medication for most elders. The following are suggestions to help improve quality and quantity of sleep:

- Plan a regular bedtime and wake-up schedule.

- Do hobbies and physical activities; an early evening walk is especially helpful.

- Avoid daytime napping.

- Avoid over-the-counter medications such as allergy medicines.

- Avoid tobacco products.

- Avoid caffeine after 4 PM (coffee, colas, tea, or chocolate), earlier if possible.

- Avoid alcohol.

- Keep bedroom quiet, dark, cool and comfortable, with good mattress and comfortable pillows.

- Take a warm bath in the evening, drink warm milk at bedtime

- Use quiet music and avoid television watching in bed

In order to find the cause of sleep problems a sleep log may be necessary to document when awake, when asleep and when tired. The Pittsburgh Sleep Quality Index (PSQI) is an effective instrument used to measure the quality and patterns of sleep in the older adult (Buysse, Reynolds, Monk, Berman, & Kupfer, 1989). Persons who fall asleep while driving need immediate assessment by a physician. In long term care facilities, care should be taken by night staff to avoid disturbing residents sleep. Keeping voices and lighting down and individualizing night care for toileting and changing wet clothing works better than checking every resident every two hours. Also consider thirst, hunger, fear and loneliness as barriers for sleep in this setting. Soft music or sitting and reading to a frightened resident often promotes sleep.

DEPRESSION

It is estimated that the incidence of depression in older adults living in long-term care facilities can be as high as 25% and is the most common mood disorder of late life (Lyketsos, et al., 2000). Depression often goes undiagnosed and therefore untreated (Teresi, et al., 2001). Diagnosing depression in this group is often difficult as older persons may exhibit non-specific somatic complaints rather than DSM-IV classified symptoms of depressed mood (Gallo & Rabins, 1999). Minor depression often becomes a chronic illness in this group but is not a part of normal aging. Depression may be associated with side effects of medications or compounded by medical conditions such as a cerebral vascular accident, Parkinson's or heart disease. It may be caused by a multitude of psychological conditions such as coping with chronic illness and frequent pain, gloomy institutionalized environments, and an assortment of losses including function, independence, social roles, friends and relatives, and past leisure activities. See Table 9-3 for factors that may contribute to depression. Many depressed people actually feel physiological symptoms. For some it is a churning feeling, particularly in agitated depression. Others experience a sensation of heaviness with lethargy and even physical pain. Some have difficulty digesting food. Brain neurotransmitters have an impact on a person's mood such as serotonin, norepinephrine, and dopamine. Depression appears to involve a reduced amount of one or more of these, hindering brain signals and in turn causing the various symptoms of depression. MRIs and brain tissue samples of depressed patients

---

TABLE 9-3: FACTORS CONTRIBUTING TO DEPRESSION

Medication Usage: Some antihypertensive, hormonal, and neuroleptics agents, Carbidopa/levodopa, Beta blockers, Clonidine, Benzodiazepines, Barbiturates, Anticonvulsants, Histamine-2 blockers, Calcium channel blockers, Thiazide diuretics, Digoxin, narcotics, and polypharmacy defined as 3 or more medications per day.

Medical Causes
Chronic illness: Late-life mental disorders are often detected in association with somatic illness. The prevalence of clinically significant depression in later life is estimated to be highest, approximately 25 %, among those with chronic illness, especially with ischemic heart disease, stroke, cancer, coronary artery disease, diabetes, chronic lung disease, arthritis, Alzheimer's and Parkinson's diseases.

Other: Persistent insomnia, impaired vision, impaired hearing, pain, posttraumatic stress disorder, or impaired physical functioning.

Psychological conditions: Educational attainment less than high school, female gender, personality types: low self-esteem, family history, heavy alcohol consumption.
Social Isolation, bereavement, frustration with memory loss.

Losses: Correlations have been found between depression and a variety of losses including loss of family home, friends, social activities, volunteering, financial security, and marital harmony.

---

shows that these neurotransmitters are below normal. Depression is associated with functional decline and excess mortality and therefore should be treated vigorously (Furlanetto, von Ammon Cavanaugh, Bueno, Creech, & Powell, 2000). Depression is associated with increased falls (Arthur, Matthews, Jagger, & Lindesay, 2002) and has been demonstrated to spread from one person to another in a phenomenon known as emotional contagion (Joiner & Katz, 1999).

The short-form Geriatric Depression Scale (GDS) (Sheikh & Yesavage, 1986) is a widely used screening tool for assessment of depression in persons over the age of 55 (Table 9-4). It is especially useful in clinical settings to facilitate assessment of depression in older adults, especially when baseline measurements are compared to subsequent scores. The GDS may be used with healthy, medically ill, and mild to moderately cognitively impaired older adults. It has been extensively used in community, acute and long-term care settings. This instrument is a simple 15 item Yes/No answer interview that takes relatively few minutes to complete. The questions fall into the following domains: somatic concerns, lowered affect, impaired motivation, lack of self-esteem, and future orientation. A score of five or above is strongly associated with depression.

Treatment of Depression

Depression is best treated using a combination of medication and therapy including life-style changes (Reynolds, Frank, Perel, & Imber, 1999). Unfortunately many older adults are only offered medication as a treatment for depression, as many nonpharmacological treatment modalities are not reimbursable. None of the antidepressant medications are 100% effective in treating depression and the risks of their usage are a multitude of adverse side effects. The most costly of these side effects, in terms of quality of life and dollars, is falls. Association between antidepressant medication usage and falls has been repeatedly demonstrated

TABLE 9-4: GERIATRIC DEPRESSION SCALE (GDS)

Choose the best answer for how you have felt over the past week:

1. Are you basically satisfied with your life? **YES/NO**

2. Have you dropped many of your activities and interests? **YES**/NO

3. Do you feel that your life is empty? **YES**/NO

4. Do you often get bored? **YES**/NO

5. Are you in good spirits most of the time? YES/**NO**

6. Are you afraid that something bad is going to happen to you? **YES**/NO

7. Do you feel happy most of the time? YES/**NO**

8. Do you often feel helpless? **YES**/NO

9. Do you prefer to stay at home, rather than going out and doing new things? **YES**/NO

10. Do you feel you have more problems with memory than most? **YES**/NO

11. Do you think it is wonderful to be alive now? YES/**NO**

12. Do you feel pretty worthless the way you are now? **YES**/NO

13. Do you feel full of energy? YES/**NO**

14. Do you feel that your situation is hopeless? **YES**/NO

15. Do you think that most people are better off that you are? **YES**/NO

Answers in **bold** indicate depression. Although differing sensitivities and specificities have been obtained across studies, for clinical purposes a score of >5 points is suggestive of depression and should warrant a follow-up interview. Score of >10 are almost always depression.

Note. From Sheikh, J., & Yesavage, J. (1986). Geriatric Depression Scale (GDS): Recent evidence and development of a shorter version. *Clinical Gerontology: A guide to assessment and intervention,* 165-173, New York: The Haworth Press.

(Joo, et al., 2002). Because of the serious side effects of these medications and sensitivity of older persons to these effects, it is safest to try non-pharmaceutical interventions on mild to moderately depressed clients. Research indicates that mild to moderate depression often can be treated successfully with non-pharmacological interventions alone (Hyman & Rudorfer, 2000). Non-pharmacological interventions may provide a feasible, safe alternative or complementary intervention to the current treatment modality for this population.

Non-Pharmacological Treatment of Depression

Psychosocial interventions may be preferred for some older adults, especially those who are unable to tolerate, or prefer not to take, medication or who are confronting stressful situations or low degrees of social support (Lebowitz et al., 1997). The benefits of psychosocial interventions are likely to assume greater prominence as a result of population demographics (U.S. Department of Health and Human Services, 1999). As the number of older people grows, the number in need of mental health treatment increases. This is especially true of the very old as they are expected to be suffering from greater levels of comorbidity or dealing with the stresses associated with disability. Psychosocial interventions not only can help relieve the symptoms of a variety of mental disorders and related problems but also can play more diverse roles: They can help strengthen coping mechanisms, encourage (and monitor) patients' compliance with medical regimens, and promote healthy behavior (Klausner & Alexopoulos, 1999). This type of therapy is usually performed in groups. Being with other people is very important in the process of successfully dealing with depression. Some of these groups are merely discussion-type support groups while others are more specific. Many of these type programs are designed to address outcomes other than depression but also have a positive impact on mood (Buettner & Fitzsimmons, 2003). These types of interventions are usually set up and run by recreational therapists, social workers, nursing, and other disciplines and are the safest treatment to try first. These include:

Feelings-based: Memory tea, life stories, bibliotherapy

Relaxation Based: Guided imagery, meditation, positive affirmations

Nurturing Programs: Pet therapy, intergenerational programs

Adventure Based: Wheelchair biking, travel, camping

Physical Based: Ambulation/walking program, social dance club, exercise for function, aquatic therapy, tai chi

Life Roles: Sensory cooking groups, community re-intergenerational, penpal programs

Cognitive Programs: Newsletters, chess club, re-motivation, cognitive therapy, problem-solving skills, coping skills training, current events.

Sensory-Based Programs: Reminiscing, sensory integration

Expressive Arts: Group drumming circles, choral club, photo therapy, flower club, humor group, woodworking

Psychosocial based: Bird watchers, bowling league, golf, rod & reel, travel, needlecraft.

Other: Spiritual, faith-based prayer group and use of rocking chairs, significantly impact depression.

Drug Treatment for Depression

The use of antidepressant drugs for depression is a popular form of therapy. Tricyclic antidepressants (TCA) have been most frequently used; however, they are no longer recommended, due to the anticholinergic properties (amitriptyline, imipramine, nortriptyline, and others). This causes drying of secretions, constipation, urinary hesitancy, and blurred vision. These side effects can impair cogni-

tive function and worsen a dementia or delirium. Tetracyclines, Amoxapine (Asendin®), and Maprotiline HCl (Ludiomil®) should also be avoided due to lowering the seizure threshold. Heterocyclics such as Trazodone (Desyrel®) have too many side effects for use as an antidepressant but in small doses has been found to be useful as a sleep aide.

Selective serotonin reuptake inhibitors (SSRIs) such as fluoxetine (Prozac®), paroxetine (Paxil®), citalopram (Celexa™), and sertraline (Zoloft®), are especially useful in the treatment of late-life depression, because these agents are reported to have fewer anticholinergic and cardiovascular side effects than the TCAs. SSRIs — which include citalopram, escitalopram, fluoxetine, fluvoxamine, paroxetine, and sertraline — are considered the safest medications for late-life depression (Physician's Desk Reference, 2002). The most common side effect of SSRIs is nausea, which is usually mild and occurs in the first weeks of treatment (Mulchahey, Malik, Sabai, & Kasckow, 1999). Dry mouth is also common and anxiety is usually transient. Sedation can be a problem in older patients who use SSRIs, especially paroxetine (Dechant & Clissold, 1991), and some compromise cognition. Sexual function can be diminished by SSRIs; the most common sexual side effects are anorgasmia and delayed orgasm. Abrupt discontinuation of some SSRIs can lead to withdrawal side effects, such as dizziness, fatigue, and nausea. Nurses should instruct their clients not to suddenly stop taking these types of medications. There are many potential drug-drug interactions with the individual SSRI, requiring care when adding any new medication (Kasckow et al., 2003).

Monoamine oxidase (MAOI) inhibitors clinical use is often restricted to patients who are refractory to other antidepressant drugs. This is due to potentially life-threatening pharmacodynamic interactions with sympathomimetic drugs or tyramine-containing foods and beverages. The sympathomimetic amines (e.g., phenylpropanolamine and pseudoephedrine) may be present in over-the-counter decongestant products that older patients are prone to self-administer. An additional concern is the risk of orthostatic hypotension, which occurs even at therapeutic doses.

In summary, many drugs can be very effective in helping elders cope with severe depression. However, care must be taken that side effects of the medications do not cause a worsened cognitive state; excessive sedation; intolerable anticholinergic drying of mucous membranes; urinary retention; or constipation. "Start low and go slow" is the best practice for the use of antidepressants in the elderly. They must realize that relief of symptoms takes up to 6 weeks.

Electroconvulsive therapy (ECT) is regarded as an effective intervention for some forms of treatment-resistant depression across the life cycle. ECT entails the electrical induction of seizures in the brain, administered during a series of 6–12 treatment sessions on an inpatient or outpatient basis. Practice guidelines recommend that ECT should be reserved for severe cases of depression, particularly with active suicidal risk or psychosis; patients unresponsive to medications; and those who cannot tolerate medications. ECT is advantageous for some older adults with depression because of the special problems they encounter with medications. The older adult has a slower response to antidepressant medications, which may render the faster onset of action of ECT another advantage in select cases. Although the clinical effectiveness of ECT is documented and acknowledged, the treatment often is associated with troubling side effects, principally a brief period of confusion following administration and a temporary period of memory disruption. There may also be longer-term memory losses for the time period surrounding the use of ECT. Although the exception rather than the rule, persistent memory loss following ECT is reported. There are no absolute medical contraindications to ECT. However, a recent history of myocardial infarct, irregular cardiac rhythm,

or other heart conditions suggests the need for caution due to the risks of general anesthesia and the brief rise in heart rate, blood pressure, and load on the heart that accompany ECT administration.

Depression in Long-Term Care Facilities

Social interactions and pleasurable experiences are ways of providing older adults with opportunities to attain happiness, purpose, and quality of life. The ability to reach this mood state level is often out of reach to older adults especially those residing in long-term facilities. This group frequently has compounding constraints to leisure in the form of multiple chronic conditions such as cognitive and mobility impairments and numerous medical diagnoses. Recreational therapists are specifically trained to help individuals with disabilities overcome such complex constraints. Recreational therapy is an important, yet often overlooked treatment option for long-term care residents with depression.

Depression and Failure to Thrive

Depression is a common and serious illness in the elderly that sometimes leads to suicide. Indirect self-destructive behavior, such as not eating and medication noncompliance, is much more common than suicide, and has been associated with decreased survival. Failure to thrive in the elderly is a clinical syndrome encompassing a number of biologic and psychosocial problems associated with increased morbidity and mortality that occurs near the end of life. It may be defined as an unexplained decrease in function, structure, or metabolic process occurring in excess of that expected for age. The easiest measurement to define this syndrome is "unexplained weight loss," though loss of function and loss of lean body mass may also be seen. Although failure to thrive is not clearly understood, its association with depression appears to be very significant.

The incidence of suicide increases with age, with the highest rates being for males over the age of 85 (Glaser, 2000). Persons in this cohort tend to use extremely lethal means and have more "success" than any other age group. It is sometimes very difficult to determine whether such deaths are the result of carefully thought-out, rational decisions in the face of loss of independence or anticipated pain or the result of a reversible depression. Suicide is seldom a cry for help in the older adult, but reflects a serious desire to end one's life. As dramatic as the suicide statistics are for older adults, they most likely hugely underestimate the true enormity of the problem. Reasons for this are not listing suicide as the actual cause of death on death certificates and not recognizing passive suicide, such as abusing alcohol and mixing deadly combinations of medications, accidental overdoses of medications, or failure to thrive.

While much controversy exists over the right of individuals to end their lives, most people would agree that suicide resulting from a depression is an unfortunate tragedy. Nurses can encourage people who seem depressed to seek treatment from physicians, nurse practitioners, therapists, or psychiatric nurses. By conveying a belief in the reversibility of depression, nurses can help older clients look for affirmative choices rather than succumb to feelings of hopelessness and helplessness.

ANXIETY

Although some anxiety is a normal human experience, abnormal levels of anxiety can cause severe distress to older adults. Women tend to be affected more often than men. Total anxiety rates for the elderly vary across studies, depending upon setting, to average about 10.1% (Lantz, 2002). Anxiety can be combined with dementia, psychosis, or depression and change the therapeutic approach from what would be needed for any of these problems individually. Anxiety-induced disorders in later years include panic disorder, phobic disorder, generalized anxiety, agoraphobia, obses-

sive-compulsive disorder, and posttraumatic stress disorder.

Panic disorder is characterized by acute panic attacks unrelated to actual physical danger. Panic attacks are periods of intense fear accompanied by physical signs and symptoms such as choking, dyspnea, dizziness, tachycardia and chest pain, trembling, sweating, nausea, numbness or tingling of extremities, flushing or chills, and fear of losing control or of dying. Phobic disorders occur when exposure to a certain identifiable stimulus provokes an anxiety attack. Phobic disorder is the most common anxiety disorder for persons of all ages, including elderly persons, and the male-to-female ratio is 1:2. In fact, phobia is the second most common psychiatric disorder after cognitive impairment and depression in individuals 65 years and older (Flint, 2001).

Generalized anxiety is similar to panic disorder except that the anxiety tends to focus on specific life circumstances, such as health, finances, and children. Indications include increased motor tension; increased vigilance; and signs and symptoms of a fight-or-flight response, such as dyspnea, tachycardia, dry mouth, or dizziness. Agoraphobia is the fear of being in public places such as standing in line or sitting in a bus. It can be severe enough that the person is unable to leave home or go to the hospital. Obsessive-compulsive neurosis is more acute than an obsessive-compulsive personality disorder and is characterized by repetitive thoughts that are not wanted by the person experiencing them and may be suppressed. The repetitive, ritualistic behavior that is performed excessively is an attempt to neutralize the obsessive thoughts. The behaviors include checking rituals, such as confirming that the stove is turned off numerous times, and cleaning rituals, such as washing the hands repeatedly after they become "contaminated."

Posttraumatic stress disorder (PTSD) can result when a person has experienced a trauma outside the range of normal human experience. It is characterized by recurrent unwanted recollections of the event, unrealistic anxiety about one's current safety and/or "flashbacks." Symbolic events, such as anniversaries, can be greatly anxiety provoking. In the effort to avoid thoughts connected with the trauma, a person may start to avoid stimuli and people that are only remotely or symbolically connected with it and live in a detached, low-emotion, protective cocoon. Alternatively, the person may demonstrate increased vigilance and arousal, as if to prevent the trauma from recurring. People who have lived through wars and natural disasters can retain anxiety from PTSD indefinitely. Nurses providing care to refugees, veterans, and other "survivors" need to be aware of the long-lasting effects that such experiences can have.

Drug Treatment

Drug treatment of anxiety has changed significantly over the years. Bromide was replaced in the 1950s with phenobarbital and other barbiturates, and in the 1960s with benzodiazepine antianxiety medications. After several years of enthusiastic use of benzodiazepines, however, long-term effects of addiction emerged. For the elderly, the side effects include sedation with increased prevalence of falls and injury and impaired memory. Whereas these drugs can work well to reduce anxiety, their long-term use can create dependency and severe withdrawal effects. Research demonstrating benzodiazepine safety for younger people is not applicable to older patients because of the longer half-life of these medications in older persons. Nurses need to evaluate the efficacy of antianxiety medications. Nurses also need to watch for unwanted side effects such as sedation, confusion, impaired coordination, dizziness, and blurred vision. Abrupt withdrawal should be avoided, because it can result in severe signs and symptoms, which are anxiety, irritability,

insomnia, fatigue, muscle twitching and sweating. Buspirone (Buspar) has had few studies supporting its efficacy but has been found to be well tolerated by the elderly (Small, 1997). Buspirone is unrelated to the benzodiazepines and has little sedation and no anticonvulsant or musculoskeletal side effects. Sedative-hypnotic antianxiety medications can exacerbate an underlying depression or cause disinhibition in patients with dementia thus causing more inappropriate behavior.

Non-Pharmacological Therapy for Anxiety

Non-drug treatment of anxiety includes having the patient discuss and ventilate anxieties in a safe and reassuring environment. Since elderly persons may be reluctant to discuss psychological problems, education about the biological basis of anxiety may be helpful. At times the environment can be changed to reduce or eliminate factors that precipitate anxiety, such as sensory overload. Relaxation techniques can also be helpful. These include: guided imagery, meditation, prayer, yoga, massage, music, a warm bath, and many others. It is important to allow older adults to choose what they would like to try rather than to decide for them. Another technique that is used for phobias (such as agoraphobia) is progressively greater exposure to the phobic item, which can result in desensitization. There are self-help groups for persons with agoraphobia that involve support and desensitization by people who are recovered agoraphobic themselves. Minimizing polypharmacy may improve or even remove symptoms. Nurses are in a critical spot and role to help identify and amend the adverse effects of polypharmacy. Nurses should not hesitate to refer a patient for psychiatric evaluation if the patient continues to have distressing signs and symptoms of anxiety.

BIPOLAR DISORDER

A bipolar affective disorder, referring to characteristic emotional mood swings between mania and depression, may also be referred to as manic-depressive disorder. This disorder usually begins between 30 and 50 years of age and almost never begins after age 60. The disease that begins earlier usually lasts into old age so geriatric nurses may see patients who have this problem. The treatment for the disorder is the drug lithium carbonate, which prevents manic episodes and improves the intermittent depression. It is important for the patient to receive a thorough evaluation before starting lithium so that reversible causes of mania such as drugs (steroids, isoniazid, procarbazine, levodopa, or bromide), metabolic disturbances (hemodialysis, postoperative state), infection, neoplasm, or epilepsy can be ruled out. To assure the safety of lithium treatment in elderly patients, kidney or thyroid function, and ECG should be evaluated. Lithium may have many side effects, even at therapeutic levels. Patients may be tempted to discontinue the drug when they are feeling good but should be encouraged to continue taking it. Lithium doses are titrated by measuring lithium levels in blood serum. As with most drugs, the elderly are more easily and more severely affected by the toxic effects of lithium than younger persons are (Sajatovic, 2002).

Side effects of lithium at therapeutic levels are

- Tremor, urinary frequency, or mild nausea.

Early indications of toxic levels are

- Increasing tremor, ataxic gait, weakness, slurred speech, blurred vision, tinnitus, drowsiness, or excitement.

Severe toxic effects include

- Increased deep tendon reflexes, nystagmus, confusion, lethargy that may progress to stupor, seizures, or coma.

PERSONALITY DISORDERS

When people with a predominant character type become ill, the physical and psychological stress can result in inappropriate coping patterns. Several of these personality types are described:

Oral Personality. Coping tends to be dependent and demanding. Patients with this personality type may act is if the caregiver has unlimited time and may become angry and reproachful when their unreasonable demands are not met. Depression and addictive tendencies often accompany this character pattern. Nurse management involves setting firm limits while communicating a positive regard. Short, frequent contact may be more effective than infrequent, longer visits.

Compulsive Personality. Behavior is very controlled, reserved and rational, often focusing on detail without being able to see the larger context of a situation. These patients tend to have a rigid moral system. They are self-controlled and conscientious and usually have great difficulty in situations where they cannot be in control. Nurses can help most by explaining carefully what they are doing, by encouraging the patient to participate in his or her care, and by accepting the patient's desire to be in control.

Hysterical Personality. These patients tend to be charming and imaginative, and they try to form close personal relationships, often inappropriately so. They attach great importance to their attractiveness and may feel this is threatened by their illness. Nurses can be most helpful by providing reassurance, allowing ventilation of feelings. Since these patients can feel overwhelmed by details, nurses need to be alert to cues that the patients do not want thorough explanations.

Masochistic Personality. These patients are characterized by having a history of repeated suffering combined with an exhibitionistic display of suffering. They tend to be self-sacrificing. Illness may be either a proof of their lack of self-worth or the only way to justify being cared for by others. They may get a sufficient secondary gain from their illness that makes them resist therapies that may improve their health. The best nursing approach is to acknowledge their suffering and their self-sacrifice while continuing to have a positive expectation that they will help themselves.

Schizoid Personality. Behavior tends to be remote, reserved and isolated. When these patients become ill, they must interact with others, which can be so threatening that they may refuse to acknowledge they are ill. Nursing care should include accepting the person's high need for privacy and refraining from intruding whenever possible. It is unlikely that these patients will respond well to attempts to "get to know them," and the truly empathic response is to give them the privacy that helps them feel more secure.

Paranoid Personality. Behavior is fearful and suspicious, oversensitive to criticism. They expect the worst in others and may act in a manner that brings out the worst in others, creating a self-fulfilling prophecy. Often when older people start to forget things, they explain their memory lapse by attributing evil intent to someone else, either real or imaginary. The woman who cannot find the dishes she wants accuses her daughter of stealing. The woman who moved into her son's house, losing most of her personal possessions, repeatedly accuses an imaginary intruder of taking her things. Nursing management of paranoid reactions can focus on the patient's underlying feeling of threat or loss, acknowledging the validity of the feeling without participating in the paranoid delusions.

Narcissistic Personality. To protect a fragile self-esteem, these patients react by acting grandiose, arrogant, and vain. Illness is a threat to their imagined self-perfection. They may react to caregivers with idealization — "my nurse is the best" — or with denigration — "I'm better than you." Nurses

need to realize the fragile foundation of such people and communicate acceptance of the individual and support autonomy whenever possible.

Many patients may have more than one of these character patterns. Evidence for nurses that they are dealing with a personality disorder is when the nurse has a strong emotional reaction to the patient, often out of proportion to the situation at hand. When a nurse notices such a reaction, he or she can pause and analyze what is going on, why the patient feels the need for self-protection, and what the nurse can best do to provide a therapeutic environment. Needless to say, this requires patience and takes practice.

PSYCHOTIC DISTURBANCES OF THOUGHT AND BEHAVIOR

Besides severe depression and manic-depressive illness, a major psychotic illness is schizophrenia. Psychotic behavior is characterized by agitation, delusions, hallucinations, a poor sense of self with resulting self-neglect, poor insight, and incoherent thought patterns. Psychotic people can live to old age. With the closing of many state mental institutions, elderly psychotic people often live in nursing homes, in single-room occupancy hotels, or as homeless street people.

Schizophrenia is a psychotic disorder that is neither manic-depressive nor depressive. It is a fluctuating disease, with prodromal, active, and residual phases. The prodromal phase in the older adult may be difficult to differentiate from organic diseases such as senile dementia of the Alzheimer's type, Huntington's disease, or drug side effects. Increased delusions, agitation, combativeness, paranoia, and hallucinations characterize the active or positive phase. The residual or negative phase is a time of blunted emotional reactions, impoverished speech, lack of spontaneity, and anhedonia.

Magical thinking, peculiar behavior, and an inability to maintain functional roles can characterize both the prodromal and residual phases, making it difficult for schizophrenics to deal effectively with their society even when not in an active phase of the disease. Overall, psychotic symptoms interfere with understanding of internal and external stimuli. In older adults, acute symptoms usually arise from noncompliance with prescribed medications or a failed treatment regimen.

Drug Therapy for Schizophrenia

The major treatment for schizophrenia is drug therapy with a class of drugs called neuroleptics. These drugs all block dopamine, which is a neurotransmitter. Because a lack of dopamine is the cause of Parkinson's disease, one effect of neuroleptics is to cause extrapyramidal side effects (EPSE) and parkinsonian signs and symptoms; these side effects are related to the strength of the dose of neuroleptic. Other side effects include sedation and the anticholinergic effects of dry mouth, constipation, and urinary retention. A life-threatening complication of antipsychotic use is neuroleptic malignant syndrome. Symptoms include muscular rigidity and dystonia. Autonomic symptoms are fever (up to 107° F), increased pulse and increased blood pressure. The treatment is to immediately discontinue the antipsychotic and aggressively treat the symptoms. High-potency neuroleptics such as haloperidol (Haldol), thiothixene HCl (Navane®), and risperidone (Risperdal®) are given in very low doses to maximize the antipsychotic effect while minimizing sedation and anticholinergic effects. Unfortunately, along with maximizing the antipsychotic effect, these doses cause the maximum parkinsonian side effects except when given with Cogentin® (benztropine). Another disturbing side effect of neuroleptics is irreversible movement disorders such as tardive dyskinesia (TD), which is characterized by involuntary movement of the tongue, lips, mouth, and jaw. This

affects self-esteem, ability to communicate, and eat, and diminishes quality of life. It may also occur as truncal dyskinesia and manifest involuntary movements of the trunk. TD occurs in as many as 31% of elderly neuroleptic users after 43 weeks (Antai-Otong, 2000). The Abnormal Involuntary Movement Scale (Guy, 1976) helps evaluate for early symptoms of TD (see Table 9-5). Considering the side effects of these medications, atypical neuroleptic agents have become the first-line drugs for treatment. These include clozapine (Clozaril®), risperidone, quetiapine (Seroquel®), and olanzapine (Zyprexa®). These agents are associated with fewer side effects while producing positive long-term treatment outcomes.

Nursing Intervention for Schizophrenia

Although the prognosis for cure of chronic schizophrenia is poor, many of those with the disease can be treated as outpatients for much of their lives. In the healthcare setting, appropriate nursing interventions can minimize the nurse's stress in caring for such patients and maximize the patients' ability to cope. First, nurses need to be aware of their own feelings. Discouragement and frustration are common. Besides administering drugs and evaluating their effect, nurses can help create a therapeutic environment that minimizes anxiety. Consistent care from all members of the healthcare team will help establish trust, as will small efforts at meeting the patient's immediate needs, such as lighting a cigarette or listening to his or her fears. Establishing a relationship is difficult, because the patients tend to remain withdrawn even while expressing dependency needs. With a trusting relationship beginning, nurses can encourage the withdrawn person to become more involved with others. This process can be very slow, with repeated false starts and regressions. It is important to give the patient sufficient distance; pushing will only increase anxieties and distrust. Throughout the process, the nurse needs to remain open to involvement and caring toward the patient. Because of the

TABLE 9–5: ABNORMAL INVOLUNTARY MOVEMENT SCALE (AIMS)

Examination Procedure

- There are two parallel procedures, the examination procedure, which tells the patient what to do, and the scoring procedure, which tells the clinician how to rate what he or she observes.
- Either before or after completing the examination procedure, observe the patient unobtrusively at rest (e.g., in the waiting room).
- The chair to be used in this examination should be a hard, firm one without arms.

1. Ask the patient if there is anything in his/her mouth (gum or candy) and, if so, to remove it.
2. Ask about the *current* condition of the patient's teeth. Ask if he or she wears dentures. Ask whether teeth or dentures bother the patient now.
3. Ask whether the patient notices any movements in his or her mouth, face, hands, or feet. If yes, ask the patient to describe them and to indicate to what extent they currently bother the patient or interfere with activities.
4. Have the patient sit in chair with hands on knees, legs slightly apart and feet flat on floor. (Look at the entire body for movements while the patient is in this position.)
5. Ask the patient to sit with hands hanging unsupported — if male, between his legs, if female and wearing a dress, hanging over her knees. (Observe hands and other body areas).
6. Ask the patient to open his or her mouth. (Observe the tongue at rest within the mouth.) Do this twice.
7. Ask the patient to protrude his or her tongue. (Observe abnormalities of tongue movement.) Do this twice.
8. Ask the patient to tap his or her thumb with each finger as rapidly as possible for 10 to 15 seconds, first with right hand, then with left hand. (Observe facial and leg movements.) [±activated]
9. Flex and extend the patient's left and right arms, one at a time.
10. Ask the patient to stand up. (Observe the patient in profile. Observe all body areas again, hips included.)
11. Ask the patient to extend both arms out in front, palms down. (Observe trunk, legs and mouth.) [activated]
12. Have the patient walk a few paces, turn and walk back to the chair. (Observe hands and gait.) Do this twice. [activated]

Scoring Procedure

- Complete the examination procedure before making ratings.
- For the movement ratings (the first three categories below), rate the highest severity observed. 0 = none, 1 = minimal (may be extreme normal), 2 = mild, 3 = moderate, and 4 = severe. According to the original AIMS instructions, one point is subtracted if movements are seen only on activation.

Facial and Oral Movements

1. Muscles of facial expression, e.g., movements of forehead, eyebrows, periorbital area, cheeks. Include frowning, blinking, grimacing of upper face. 0 1 2 3 4
2. Lips and perioral area, e.g., puckering, pouting, smacking. 0 1 2 3 4
3. Jaw, e.g., biting, clenching, chewing, mouth opening, lateral movement. 0 1 2 3 4
4. Tongue. Rate only increase in movement both in and out of mouth, not inability to sustain movement. 0 1 2 3 4

Extremity Movements

5. Upper (arms, wrists, hands, fingers). Include movements that are choreic (rapid, objectively purposeless, irregular, spontaneous) or athetoid (slow, irregular, complex, serpentine). Do not include tremor (repetitive, regular, rhythmic movements). 0 1 2 3 4
6. Lower (legs, knees, ankles, toes), e.g., lateral knee movement, foot tapping, heel dropping, foot squirming, inversion and eversion of foot. 0 1 2 3 4

Trunk Movements

7. Neck, shoulders, hips, e.g., rocking, twisting, squirming, pelvic gyrations. Include diaphragmatic movements. 0 1 2 3 4

Global Judgments

8. Severity of abnormal movements. 0 1 2 3 4   based on the highest single score on the above items.
9. Incapacitation due to abnormal movements.
    0 = none, normal   1 = minimal   2 = mild   3 = moderate   4 = severe
10. Patient's awareness of abnormal movements.
    0 = no awareness   1 = aware, no distress   2 = aware, mild distress
    3 = aware, moderate distress   4 = aware, severe distress

Dental Status

11. Current problems with teeth and/or dentures? 0 = no   1 = yes
12. Does patient usually wear dentures?   0 = no   1 = yes

Note. From Guy, W. (1976). *ECDEU Assessment Manual for Psychopharmacology,* revised ed. Washington, DC, U.S. Department of Health, Education, and Welfare.

chronicity of schizophrenia, family-oriented treatment is paramount to successful outcomes. Education, stress management, and supportive therapy are the basis of treatment for the family. Older adults with schizophrenia challenge nurses to develop holistic plans of care. The overriding goal of treatment is to improve quality of life and functioning levels through the appropriate management of symptoms.

SUBSTANCE ABUSE: ALCOHOL AND DRUGS

Despite numerous studies, the extent of alcohol abuse in older adults is unclear, as alcohol and other drug abuse by the elderly is a largely hidden problem. It is known that older women drink less than men and that there is a general decline in alcohol use with age. Large studies have reported alcohol use ranging from 39% to 60% with approximately 7% of these to be at-risk drinkers (Resnick, 2002). At-risk drinkers are females who consume 9 or more drinks per week, or men who consume 12 or more drinks per week.

The most commonly held perception of drug abuse is that of illegal drugs, with young people or middle-aged people coming to mind as the most common drug abusers. Many do not think of senior adults as abusers of illegal drugs as relatively few chemically dependent elderly are treated in chemical dependency programs. Consequently, the issue of illegal drug use among senior adults is underresearched, and many researchers believe that the number of seniors who abuse illegal drugs is much higher than most in society believe. There is some evidence of elderly illicit drug use involving marijuana, LSD, opiates, and polydrug abuse. The older adult may use alcohol in combination with psychoactive drugs, amphetamines, or barbiturates. The federal government's National Household Survey on Drug Abuse estimates that 568,000 people aged 55 or older used illegal drugs in the past month

(SAMHSA, 2001). During the next decade, as the baby boomers age, that number is expected to increase significantly. The reason is that the boomer generation used more illicit drugs and alcohol than previous generations and many are bringing those habits with them into their later years.

The most common drug dependency problems among older adults result from the misuse of prescription drugs. This may be from lack of knowledge or lack of adherence or may be from receiving prescriptions from multiple providers.

Another category of substance abuse in the elderly population is the overuse of over-the-counter (OTC) drugs. One third of all money spent on medicine by the elderly was spent on OTC drugs such as analgesics, laxatives, sedatives, cold and allergy remedies, alcohol-based cough medicine, and caffeine. These OTC medicines can become a problem when they are used excessively. Daily laxative use, for instance, can cause dependency, with loss of normal bowel tone as well as electrolyte disturbances. Some of these drugs can interact in unhelpful ways with prescribed medications. When taking a nursing history, nurses should ask about OTC medications and how often the drugs are used.

Alcohol is the most common substance abused, with sedatives and antianxiety medications accounting for most of the rest. It is difficult to estimate accurately the prevalence of substance abuse in the elderly, partly because it is apparently an underdiagnosed problem. Physicians and counselors also find it hard to differentiate between chemical dependency problems and what would be normal physical and mental ailments for this age group.

The stigma attached to chemical dependency problems in older persons fosters denial and makes it difficult to determine the extent of dependency. Individuals often enable their chemically dependent spouses out of a sense of duty, thus increasing the likelihood of denial.

The clinical manifestations of alcoholism may be nonspecific, with patients appearing to have dementia, depression, or physical illness. Nonspecific signs and symptoms such as falls, injuries, unusual behavior, malnutrition, self-neglect, incontinence, diarrhea, and hypothermia can all be indications of an underlying problem with alcoholism. Accurate diagnosis of alcoholism in the elderly becomes even more difficult when a misdiagnosis of dementia is made. Several screening tools exist that can help health workers recognize patients who have difficulty dealing with alcohol. One is the CAGE questionnaire:

1. Have you ever tried to Cut down on your drinking?

2. Are you Annoyed when people ask you about your drinking?

3. Do you ever feel Guilty about your drinking?

4. Do you ever take a morning Eye-opener?

A yes answer to even one of these questions means that a more careful evaluation of the person's alcohol consumption is needed (Zimberg, 1996).

Alcohol can cause a wide range of problems, including intoxication, potential for injury, and physical withdrawal symptoms that may include delirium and hallucinations. Chronic alcohol abuse can also cause illnesses such as liver disease, ulcers, esophageal varices, damage to heart muscle, arrhythmias, and central nervous system (CNS) damage, such as memory loss and loss of coordination. Sedatives and anxiolytics, particularly the benzodiazepine tranquilizers, can cause problems of intoxication as well as withdrawal signs and symptoms ranging from malaise and insomnia to tachycardia, orthostatic hypotension, and delirium.

One of the major consequences of alcohol abuse is the development of liver disease. For the elderly with liver damage, many of the drugs used are metabolized at different rates. When alcohol is taken with other sedating drugs, a dangerous CNS depression can develop. For those with memory problems and loss of motivation for self-care, medications are often not taken as directed. For elderly alcoholic patients all these mechanisms combine to cause difficulties with prescribed drugs and the management of concurrent illness.

Other problems associated with drug and alcohol abuse that may negatively impact family and friends are depression, aggression, malnutrition, and economic difficulties. Legal problems can be numerous and may include criminal charges, revocation of driver's license, increased auto insurance rates, loss of the determination of capacity in guardianship and conservatorship proceedings, as well as in the execution of documents such as wills, durable powers of attorney for healthcare decisions, and living wills. Typically, only a "fair preponderance of the evidence" is necessary to prove incapacity, and many states include drug and alcohol abuse as a qualifying disability. Legal issues may also arise in dealing with agencies such as the Social Security Administration and insurance companies. Abusing alcohol or drugs may affect an individual's ability to collect particular benefits, or it may affect the manner in which they may collect benefits. Eligibility for certain welfare programs may be affected by alcohol or drug abuse. Supplemental Security Income (SSI), a federal welfare program administered by the Social Security Administration, cannot be administered to medically diagnosed alcohol or drug addicts unless they are undergoing appropriate treatment for their condition.

Alcohol or drug abuse may also affect life insurance claims. The amount that a beneficiary receives may depend on whether the policy contains a clause that precludes an alcohol or drug abuse-related death from qualifying as an accidental death. Alcohol or drug abuse may affect an individual's employment opportunities. Some employers may require a drug screening to determine if employees abuse alcohol or drugs be performed in order to secure or retain employment, affecting ability to become or remain employed.

Treatment of Abuse Problems

A trusting, non-judgmental relationship is the first step in treatment. The next is admission of the problem. The nurse's role is to assist the older adult in admitting and then seeking help with their problem. This is not often easy and sometimes has to be done in an indirect manner. Many life-changing events place the older adult at risk for chemical dependency. Aging brings on losses of life roles, family, friends, function, and self-identity. Coping with illness, pain, and financial constraints may limit their social and recreational options. These contribute to lower self-esteem, isolation, and depression, which increase the likelihood of alcohol and other drug abuse. The older adult may not be ready to admit to a alcohol or drug problem but may be open to learning positive coping methods.

The older adult is often viewed as a poor treatment risk because society sees them as physically, mentally, and economically unstable. However, successful treatment and recovery are highly possible for this population if interventions and treatments are positive and get to the root of their problems. During intervention and treatment, it is important to build social support networks for the elderly. Programs that reinforce skills and focus on reducing isolation decrease the risk of relapse. Involving spouses and other family members in the treatment and aftercare process helps to educate them about the effects of chemical dependency on the older person and on relationships within the family.

Group treatment, such as Alcoholic Anonymous (AA) meetings, raises levels of social interaction among individuals and helps them get positive support from peers. Some older adults prefer to be with those in their age group, while others may prefer to participate in multi-age groups. Churches, the community, and family are of central importance and can provide excellent support networks. These can be an integral part of a successful treatment and recovery process.

GAMBLING ADDICTIONS

Pathologic gambling and problem gambling affect approximately 5 to 15 million Americans and are identified in every social class and age (Unwin, Davis, & Leeuw, 2000). People with these conditions are unable to control their impulses to gamble and end up losing money, family, work, and social relationships. Many experts think that pathologic gambling is an addiction because of the "rush" felt when a person wins and loses money. Past experiences and personality type also play a large part. In recent years, the majority of states have legalized some form of lottery or casino gambling as an alternative means to raise tax revenues. Gambling has gone from a sin or a vice to government-condoned, mainstream entertainment. Competition for the ever-increasing number of players has resulted directly in the implementation of aggressive advertising tactics in order to maintain a profitable customer base by the gaming industry. As such, casinos and lotteries shift much of their focus to their most vulnerable and reliable spenders, the older adult.

Lured by freebies — bus rides, gambling chips and buffet lunches — seniors are filling casinos. They are also involved in many other types of gambling avenues: lotteries, especially scratch-offs, race tracks, bingo parlors, Internet casinos, jai alai, dog and horse tracks, illegal sports betting, and the stock market. Although seniors are responsible for at least 38% of all gamblers, they contribute a higher percentage of the profit, about 65%. The average individual gambling debt reported to a gambler's help line was $35,185. Data varies as to the extent of the problem, or the number of those meeting the criteria for pathological gambling, but although it is suggested it is not significant, all agree it is a growing problem (Petry, 2002).

Reasons Seniors Turn to Gambling

- Many seniors have disposable incomes.

- Some have limited financial resources or are looking for that big payoff to compensate an ever-shrinking limited retirement income.

- Opportunity and availability for elderly to gamble.

- Some are bored with lots of time on their hands after retirement.

- Health changes and psychological losses create the inability to participate in past leisure time activities. In the resulting void, gambling offers excitement.

- Some are lonely, have lost a spouse, close friends, or moved from other parts of the country to a new area of retirement, leaving family and friends behind.

- Limited alternatives for socializing.

- Seniors are subject to peer pressure and some are just looking to be with their peers in an exciting and fun activity.

With increasing numbers of older adults, gambling will become an increasing problem. There are many reasons for participation in gambling as seen above. In moderation, it can be an enjoyable avenue of socialization and fun, but for some it becomes an addiction. As the older adult is generally reluctant to divulge personal problems, they usually do not seek help on their own until it is too late: They lost everything — their homes, their life's savings, their families, their dignity, their self-respect, and their hope. They often gamble away their retirement savings, social security, and pensions at a time in life when this money cannot be recouped, leaving the person destitute and often suicidal. Depression, drinking, and taking drugs often go along with pathological gambling, adding to their problems.

Gambling Warning Signs

In an attempt to reach pathological gamblers before their lives, and the lives of their families are ruined, it is suggested that older adults should be screened, during regular visits, for their potential to become gambling addicts. The following warning signs are frequently seen as an adult develops a gambling problem:

- Loss of interest in meaningful activities such as work, hobbies, recreation, or religious activities.

- No longer attending routine family and social activities.

- Changing from gambling with others to gambling alone.

- Secrecy or deception when asked about gambling or financial activities.

- Intense interest in gambling-related matters, manifested in statements of repeated winnings, more frequent gambling trips, or spending more time and money gambling.

- Moodiness, irritability, anxiety, or depression, or expressions of hopelessness, and reference to death and suicide.

- Worsening of chronic health problems, including cardiac and respiratory problems, gastric distress, or more frequent minor illnesses.

- No longer using prescribed medications because money is used to gamble or pay gambling debts.

- Increased difficulty living within a household budget.

- Late notices of bills or telephone calls from creditors.

- Borrowing money, especially if the reason is unclear or seems inappropriate.

- Missing personal or household items.

- Liquidation of assets and/or the onset of bankruptcy proceedings.

- Neglect of self or home.

Many of these signs are seen in non-problem gambling adults. In the absence of outright gambling concerns voiced by the older adult and/or their family members, gambling problems can be overlooked! Advice to give to older adults who do enjoy gambling:

- Gamble only what you can afford to lose.

- Avoid "chasing" lost money.

- Accept loss as part of the game.

- Past results do not predict future results.

- Balance: time, money, and energy.

- Don't gamble to solve problems.

If a problem is suspected, assess the older adult by asking the following questions. A yes to any question after number 1 usually indicates a problem.

- Do you ever gamble?

- Have you ever felt the need to cut down on gambling?

- Have you felt annoyed if criticized about your gambling?

- Do you ever feel guilty about your gambling?

- Have you ever borrowed money to gamble?

- Have you ever gambled until your money was all gone?

The first step in treating gambling is admission of a problem. Self-help groups such as Gamblers Anonymous are useful for the gambler while Gam-Anon is useful for the family and/or friends of a gambler. There are also counselors specifically trained to assist dealing with gambling problems.

SUMMARY

Two categories of mental and emotional problems exist in geriatric populations: those that develop in older age, and those that develop earlier and have become "chronic" by later years. Although nurses may have more success in their

efforts to affect less chronic problems, Jenicke (1989) outlines four principles that form the basis for nurses' approach to elderly people with any type of mental or emotional problems:

1. Fostering a sense of control, self-efficacy and hope.

2. Establishing a relationship.

3. Providing or elucidating a sense of meaning.

4. Establishing constructive contingencies in the environment.

One technique that can help to accomplish much of this approach is the life review. Even in short patient-nurse interactions, reminiscing and life review can help the patient feel known, respected, and cared about. Therapeutic reminiscing is not just idle conversation; it involves a review of all the varied elements that contribute to the development of that individual. Life review is a way of looking back that allows comforting memories to be reexamined and sharing with others the commonality of experiences while recognizing the individual's uniqueness. Exploring the memories of the past with a group of elderly or an individual can help the person reconstruct their reality today through the examination of the past.

Finally, in dealing with patients with emotional and psychological problems, nurses need to remain constantly aware of their own emotional well-being. It is essential not to get drawn into emotional reactions that may be counter-therapeutic. It can be very challenging for a nurse to remain caring, involved, and therapeutic. If a nurse is unaware of feelings in reaction to a patient, it is difficult to focus on meeting the patient's need. For instance, nurses who have unexamined needs for control will have difficulty fostering a sense of autonomy in their patients. A nurse who holds negative beliefs about substance abusers will be unlikely to deal objectively with a person with a history of substance abuse. But a nurse who knows the limits of his or her own compassion and empathy will be much more likely to provide care according to patients' varied needs.

RESOURCES

American Schizophrenia Association:
  1-407-393-6167

Center for Substance Abuse Treatment, National Treatment Hotline:
  1-800-662-HELP

Cocaine National Hotline:
  1-800-COCAINE

Emotional Distress Hotline:
  1-800-LIFENET

Gamblers Anonymous:
  1-213-386-8789
  Web: http://www.gamblersanonymous.org/

Mental Health Infosource:
  1-800-447-4474

NAMI (National Alliance for the Mentally Ill) Helpline:
  1-800-950-NAMI (6264)
  Web: http://www.nami.org/

National Clearinghouse for Alcohol and Drug Information:
  1-800-729-6686
  Web: http://www.health.org

National Council on Problem Gambling:
  1-800-522-4700
  Web: http://www.ncpgambling.org/

National Institute of Mental Health (NIMH):
  1-866-615-6464
  Web: http://www.nimh.nih.gov/

National Institute of Mental Health Panic Disorder Helpline:
  1-800-64-PANIC
  Web: http://www.nimh.nih.gov/anxiety/
    anxietymenu.cfm

National Obsessive Compulsive Disorder (OCD) Information Hotline:
  1-800-NEWS-4-OCD
  Web: http://www.nimh.nih.gov/publicat/
    ocdmenu.cfm

National Senior Gambling Task Force:
  1-800-522-4700
  Web: http://www.seniorgambling.org/index.asp

National Sleep Foundation:
  1-202-347-3471
  Web: http://www.sleepfoundation.org/

Suicide Hotline:
  1-800-SUICIDE (784-2433)

EXAM QUESTIONS

CHAPTER 9
Questions 59-70

59. The mind-body connection

    a. is not clearly defined for depression.

    b. has not received much attention for affective disorders.

    c. explains why healing can occur through power of thought.

    d. may cause physical symptoms in a depressed person.

60. You are concerned about your 95-year-old client's ability to achieve ego integrity as you have noticed that he

    a. is flexible in adapting to the environment.

    b. makes as many decisions as possible independently.

    c. knows, and accepts, what he can and can not physically do.

    d. has been rude and insensitive towards his neighbors.

61. The use of coping mechanisms tends to remain stable throughout life. Older adults generally cope with common life events based on

    a. the number of losses they have experienced.

    b. avoiding stress and keeping feelings bottled up inside.

    c. the number of personal friends and support systems.

    d. experiencing stress and learning useful ways to react.

62. A good question to start with during a mental health assessment is to ask the client

    a. how are you feeling today?

    b. what do you do when you are feeling stressed?

    c. who do you go to when you need help?

    d. do you belong to any support groups?

63. Delirium is characterized by

    a. slow onset.

    b. acute onset.

    c. progressive course.

    d. excess sleeping.

64. Sleep patterns in the older adult

    a. are stable throughout adult life.

    b. increase in both quality and quantity.

    c. may be improved without using medications.

    d. are disturbed in less than 50% of older adults.

65. A safe first treatment for the mildly depressed older adult is

    a. increased physical activity.

    b. enteric-coated tablets.

    c. short course ECT.

    d. MAOIs.

66. The patient with the highest risk for suicide is the

    a. 18-year-old female, failing college.

    b. 30-year-old executive, recently divorced.

    c. 90-year-old man, facing moving to a nursing home.

    d. 22-year-old male homosexual, coming out to parents.

67. Anxiety induced disorders include

    a. bi-polar disorders.

    b. personality disorders.

    c. obsessive-compulsive disorders.

    d. schizophrenia.

68. A male nursing home resident has symptoms of moderate anxiety. To reduce his anxiousness you would

    a. provide lively music with kindergarten group.

    b. ignore the anxiety as he is probably seeking attention.

    c. give PRN medication and use physical restraint if needed.

    d. provide choice of relaxation intervention.

69. Alcohol usage in the older adult

    a. is very easy to detect in this population.

    b. may be hard to distinguish from other age related conditions.

    c. has little impact on the older adult, his/her family or society.

    d. is very rarely a problem that needs attention.

70. Excessive gambling in the older adult is

    a. limited to those who can afford to lose the money.

    b. only a problem to those who have access to casinos.

    c. a growing problem caused by a variety of reasons.

    d. a good means to supplement their incomes.

CHAPTER 10

PSYCHOSOCIAL ISSUES OF THE OLDER ADULT

CHAPTER OBJECTIVE

After studying this chapter, the reader will be able to discuss how social factors affect an older adult's psychological well-being.

LEARNING OBJECTIVES

After studying this chapter, the learner will be able to

1. discuss the impact social support has on the physical and emotional health of older adults.

2. explain the 5 stages of grief as they pertain to coping with the multiple losses of aging.

3. explain the various types of abuse of older adults and factors that make them vulnerable to abuse.

4. discuss barriers and myths as they pertains to sexuality in the older adult.

5. describe the meaning of spirituality as it applies to older adults and identify symptoms of spiritual distress.

INTRODUCTION

Psychosocial issues are factors involving the relationship of the older adult's role and status to that of a group or community. These factors are developed through past experiences that effect emotions, behavior, thoughts, attitude, and how a situation may be perceived and understood. Older adults and their family members and caregivers often encounter new and challenging psychosocial issues that accompany aging. The topics in this chapter are significant, as they may exert a positive or a negative force in successful aging.

SOCIAL FUNCTIONING AND SUPPORT

Humans are social creatures that intrinsically give and receive support to others. Social functioning and support is critical for the older adult for several reasons. First, it correlates with physical and mental functioning. Secondly, social well-being enhances the ability to cope with health problems and to maintain autonomy. Third, it increases social activity participation.

Social Support

The term social support is any action or behavior that serves to assist another in meeting his or her personal goals or in dealing with the demands of a situation. This can be in the form of emotional support, (empathy, love, understanding, listening, advocating), instrumental support (tangible aid and help such as money, transportation, food) and informational support to aid with coping or managing. A social network is the means by which social support is distributed and exchanged, and is made up of individuals and groups. The two types of

171

social support are formal and informal. Despite the existence of an extensive formal support system in this country, older adults receive the bulk of their support informally. This type of support is given by family, friends, neighbors, and group affiliations with groups such as a church. These types of support are what allow many older adults, who live alone, to remain independent. This also removes a tremendous amount of burden off of the healthcare system in general.

Social support is a dynamic phenomenon that changes in intensity, frequency, number, and complexity over time. Family composition, marital status, ethnicity, gender, and home setting all play an important role in shaping support systems. Although social support is considered essential for survival, its role for older adults is critical. When an older adult does not have enough informal support to fulfill his or her needs, then formal support is necessary. An example of this is an older adult who has no family or friends to set up medications for the week. This person would need formal in-home services to provide this service in order to maintain independence and remain in his home. Unfortunately, some forms of support have a negative impact on the older adult. This might be a friend that encourages maladaptive coping mechanisms, such as drinking one's problems away. This might be a well-meaning trusted neighbor whose advice is based on limited or inaccurate knowledge. It could also be the helpful person that is actually taking advantage of the older adult's vulnerability. Examples of informal support that may be given:

- Yard/house work/laundry/cooking/cleaning etc.

- Record keeping, finances, correspondence, advocating, representing.

- Transportation, attending community events, shopping, meals, assistance with medications.

- Help with ADLs, respite, financial assistance.

- Emotional support, listening, advising, helping to cope, love, companionship.

Assessing informal social support is important, especially for the patient who lives at home. It helps determine what formal services are required to keep them in their communities. It is important to ask directly about loneliness, as a patient can have support systems in place but still feel lonely. Particular attention should be paid to widowers as they have significantly fewer social resources and contacts (Fry, 2001). Many older adults find it hard to admit that they are lonely. When assessing support:

- Ask about types of informal support: who provides, what type of support, how often.

- Identify the major support of the individual.

- Identify recent losses or additions to support system.

- Identify conflicts within system: who involved, nature of conflict.

- Determine the amount of support needed versus amount available.

- Identify any negative emotional impact from needing support such as on self-esteem, depression, helplessness, identity, role in family.

- Are there other potential support currently available but not being utilized.

- Ask if they feel lonely. Have enough friends. Or are feeling bored or isolated.

If the older adult lacks services that cannot be arranged informally, then formal services will need to be provided. For clients who feel lonely, provide with community opportunities to engage in hobbies, volunteer, join clubs of interest and senior centers. For the older adult who is home bound, senior companion programs, pet therapy visits, and intergenerational and church based programs are all possible options to bring more contacts into the home. A referral to a recreational therapist is a good method of improving social contacts and reintegrating the older adult into the community.

Social Isolation Older adults who continue to interact with others tend to be healthier, both physically and mentally. Advances in medicine enable more Americans to live longer. But, unfortunately many older adults are living lonelier as increasing numbers of older people outlive partners in important social relationships. For many, the golden years are becoming cold years of social isolation and loneliness. Social isolation has been linked to a variety of adverse health outcomes, including depression and cardiovascular disease (Sorkin, Rooks, & Lu, 2002). Social isolation is not having enough opportunities to interact and engage other people. There are numerous reasons for this, a few being: transportation difficulties, immobility, decreased cognitive or physical functioning, lack of finances, poor health, sensory impairments, difficulty communicating, loss of family and friends, transfer to a new environment, and depression. A person may live with numerous other people and yet still be socially isolated. Many of the characteristics of long-term care facilities have the potential to facilitate social networks, such as activity programs, group dining, and common living areas. Unfortunately, these characteristics are not always successful, as many older adults in this setting feel isolated. Three factors have been found to increase levels of loneliness among elderly individuals residing in a nursing home: lack of intimate relationships, increased dependency, and loss. Loneliness in this setting is associated with social isolation, cognitive deterioration, hopelessness and the inability to perform independent activities of daily living (Hicks, 2000). In a 2001 study it was found that 35% of residents in assisted living centers met the criteria for social isolation compared to 17.5% of those living at home (Tremethick, 2001). Interventions to assist older adults in long-term care facilities to reduce social isolation are:

- Educating staff members in all departments to be aware of the socialization needs of all residents.

- Assisting residents in maintaining contact with important relationships, on the outside. This could be through telephone calls, assisting to write letters, and/or arranging visits. (Relationships with friends do not necessarily require face to face visits. Emotional benefits do not depend on the number of contacts, but rather on the quality of intimacy.)

- Facilitate opportunities to meet and make new friendships. This could be through introductions, dining room seating arrangements, clubs and activity participation, support groups, and others. Activities that offer the opportunity to talk about the past and that offer choices and control provide good opportunities for friendships.

- Residents with dementia and those with very low functioning also need social contacts and can benefit from being read to by other residents or included in discussion groups.

- Don't forget the opportunity to make friendships with persons of other generations or cultures. Many local schools have community service requirements of their students or have clubs that engages in these types of activities.

- For residents with isolation, depression, or apathy, obtain a physician order for recreational therapy to evaluate and treat. This is the most effective method of insuring that this gets carried out.

Coping with Losses

One of the many difficult situations that older adults have to face, as they grow old, is loss. This may be loss due to the death of a spouse, pet, close friend, relative, or other important person. It could be the loss of function such as no longer having the ability to walk independently, to be incontinent or lose one's hearing or vision. It may be a loss of a role such as no longer having an occupation or no longer earning money. Or perhaps there has been a role reversal with the adult child taking care of the parent. It may mean the loss of independence, giving up driving or another important hobby, giving up the family home, giving up alcohol or smoking, or life-long favorite foods. Older adults do not cope as well as young people. This is due to the added years of meaning behind the loss, fewer years with which to move on, and fewer options for replacing the loss. Losses can have multiple ramifications—psychological and social, as well as physical. The loss of a driver's license due to physical or cognitive health can gravely affect a person's self-esteem, sense of responsibility, and independence. It means much more than just giving up a license.

Bereavement is considered to be one of the most traumatic experiences in one's life at all ages. Each year 800,000 people become widowed, adding to the 10.5 million existing older adults in widowhood (Prigerson, Maciejewski, & Rosencheck, 2000). The death of a spouse can affect all aspects of the surviving spouse's present and future functioning. Many older adults never fully recover from death of a spouse or a close friend. Loss and bereavement usually produce intense feelings of grief and depression. Death of persons who previously had provided them with an important source of interpersonal intimacy produces feelings of isolation and loneliness. Many losses are predictable and family and caregivers can assist in helping the adjustment go smoothly.

Interventions for grieving older adults

Provide the older adult with plenty of opportunities to express their emotions and concerns both before and after any loss, no matter what they are feeling. It can not only be cathartic but also lead to greater personal insight.

- Listening offers direct comfort and support.

- Loss of the work role due to retirement, and the identity crisis that may accompany retirement, can be eased through pre-retirement counseling, activity planning, volunteer work, and encouragement to pursue leisure interests.

- Research shows that older adults who find comfort from prayer and church attendance, will adjust to widowhood easier (Fry, 2001). Offering spiritual opportunities before and after losses.

- Include a wide variety of social support: family, peers, informal relationships, neighbors, formal support groups and opportunities for new productive and meaningful social roles.

- Encourage initiating the readjustment process as early as possible by trying to get back to normal routine activities.

- Help identify areas and activities of interest in which one can get physically and mentally involved.

- Assist in re-establishing contacts/relationships with friends/relatives with whom one can relate well.

- Encourage participation in social activities.

- Provide opportunity to participate in support group meetings.

- Assess for depression and suicide ideation.

Initially, when a person dies, loved ones go through a stage of shock and numbness, even when the death was expected. (See Table 10-1.) As the numbness wears off, it is usually followed by a period of yearning and holding on to memories of the deceased. This period may also be characterized by protest, with feelings of guilt, loneliness, anxiety, fear, and irritability. The bereaved can also have ambivalent feelings about the deceased, having anger at being left behind. Another form of ambivalence can occur when the family had a poor relationship with the deceased. For some women, for instance, widowhood can be a release from the stressors of a difficult marriage and a chance to explore and meet their own needs. Such ambivalent feelings can increase feelings of guilt. Nurses can support the bereaved by accepting all of the

TABLE 10-1: THE STAGES OF GRIEF

The process of grief is not a cut and dried process that can be subdivided into strict categories. Rather, the grief process is a continuum, with each person experiencing it in a different way and in a different order. Dividing the grief process into "stages" helps the grief stricken person to understand that their experiences and emotions are normal. It also helps caregivers understand their client's needs better. Some people will quickly progress through all the phases, while others appear to get "stuck" in a particular phase. Briefly, the stages of grief are as follows:

1. **SHOCK AND DENIAL:** The reality of death has not yet been accepted by the bereaved. He or she feels stunned and bewildered-as if everything is "unreal."

2. **ANGER:** The grief stricken person often lashes out at family, friends, themselves, God, the doctor, the hospital or the world in general. Bereaved people will also experience feelings of guilt or fear during this stage.

3. **BARGAINING:** In this stage, the bereaved asks for a deal or reward from either God, the hospital, doctor or the Clergy. Comments like "I'll go to Church every day, if only my husband will come back to me" are common.

4. **DEPRESSION:** Depression occurs as a reaction to the changed way of life created by the loss. The bereaved person feels intensely sad, hopeless, drained, and helpless. The deceased is missed and thought about constantly.

5. **ACCEPTANCE:** Acceptance comes when the changes brought upon the person by the loss are stabilized into a new lifestyle. The depth and intensity of the mourning process depends on many factors. Age, circumstances surrounding the death, relationship of the deceased to the survivor and to other family members, are all significant. Recently experiencing the death of another significant person in the owner's life can also affect how the current death is handled.

(Kubler-Ross, 1997)

bereaved person's feelings and allowing him or her to explain those feelings, without advance expectations by the nurse. Persons may report dreams and visualizations and even hallucinations of the loved one and preoccupation with possessions of the dead person, with places and experiences shared. Physically, survivors often experience many symptoms such as nausea, restlessness, sleep disturbances, and appetite changes. Symptoms of grief may lead to false labels of dementia (Hegge, & Fischer, 2000). Socially, the bereaved may withdraw or may enter into a frenzied period of activity. Usually, there is a gradual decline in mourning and a return of interest in life, a resumption of previous patterns of living. Sometimes bereavement is prolonged. Major indicators of this include:

- Severe identification phenomenon, incorporating traits of the deceased.

- Multiple physical signs and symptoms without apparent illness.

- Prolonged social isolation.

- Self-destructive behavior such as excess drinking or inadequate food consumption.

- Severe insomnia and/or anorexia.

- Prolonged feelings of depression, despair, worthlessness, or guilt.

- Denial of grief feelings.

The nurse's role in the case of prolonged grief is to encourage the grieving person to get help, both in terms of professional therapeutic help and from the person's informal support system. Hospice nurses often remain actively involved with families during the period of bereavement. If nurses are aware of the losses their patients have suffered and understand the emotional, social, and physical effects of bereavement, they can adapt their plans of care to focus on the needs of the grieving patient and family. One caution is that a bereaved person may say he or she is fine because that is the socially expected response when, in fact, the person is still deep in the process of grieving. Nurses can help in such instances by accepting the bereaved person's sad and angry thoughts, by giving the person social permission to grieve. It is never helpful to tell a grieving person that he or she has grieved too long; it's better to focus on the potential of a positive outcome.

ELDER ABUSE

Elder abuse has become an increasingly visible problem and is recognized as a legitimate concern of nurses as healthcare providers. Elder abuse, a social atrocity that can lead to death, remains deeply shrouded in the secrecy that surrounds family violence. Estimates range from 1.5 – 2.5 million cases per year, but it is also believed that less than one case in 14 is reported to a public agency (Aravanis, Adelman, Breckman, Fulmer, Holder, Lachs, et al., 1993).

One way to look at abuse or mistreatment is to look for unmet needs of the older adult. Unmet needs may include inadequacy of nutrition, personal care, medical attention, and psychosocial needs. This way of looking at abuse and neglect enables the healthcare practitioner to remain non-judgmental while helping the individual meet those needs. Generally 5 categories of elder abuse and mistreatment are recognized: physical abuse, neglect, emotional and psychological abuse, financial exploitation, and sexual abuse. The three domains of elder abuse are institutional abuse, domestic abuse, and self abuse. Keep in mind that it is not rare for elderly individuals to experience several types of abuse at the same time.

PHYSICAL ABUSE

Physical abuse is defined as the willful, non-accidental use of force to inflict pain, injury, impairment, or unreasonable confinement of an individual. This constitutes 15.7% of reported cases of abuse in older adults. Physical abuse or mistreatment typically includes hitting, slapping, beating, pushing, punching, shoving, shaking, kicking, pinching, and burning. The inappropriate use of drugs or physical restraints, force-feeding, and any other type of physical punishment are examples of physical abuse. It is important to assess and interview the individual privately and immediately if abuse is suspected. The following are suspicious signs and symptoms to watch for that could indicate abuse:

- The individual is brought to the hospital emergency room by someone other than the caregiver, or the person is found alone.

- There is a prolonged period between injury or illness and presentation for medical care.

- There is a suspicious history. Doctor or facility "hopping" as well as explanations of injuries that are not consistent with the injury are suspect.

- There is noncompliance with prescribed medications or suggested treatments.

- Cuts, lacerations, abrasions, puncture wounds, fractures, and dislocations.

- Bruises, welts, or discoloration on face, upper arms, or ankles.

- Burns from cigarettes, acid, friction of ropes or chains, etc.

- Injuries to head, scalp, face, absence of hair and/or hemorrhaging below scalp.

- Injury not properly cared for or hidden, or signs of old injuries.

- Loss of weight, dehydration or malnourishment without etiology.

- Soiled, torn clothing.

NEGLECT
(ACTS OF OMISSION)

Frequently emergency rooms are the primary point of entry to the healthcare system for the elderly abused or neglected person. Neglect refers to "omissions" either by self or others. It describes situations in which the basic needs of an elder are not being met. This is the largest category of reported abuse with 58.5% of the cases (Lynch, 1997; Quinn & Tomita, 1997). The lack of attention can be to the person or his environment. Neglectful actions can include lack of adequate nutrition, personal care, medications, medical attention or a safe well-maintained home or place to live. Neglect may be either intentional or unintentional. The neglect may be intentional if withholding the necessities of life and physical care is done willfully. Unintentional neglect is usually done due to lack of experience or information of the caregiver. In cases of self-neglect, the decision to intervene, following recognition of the problem, may be more difficult than in cases of caregiver neglect or physical abuse. The need to respect the person's right to self-determination may supersede your need as a healthcare provider to ensure patient safety. Assessing the functional and educational needs of any elder experiencing self-neglect is vital.

Possible Indicators of Neglect

- Inadequately clothed
- Untreated medical condition
- Rashes, sores, or lice
- Inadequately nourished or hydrated
- Fecal or urine odor
- Unsanitary and hazardous living environment
- Signs of over-medication, under-medication, or misuse of medication
- Isolated for long period of time without stimulation

EMOTIONAL AND
PSYCHOLOGICAL ABUSE

Psychological abuse inflicts emotional pain and distress on the elderly individual. It may be difficult to detect unless witnessed. Psychological abuse includes name-calling, saying unkind things about the older adult within their hearing, and mocking them (Quinn & Tomita, 1997). Threats, insults, or humiliation are psychological abuse. Ignoring or isolating an elderly person and excluding them from day-to-day activities is psychological neglect. Manifestations of this type of abuse can be confusion, disorientation, fearfulness, trembling, and fidgeting when certain subjects are discussed, changing the subject frequently and cowering when the caregiver is present. Lack of eye contact, withdrawal, and clinging are signs as well.

Possible Indicators of Psychological Abuse

- Low self-esteem
- Suicidal behavior
- Confusion or disorientation
- Over-anxious or withdrawn
- Depression
- Severe mood changes
- Denial
- Agitation
- Fear

FINANCIAL
EXPLOITATION

Financial abuse occurs when family members, caregivers, or "friends" take control of the assets of an elder either through coercion, misrepresentation, or outright stealing (Lynch, 1997). The victims often have cognitive or physical impairments. Financial abuse occurs in about 12.3% of reported cases of elder abuse.

Possible Indicators of Financial Exploitation

- Unusual activity in bank accounts

- Checks signed by an older adult who is incapable of writing

- Unmatched signatures

- Changes to will when the older adult is incapable of making those decisions

- Changes in power of attorney when the person is incapacitated

- Unusual concern of caregiver in regards to cost of care

- Overdue bills, unpaid bills, or disconnection notices

- Placement in an institution that does not correspond to estate

- Missing cash and possessions such as jewelry, furniture, art, or silverware

- Lack of basic amenities such as grooming items and clothing that exhibit disparity between assets and lifestyle

- Withdrawals of large sums of money indicating radical changes by an older adult including sudden use of ATM and credit cards

- Sudden transfer of assets to distant relatives or caregivers

- Large bills for care either not given or poorly given

- Forged signatures and documents to be signed by the older adult which they do not understand

Any allegation by an elder of financial exploitation should be taken seriously. Typically, someone who the older adult trusts is handling his or her finances with or without authorization. The financial abusers have strong personalities and offer the elder someone to rely on and become dependent on. The data on the extent of financial exploitation are difficult to determine. Banks, lawyers, and judges, who typically see financial abuse and report to the police, are not mandated to report, in most states, to the agencies who keep the statistics about abuse and neglect.

SEXUAL ABUSE

Sexual abuse is defined as nonconsensual sexual contact with an older adult. Sexual contact with any person incapable of giving consent is also considered sexual abuse (National Center on Elder Abuse, 2002). Sexual abuse includes unwanted touching, rape, sodomy, coerced nudity, and sexually explicit photographing. An abuser needs less physical strength to subdue an older adult during a sexual assault. Intimidation may be the only threat needed to make the person submit to the abuse.

Possible Indicators of Sexual Abuse

- Torn, stained, or bloody underclothing

- Difficulty in walking or sitting

- Pain, itching, bruising, or bleeding in genital area or breasts

- Unexplained venereal disease (VD) or genital infections

- Inappropriate displays of affection by the caregiver

Miscellaneous Indicators of Abuse

The National Center on Elder Abuse (2002) has identified two important characteristics that occur in several types of elder abuse that can be seen in any practice setting. These are frequent and unexplained crying and an unexplained suspicion, or fear of a particular person in the care setting. The following are other general signs and may apply to any of the five specific categories of abuse:

- History of alcoholism or drug abuse by the caregiver.

- Caregiver refusing to allow person to speak for himself, or without the presence of the caregiver

- Obvious absence of assistance by the caregiver

- Aggressive behavior of caregiver such as threats, insults, or harassment

- Obvious indifference toward the elderly person by the caregiver

- Obvious anger toward the elderly person by the caregiver

LEGAL OBLIGATIONS

Strategies for dealing with elder abuse and neglect must balance the elderly individual's needs for safety against their need for autonomy and self decision-making. Regardless of this dilemma, most states have mandatory reporting laws which require the full disclosure of suspected elder mistreatment. State legislation addresses specific elder abuse statutes for both community and institutionalized elderly. The laws of each state indicate the age limits to be considered elderly, but it is not less than 60 years of age in any state (Capezuti, Brush, & Lawson, 1997). All 50 states have Adult Protective Service (APS) laws that outline which practitioners are mandatory reporters. In all but 8 states, mandatory reporters include medical professionals, healthcare providers, service providers, and all government agents. This would include nurses, physicians, psychologists, social workers, and pharmacists, who are required by law to report possible cases of elder abuse or mistreatment. APS or the responsible state agency is mandated to investigate all reports often within specific time frames. Civil and criminal penalties are given for failure to report. Mandatory and voluntary reporting is based on suspected abuse or neglect identified by the reporter. APS or another agency is responsible for investigation and validation of the mistreatment. APS laws provide immunity for reporting suspected abuse or neglect in "good faith." You, the nurse, must be able to show that you acted without malice

and with good intentions. Additionally, some states assure confidentiality to reporters and the reports.

All states and the District of Columbia have laws authorizing the Long-Term Care Ombudsman Program (LTCOP). The LTCOP is responsible for advocating on behalf of long-term care facility residents who experience abuse, violations of their rights, or other problems. LTCOPs are mandated in each state as a condition of receiving federal funds under the Vulnerable Elder Rights Protection Title, created by the 1992 amendments to the Older Americans Act. It addresses the need for strong advocacy to protect and enhance the basic rights and benefits of vulnerable older people. LTCOPs are an integral part of the systemic response to institutional elder abuse. LTCOPs may discover an abusive situation when responding to complaints within a facility and then, if appropriate, make a referral to an APS program, a law enforcement agency, or the agency responsible for licensing and certifying such facilities. Moreover, in some states, the LTCOP actually fulfills the role of adult protective services and has the legal authority to investigate and respond to abuse occurring within long term care facilities.

The Joint Commission for Accreditation of Health Care Organizations (JCAHO) has set standards that require emergency room nurses to make reports of elder mistreatment or domestic violence. Recent studies have suggested that a significant portion of elder abuse may be accounted for as spousal abuse that could have been occurring for years. Healthcare providers need to recognize this possibility and screen all women and persons over age 60 for possible abuse, utilizing individual facility policies and procedures. Many policies and procedures exist to promote the documentation and reporting of elder mistreatment or abuse. These procedures include:

- Call the abuse Hot Line listed in your telephone directory.

- Notify the individual in your agency or facility, usually a social worker or administrator, who has been delegated the responsibility of handling abuse problems.

- If immediate danger is suspected, call the police.

- Contact the state agency such as APS for assistance.

When documenting, include all circumstances, including name, sex, race and address of the abused, as well as the current location of the abused and the type of abuse that occurred or is suspected. Make sure your documentation is accurate, detailed, and objective. As much as possible, write down the exact words of the elder and their caregiver. All nurses should know the community resources available to the abused person and to the abuser. Know the limits on your states APS laws in regard to emergency shelter, help with basics like food or clothing, medical and psychiatric care, case management services, and legal assistance.

VICTIMS AND ABUSERS

Who are the abusers and who are the victims? The median age of victims is 77.9 years old. Of these 65.8% are Caucasian, 17.4% African American, 10.5% Hispanic American, and 6.3% for other. Female victims made up 67% of all elder abuse cases (Teaster, 2000).

Relationship to the Abused:

Adult children	47.0%
Spouse	19.0%
Other relative	9%
Service provider	4%
Grandchildren	9%
Friend/neighbor	6%
Sibling	6%

Source: Administration on Aging (1998) The National Elder Abuse Incidence Study; Final Report, 1998. Washington, DC: AOA.

THEORIES ON THE POSSIBLE CAUSES OF ELDER ABUSE

Domestic abuse is the most common form of elder abuse; 90% of all elder abuse cases involve a family member. Societal changes may play a part in the commonness of elder abuse in our time. Historically, families took care of their elders within the long-term family, with everyone sharing the responsibility. Increased mobility, strained economic times, dual-income family requirements, and smaller nuclear families forces the supervision of the older adult to fall onto a select few. Care is customarily transferred to an institution or family member who is willing to take on the task. A combination of different theories can be used to examine the cause of elder abuse incidents.

Stress of the caregiver. Caring for older people can be a stressful, exhausting, and frustrating task. The more physically or cognitively impaired, the harder and more challenging the task becomes. If the caregiver has personal problems, an underlying mental illness, a lack of understanding or knowledge of the elderly person's condition, financial burdens, unmet personal needs, or does not receive support from others, the stress may become overwhelming. Internal factors of the caregiver such as ineffective coping skills, emotional problems, and personal problems can increase the stress of the situation for the caregiver. External factors that may also increase stress to the caregiver include mental or physical impairment of the elder, financial burden, and lack of family and community support.

Impairment of dependent elders. The General Accounting Office recently published a study that found 80% of the estimated 6 million dependent elders in the United States are cared for in the domestic setting. Many of these individuals have cognitive or physical impairments. Researchers have found that elders with cognitive impairments are more likely to be abused than those who are cognitively intact (Coyne, 2001). Poor health leads to an increased dependence on the caregiver, which obviously can cause more stress.

Cycle of violence. This theory holds that some families are more prone to violence than others, and that elder abuse is a normative behavioral pattern in these families.

Personal problems of the abuser. Research has supported that abusers of older adults tend to have more personal problems than do non-abusers. Professionals have observed that adult children who abuse their parents frequently suffer from problems such as mental disorders, emotional disorders, alcoholism, drug addiction, and financial difficulties.

The significance of spousal abuse in relation to elder abuse needs to be recognized by all nurses. Although abuse in institutional settings has been recognized for many years, it is only recently that domestic violence and spousal abuse towards the elderly have become evident. Caregiver burden and stress are significant in abusive relationships in the community, but spousal abuse that has occurred for years can be much more dangerous and deadly.

WHERE ELDER ABUSE IS OCCURRING

Institutional abuse refers to any of the five categories of abuse that occur in residential facilities established for older adults such as nursing homes, foster homes, group homes, and board-and-care facilities. Perpetrators of institutional abuse are persons with a legal or contractual obligation to provide the victim with care and protection and include paid caregivers, accessory staff, and other professionals. In the institutional setting, an elder person may experience abuse from three sources: staff-to-patient abuse, patient-to-patient abuse, or visitor-to-patient abuse.

National data on institutional elder abuse is not yet available; however, a General Accounting Office report presented to the Senate Special Committee on Aging found that over 2,000 nursing homes have been acknowledged as repeatedly harming their residents. The Office of State Long-Term Care Ombudsman maintains complaint data in every state. These complaints are made by or on behalf of nursing home residents, and some data pertains to the abuse, neglect, or exploitation of older persons in the institutional setting. The Nursing Home Quality Protection Act was passed in 2001 and sets forth minimum staff requirements, sanctions for non-compliance, Internet disclosure requirements, and several other provisions for the care and safety of nursing home residents. Federal law also requires that all nursing homes have a Residents' Bill of Rights.

Studies have identified nursing assistants as making up the largest group of abusers and male employees as responsible for the majority of abuse incidents (Payne & Cikovic, 1996). The abusers justified their actions as responses to stressful situations in which they had been provoked. Administrators and owners of nursing homes must provide better working conditions, stress management techniques, and humane treatment of staff in order to provide more humane treatment to residents in long-term care. Modification of the attitudes of the staff toward the residents is imperative, as is changing staff attitudes towards anyone who abuses the elderly. Recognition of the harmful and debilitating effects of physically restraining residents in long term care settings has improved the quality of life and lessened injuries from this form of physical abuse.

Despite this disturbing occurrence of abuse in residential settings, the fact is that most abuse of the elderly occurs in their homes by their own family. However, with astonishing frequency, abuse occurs in the home by paid caregivers. Theft of personal effects is the most common problem in the home

(Ebersole & Hess, 1998). Often, older adults are accused of being "paranoid" or "confused" about where they have put their belongings. Most older adults live at home and receive care at home as they age. Most of this care is given by the family who may or may not be willing and able to assume this care. While many steps have been taken to combat elder abuse and neglect, much remains hidden and secret. Violence and neglect in the home are volatile issues. The home, especially in this country, has been seen as safe from government interference, a haven. Because behavior inside the home has traditionally been private and beyond the reach of public policy, secrecy and isolation are common in a victim/abuser relationship. The nurse may be the initial visitor in the home to recognize the problem of elder abuse. Becoming a patient advocate for individual rights and autonomy, as well as protection, requires skill and dedication.

Interventions

The first phase of intervention is identification of the elder abuse.

Since elder abuse tends to be episodic and reoccurring, review of past emergency room visits and accidents must be undertaken (Quinn & Tomita, 1997).

The risk factors for abuse that need to be considered are:

The family history:

Is there a history of violence or mental illness?

The living arrangements:

Who lives in the home? Is either person isolated?

The lifestyle of the potential victim or abuser:

What recent stressful events have occurred and what happened as a result?

What do family interactions reveal about how stressors are handled?

What are the emotional stressors in the current situation?

What is the health status of each?

What is the cognitive status of the potential victim?

The resources available:

What is the financial status of the potential victim/abuser?

How dependent are they on one another?

What social support system is available to either victim or abuser?

Some questions to consider asking:

1. Are you afraid of anyone?

2. Has anyone close to you tried to hurt or harm you recently?

3. Has anyone close to you called you names or put you down or made you feel bad recently?

4. Does anyone make you stay in bed or tell you you're sick when you know you aren't?

5. Has anyone forced you to do things you didn't want to do?

6. Has anyone taken things that belong to you without your OK?

Nurses need to overcome the barriers to recognition and intervention of abuse and violence. The barriers according to Shea, Mahoney, and Lacey (1997) are personal, social and sociocultural. Being knowledgeable about elder abuse or domestic violence does not necessarily reduce the incidence of these occurrences. Nurses who have had a personal experience with domestic violence, which many nurses have, may be acutely sensitive to caring for victims. Powerful emotions such as anger, shame and helplessness may prevent the nurse from caring and advocating for an abuse victim. Social norms about the use of physical punishment and the family's right to privacy may prevent the recognition or reinforce the conspiracy of silence fostered by the abuser. Some nurses may blame the victim for not seeking help sooner. In some institutions there may be medical, economic, political, legal, and ethical barriers to identifying abuse. There may be sanctions for your attempt to go beyond the medical aspects of care because they take time and resources that are limited. As mentioned before, JCAHO and major professional organizations such as the American Nurses Association (ANA) and the American Medical Association (AMA) have policy statements supporting the need for advocacy. Living in an abusive situation can destroy a victim's quality of life no matter when or where it occurs. Nurses have the power and privilege to restore damaged self-esteem and promote health. Interventions for elder abuse focus on stopping the exploitation of the individual while protecting their safety and autonomy. Since many victims of abuse will remain with the abuser, it is necessary to intervene with both the victim and abuser.

- Crisis intervention strategies to handle medical and legal emergencies (most procedures follow civil and criminal statutes)

- Case management

- Counseling to the abuser and the abused

- Housing assistance

- Emergency housing, food, and medical care

- Referral to counseling and support groups

- Dietary assistance

- Guardianship assistance

- Financial or legal aid

- Informal support system development

Legal interventions, specifically in a home situation, may include a guardianship or conservatorship. The focus is on using the least restrictive options with the least amount of court intrusion. While one goal is to hold the abuser accountable for his or her actions, another goal is to allow the victim the autonomy to return to the situation he or she chooses. Emergency shelters have been established in some communities to provide care during crisis situations.

Your willingness to interrupt an abusive situation by listening and asking questions may encourage elderly abused individuals to seek and accept help as nurses are often viewed as a respected and trusted member of the healthcare team. Since many elderly abuse victims are unable to ask for help due to cognitive impairment or dependence, there is an additional burden to be a proactive advocate. This is accomplished by reporting all suspected abuse of any type, recognizing the impact of spousal abuse on elder abuse, and training non-professional staff to develop skills with geriatric patients.

National Center on Elder Abuse
1201 15th St., N.W.
Washington, DC 20005-2800

(202) 898-2586

SEXUALITY

Sexual functioning is an intricate interaction involving a number of systems: endocrine, motor, sensory, physical, and sensual. Sexual activity is a component of the well-being of the individual, while sexuality is part of self-identity at any age. Sexual activity is a primary basis of human relations, and it is a basic right of every person in society. Sexuality and sexual activity are considered to be part of youth; hence, the combination of sexuality and aging is considered strange.

A number of studies support the premise that a large percentage of individuals over the age of 65 not only continue sexual activity, but are generally satisfied with sex and with their partners (Freedman, 1999). Our society has many myths regarding older adults and sex. Older adults are often stereotyped as being non-sexual and not wanting to or able to have sex.

Unfortunately, because of these societal beliefs the sexual needs of older individuals tend to be ignored by family members, healthcare workers, and society in general. For women, the experience

---

TABLE 10-2: NORMAL AGING CHANGES AND SEXUAL FUNCTION

Aging and Female Physiological Changes

- The vagina lubricates more slowly and the amount of lubrication in the vagina is decreased relative to the amount in younger years.

- The labia and clitoris are less engorged with blood during sexual arousal.

- Perceived orgasmic intensity may be lower due to fewer uterine and vaginal contractions during orgasm.

- A gradual thinning of vaginal tissue and shortening of the vaginal canal.

- The uterus and the cervix become smaller, and, in a small number of women, this may lead to painful uterine contractions with orgasm.

- Sex drive may increase as estrogen levels decrease and androgens begin to play a larger role in sexual response.

Aging and Male Physiological Changes

- Orgasm does not necessarily involve ejaculation as much as it may have in the past because the prostate has lost elasticity and does not produce as much semen.

- More frequently, erections may be "lost" before having an orgasm.

- In terms of urgency, sex drive decreases somewhat.

- It is more difficult, takes a longer time, or more stimulation to obtain an erection.

- The time it takes to have another erection after orgasm (the refractory period) increases, and may take up to 24 or 48 hours.

- It may take more stimulation than it used to for ejaculation to occur, and intercourse may be more prolonged.

- While erect, the penis is not as hard as it was in youth.

- Ejaculation is not as forceful as it was before, and the volume of ejaculate is reduced because of prostate changes.

---

of menopause should come as a time of liberation and self-actualization, but instead, our youth-oriented society encourages hormone replacement, face lifts, and many anti-aging products exacerbating women's fear of aging (Stotland, 2002).

Age-Related Changes

There are a number of age-associated changes that affect sexual functioning. For women, decline and eventual cessation of estrogen production during menopause leads to atrophy of urogenital tissues and an overall decline in genital vasocongestion and lubrication. As a result, sexual desire may decrease, orgasm may be less intense, and genital stimulation during sex may be less effective and comfortable

without the use of external lubrication. Hormone replacement therapy will reverse these changes in many women but should not be used without careful evaluation of risks versus benefits. Despite mild declines in testosterone production in men, there is no equivalent male menopause that alters sexual function or fertility to the same degree as occurs in women. Arousal in men may take longer and require more genital stimulation. The erections tend to be less durable and less reliable and the ejaculatory volume decreases and the refractory period can increase significantly. Older adults will notice changes in their bodies and in their sexual response. It is helpful to educate your clients so they are aware of what

TABLE 10-3: COMMON CAUSES OF SEXUAL DYSFUNCTION

Diabetes Mellitus	Urinary Incontinence
Decreased Hormone Production	Alcohol
Chronic Renal Failure	Radiation
Arthritis	Medications
Myocardial Infarction	Fear
Congestive Heart Failure	Shortness of Breath
Peripheral Vascular Disease	Fatigue
Liver Disease	Depression
Cerebrovascular Accident	Anxiety
Ileostomy	Pain
Colostomy	Altered Body Image
Urinary Catheter	

Note. From Barash, R. A. (1991). How Aging Affects Sexual Functioning. California Nursing. May-June, pp 25-28.

changes are normal and what need further investigating (see Table 10-2).

Sexual dysfunction does not happen to every older adult, although its prevalence certainly increases with age. For men, erectile dysfunction (ED) is the most common form of sexual dysfunction, affecting over 50% of men ages 40 to 70 and 86% of men over the age of 80 (Prins, Blanker, Bohnen, Thomas, & Bosch, 2002). There are limited data on the prevalence of sexual dysfunction in older women. Hypoactive sexual desire, inhibited orgasm, and dyspareunia (pain during sex) are the most common disorders (Renshaw, 1996).

Medical and psychiatric disorders are the most common causes of sexual dysfunction in geriatric patients. Many of these conditions are common in older adults (see Table 10-3). Fatigue, pain, and physical disability due to medical illness can make individuals feel less sexy and confident in their sexual ability. Fear may also pay a part especially after a cardiovascular event. The traditional advice for return to sexual activity was the ability to climb two flights of stairs. The newer guideline, assuming sexual activity will be with the patient's usual partner, is the ability to perform approximately five metabolic equivalents of physical activity. A physician or exercise physiologist can educate patients

and their often equally anxious partners on understanding when they meet this benchmark and provide other tips on how to safely resume sexual activity (Rashbaum, 2002).

Psychiatric illnesses, especially major depression and dementia, are associated with sexual dysfunction in late life. Low libido is a cardinal symptom of depression. Men with Alzheimer's disease suffer from high rates of erectile dysfunction, in part due to impairment in ability to maintain a cognitive focus on sexual stimulation during sex. Psychosocial stresses such as the loss of a partner due to disability or death, fears of self-injury or death due to medical conditions (e.g., history of myocardial infarction, shortness of breath), or sensitivity to loss of personal appearance or control of hygiene (e.g., due to incontinence or the presence of a colostomy) can sometimes spell the end of an individual's desire for sexual activity. The availability of partners is an acute issue for women, who outnumber men by over two to one by the age of 85. The impact of medication cannot be underestimated (psychotropic medications are common culprits) and can affect all stages of sexual function.

Nursing Assessment and Interventions

Nurses interested in promoting sexual health in older adults must be comfortable in obtaining sexual information. The nurse should project ease, openness, and have a non-judgmental manner. Nurses should examine their own values regarding sexual expression to avoid imposing them on their clients. There are many different types of sexual activities and the nurse should be comfortable talking about all of them. Of all sexual issues, masturbation is the one that still evokes defensiveness, guilt, and discomfort. In the early 1900s parents were taught to stop their children from touching themselves. As a result, older adults were taught in childhood that masturbation could cause everything from warts to epilepsy to insanity. Another type of sexual activity for the older adult is homosexuality. The number of gay and lesbians is expected to increase for several reasons: Women take a more assertive sexual role as they age, the gay liberation movement has led to increases in acceptance of homosexuals, and women outnumber men 7 to 1 after the age of 75. Unmarried couples or singles that are sexually active outside of marriage is also common in the sexually active older adult population. Do not assume that someone is sexually inactive or has no sexual desires unless they say so. Questions to ask to assess intimacy and sexuality:

- Are you satisfied with the kind and amount of intimacy you receive?

- What concerns or questions do you have about continuing to fulfill your sexual needs?

- What information or help do you think you might need?

These types of question should open the lines of communication for most elders. If their concerns are due to sexual dysfunction, arrange an evaluation with their physician or a referral to an urologist. For problems that are psychological, counseling should be arranged with a social worker or psychologist who specializes in sexuality issues. For practical problems that you feel comfortable and knowledgeable in answering:

- For vaginal dryness use a water-based lubricant such as K-Y jelly.

- Communicate with the partner about what is desired and what is not desired in a clear and positive way. Don't expect your partner to guess likes and dislikes.

- Position for comfort: Suggest using a side by side position with the man in the back. This position is effective because it allows vaginal intercourse without putting major stress on any joints or necessitating one partner to put his or her weight on the other.

- For fatigue or minor difficulties with erection, suggest making love in the morning.

- Suggest use of a vibrator to help stimulate for those who have joint pain or become easily fatigued.

- To help get in the mood, encourage basic romantic mood-setting ideas such as candles, soft music, or a body massage.

Sex in Long-Term Care Facilities

Nursing homes and institutions can mark the end of sexual freedom for the older adult. Consider the surroundings: no locks on doors, semiprivate rooms, and single beds. Sex is frowned on and this may well be because the staff have their own biases and myths surrounding later-life sexuality. They may resist any movement in this direction. Sex between consenting nursing home residents should be considered normal as long as no physical or emotional abuse is occurring.

There is much debate and discussion about sexual activities between two nursing home residents, when one or both of them have cognitive impairment. Oftentimes when this occurs, these residents are separated, chemically restrained, or transferred to a different unit or facility. These cases must be examined on an individual basis and policies should be in place for sexual activity between consenting residents. This should include the educating of all staff member on sexual rights and needs. It should also include not imposing staff values on the residents. Some facilities use "do not disturb" signs for their residents who masturbate or have sexual relationships. Progressive nursing homes have policies that include the right to seek out and engage in sexual expression, including words, gestures, movements, or activities that appear motivated by the desire for sexual gratification. Most of the nation's 17,000 facilities for older adults offer only fleeting education for staff members on the subject and few have formal guidelines or policies. For an older adult in a nursing home, an intimate relationship, or finding love again, can be an unexpected joy, and contribute immensely to quality of life.

A second problem that occurs in nursing home is the misinterpretation of the action of a resident with cognitive impairment to be one of a sexual nature. Male residents, in particular, are vulnerable to being labeled "dirty old men" when their attempts to satisfy a basic need are perceived as sexual actions. A confused male resident on a predominately female unit, could easily enter the wrong room to remove clothing, use the bathroom, or climb into bed. A urinary tract infection, or wet, soiled, or uncomfortable underclothing may prompt the removal of clothing in an inappropriate place. These incidents should be evaluated carefully to determine if there is an underlying cause before it is concluded the resident was acting out sexually. Other actions, which are sexual in nature, also may occur. Misidentification of another resident as a spouse can easily transpire due to agnosia and/or or visual impairments. Masturbation in public areas due to lack of inhibition may also be problematic. Providing privacy for self-stimulation is essential. For the resident with cognitive impair-

ment and problematic sexual behavior, see Chapter 6 for information on dementia.

SPIRITUALITY

Spirituality is that which gives meaning to one's life. Spirituality is a broad concept that has a different meaning to each individual, who may express it in many different ways. Some of the more common practices associated with spirituality are religion, meditation, voodoo, therapeutic touch, sex, new age, healing, special powers, Extrasensory perception (ESP), out of body experiences, and nature. Spirituality is a universal human phenomenon, yet conceptual confusion, ambiguity, and scientific skepticism have prevented adequate investigation into its potential effects. The lack of conceptual clarity and absence of a precise theoretical definition prevent recognition of spiritual distress and, hence, appropriate intervention. Spiritual needs change during different phases of life and during times of illness. Religion is one type of expression of spirituality and is the one that has been given the most research attention. It is also the most commonly practiced method of spirituality among older adults (Weaver, Flannelly, & Flannelly, 2001). Other expressions may include prayer, meditation, interactions with others or nature, and relationship with God or a higher power. Native Americans and others have high spirituality connectiveness with nature, which embraces the protection of the life-giving elements of soil, water, and air.

Researchers have found common themes among older adults and spirituality: God exists and acts in the lives of persons, God calls them to action and is a source of connection in times of loss (Lowry & Conco, 2002). This study also found that spirituality positively affects attitude, particularly as health declines (Lowry & Conco, 2002). Large reviews of research suggest that most patients have a spiritual life and regard their spiritual health and physical health as equally important (Mayo Clinic, 2001). Furthermore, people may have greater spiritual needs during illness. Most studies have shown that religious involvement and spirituality are associated with better health outcomes, including greater longevity, coping skills, and health-related quality of life (even during terminal illness) and less anxiety, depression, and suicide. Several studies have shown that addressing the spiritual needs of the patient may enhance recovery from illness (Mueller, Plevak, & Rummans, 2001).

Assessment of Spiritual Needs

Spirituality is highly personal and must be approached in a non-obtrusive and sensitive manner. What is most important to understand is that spirituality is of paramount importance in the lives of many older adults and it is unique and individual to each person. Do not attempt to place your values on others. Respect the values of others even if you do not believe in them or if they go against your religion or beliefs. Older adults expect respectful and empathic healthcare providers who meet both their physical and spiritual needs. As nurses are often the ones interacting with the older adult in times of healthcare crisis, they are in the ideal position to ensure that spiritual needs are being met. When assessing needs use open-ended questions to allow the older adult to describe their perceptions of spirituality, religion, health, and the role of spirituality in helping them cope, such as:

1. Are your spiritual needs being met?

2. Are you at peace?

3. Do you have spiritual pain?

4. Are you hopeful or do you despair?

5. How do you express spirituality: prayer, religious commitment, personal faith, relationship with others, nature, or something else?

6. Do your beliefs help you cope with anxiety, pain, and achieving peace?

Spiritual Distress Symptoms

Some older adults are not able to express, or have not received the opportunity to express spiritual distress. These are some signs that may indicate distress:

• Expresses concerns with meaning of life and death or belief system (critical factor)

• Displays anger towards God

• Questions meaning of suffering

• Verbalizes inner conflicts about beliefs

• Verbalizes concern about relationship with deity

• Questions meaning of own existence

• Is unable to participate in usual religious practices

• Seeks spiritual assistance

• Questions moral or ethical implications of therapeutic regimen

• Gallows humor

• Displacement of anger

• Displays signs and symptoms of depression

Interventions for Meeting Spiritual Needs

• Programs or opportunities to develop their spirituality through prayer, art, writing, reflections, guided imagery, religious or spiritual readings, ritual, or connection to others or God

• Weekly nondenominational prayer services

• A prayer corner in the facility

• Availability of religious reading material, music and bible and other readings on tape

• A monthly calendar placed in each patient's room listing the holy days of many different religions and other spiritual experiences such as meditation

• Chaplins, priests, and other religious leaders

available both for in-home and facility needs

- A book of prayers and meditations placed at the bedside in each room

- Meditation or quiet rooms available

- Volunteers, friends, staff and others to read passages, affirmations, and other materials

- Videotapes with spiritual theme

SUMMARY

Care for the older adult means much more than diagnoses and treating illness. It means addressing the psychosocial issues that reduce quality of life. Maintaining and improving quality of life requires the holistic care approach that is the foundation of nursing care and what sets nurses apart from the medically modeled trained physician. These basic human needs and issues such as support, coping with losses, feeling safe, and sexual and spiritual satisfaction are paramount for this population.

EXAM QUESTIONS

CHAPTER 10
Questions 71-75

71. An older adult is most likely to receive social support from

    a. state Medicare programs.

    b. local senior citizens agencies.

    c. Administration on Aging.

    d. a next door neighbor.

72. In order to accept a loss a person goes through five stages of grief. The older adult

    a. tends to cope better than younger people.

    b. always go through the stages in the same order.

    c. should be encouraged not to express their pain.

    d. may sometimes get stuck in a particular stage.

73. The person most likely to abuse an older adult is

    a. a nurses' assistant in a nursing home.

    b. a home repair scam artist.

    c. an adult child of the abused.

    d. their spouse.

74. Sexuality and older adults

    a. is rarely a problem as they have little interest in sex.

    b. is not conducive in the nursing home setting.

    c. is not an issue for nurses to be involved in.

    d. consists only of heterosexual relationships.

75. The most common expression of spirituality is

    a. religion.

    b. meditation.

    c. nature.

    d. therapeutic touch.

CHAPTER 11

PREVENTION
AND REHABILITATION

CHAPTER OBJECTIVE

After studying this chapter, the reader will be able to discuss the implications of prevention on the health of older adults and how rehabilitation and various therapies assist in returning to or maintaining maximum levels of functioning.

LEARNING OBJECTIVES

After studying this chapter, the reader will be able to

1. describe the differences between the three levels of prevention.

2. explain the importance of immunization and health promotion screening for older adults.

3. understand the principles of rehabilitation.

4. describe the roles of physical, speech, recreational, and occupational therapies for the older adult.

5. discuss how physical activities may be used in promoting wellness in the older adult.

INTRODUCTION

Illness prevention and methods of maintaining or regaining function are vital areas of health care for older adults. Nurses provide care at three levels of prevention. Primary prevention is aimed at detecting and reducing risk factors that predispose people to disease. Immunization and exercise programs for falls prevention are examples of primary prevention. Secondary prevention involves early detection of a disease before the disease becomes dangerous or disabling. Early detection of hypertension or elevated blood sugar is an example of secondary prevention. Tertiary prevention consists of detecting a disease that is symptomatic and taking action to maximize recovery. Teaching a diabetic patient to self-administer insulin or providing fluid to a dehydrated patient in a nursing home are examples of tertiary prevention.

In all phases of prevention, nurses assess patient needs, plan the care needed, and implement the plan. Implementing the care plan includes hands-on caregiving and coordinates with other disciplines to get the necessary care. Understanding what other disciplines offer in the area of prevention and rehabilitation is necessary in order for the nurse to select the most appropriate therapies and interventions for his or her patients. This chapter discusses the role of immunizations, screening, exercise, and other disciplines for health optimization and rehabilitation.

IMMUNIZATIONS

More than 30,000 adults die each year from diseases that vaccinations could have prevented, usually from complications of influenza and pneumonia. The Federal Center for Disease

Control and Prevention has issued their first adult immunization schedule:

- Flu shot: One each year (McElhaney, 2002).

- Pneumococcal vaccine: For everyone over the age 65, a one-time dose. If last vaccination was more than 5 years ago, re-vaccinate.

- Tetanus/diphtheria: One booster dose every 10 years.

- MMR (measles, mumps, rubella), meningitis, hepatitis A and B: Vaccines are considered on an individual basis based on exposure, childhood immunization record, and current diagnoses and disease state.

- More information is available at the National Immunization Hotline: 1-800-232-2522.

SCREENING

General recommendations for screening disease states and conditions change frequently and may vary greatly depending on factors such as geographic location and ethnic mix. Learn the recommendations for the area where you work based on the specific population you work with. This information may be obtained from local, regional, or state boards of health. From the Mayo Clinic Rochester Department of Internal Medicine Division of Geriatric Medicine comes the following recommendations:

Blood Pressure: Persons thought to be normotensive should receive blood pressure measurements at least once every 2 years.

Skin Cancer: Skin inspection, a simple examination without risk, is the principal screening test to detect skin cancer. The primary risk factors for skin cancer are a previous history of precancerous lesions, a family history of melanoma, and sun exposure. There is little evidence supporting the effectiveness of physician-performed screening over self-recognition. However, visual impairment

(common in the elderly) may reduce the ability to self-inspect. Recommend annual inspection of patients with a family or previous history of skin cancer, precursor lesion, and those with increased sun exposure.

Hearing: Simple accurate tests of hearing are available at low cost. Recommendation is for periodic/annual hearing assessment and otologic examination of all older adults. Formal audiometry not advised if the patient is unwilling or unable to use appropriate assistive devices.

Vision: Annual testing of visual acuity and for glaucoma.

Dental: Periodic dental visits, daily brushing and flossing.

Oral Exam: Risk factors for oral cancer include age greater than 60 years, excessive alcohol consumption, and tobacco use. Inspection and palpation of the oral cavity are the screening tests available for oral cancers. Screening recommended only to those individuals considered at high risk, which would mean screening all persons over age 60.

Prostate Cancer: Age is a major factor in the incidence of prostate cancer. Over 80% of all cases of prostate cancer occur in men over the age of 64 years. Three screening techniques are in clinical use: the digital rectal examination (DRE), transrectal ultrasound, and prostate specific antigen (PSA). The positive predictive value for the DRE is 22–31%, transrectal ultrasound, 17–41% and prostate specific antigen (PSA) 35%. The transrectal ultrasounds are used only after a positive DRE or PSA. These positive predictive values are too low to be clinically useful. There is insufficient evidence to recommend for or against routine digital rectal examination as an effective screening test for prostate cancer in asymptomatic men.

Ovarian Cancer: Currently there are three broad categories of screening techniques available: pelvic examination, ultrasound and other imaging techniques, and carcinoembrionic antigen (CMA) 125 and other tumor markers. In general, ovarian malignancies have disseminated by the time they are palpable. There is no recommended screening of asymptomatic women for ovarian cancer.

Uterine/Cervical Cancer: Current screening modalities include bimanual pelvic examination, Papanicolaou smear, endocervical aspiration, and endometrial sampling. All four modalities are unreliable and inaccurate "in older women." Most importantly, early detection in asymptomatic women has not been shown to decrease the mortality from uterine cancer. However the American Geriatric Society recommends screening annually, reducing to every 2–3 years after 3 negative screenings. Specifically for cervical cancer it is recommended to discontine Papanicolaou smears at age 65 if previous Papanicolaou smears have been regular and consistently normal (Stekler & Elmore, 2002). For under-screened elderly women, screening with Papanicolaou smear at least once is recommended if patient's functional status and medical condition are sufficient to withstand therapy for any lesion discovered.

Feet: Annual assessment of foot care by history and physical examination. Health care providers can identify foot problems by simply examining the feet, asking about the presence of pain, and ability to perform needed foot care. High-risk populations and patients with diabetes should have routine inspection.

Gait and Falls: Periodic evaluation of gait and balance and inquire about history of falls and fear of falling.

Cognitive Function: Without screening tools, early or mild dementia can remain undetected. The Mini-Mental Status Examination is adequate for detecting cognitive impairment, establishing a baseline, and measuring decline over time. However, there is insufficient evidence to determine whether routine screening for cognitive impairment should be included or excluded in the periodic examination of the older adult. Screening is best targeted to persons over age 80, individuals entering long-term care facilities, hospital inpatients (e.g. pre-operatively), and in those demonstrating functional decline.

Osteoporosis: Age is the greatest risk factor for osteoporosis. For women who live to be 85, approximately 50% will have an osteoporosis-related fracture during their lives, 25% will develop an abnormality of the spine, and 15% will fracture their hip. It is recommended that women 65 and older be routinely screened for osteoporosis and begin treatment if necessary to reduce the risk of fracture and spinal abnormalities often associated with the disease. Screening should begin at 60 for those women identified at high-risk because of their weight or estrogen use.

Thyroid Disease: Thyroid dysfunction increases with age, particularly in women over age 50; therefore, periodic testing is advised.

Lung Cancer: Lung cancer is the leading cause of cancer death in both men and women; however, screening asymptomatic persons (with or without a history of smoking) for lung cancer by performing routine chest radiography or sputum cytology is not recommended. Periodic auscultation of lungs is recommended.

Breast Cancer: Several screening strategies have been recommended for detection of breast cancer, including: breast self-examination, clinical breast examination and mammography. Breast self examination has a low sensitivity — between 20 to 30% — which is even lower among elderly women. A biennial mammography for average risk women over age 65 is recommended. The upper-age limit to conclude screening should occur when a woman is expected to die within 6 years from a non-breast cancer cause.

Colorectal Cancer: Colorectal cancer is the second most common cause of cancer mortality. The present tests available for colorectal cancer screening are digital rectal examination, fecal occult blood test, sigmoidoscopy, barium enema, radiography, and colonoscopy. It is recommended to screen average risk individuals over 65 who are expected to live an additional 13 years with flexible sigmoidoscopy every 5 years. Since the average life expectancy at 75 years is 12 years, this would mean discontinuing screening at age 75 years in most elders.

Lipids: Coronary heart disease (CHD) is the number one cause of death in individuals over 65 years of age. Periodic screening and treating high blood cholesterol in adults younger than 70 years of age who already have manifestations of atherosclerotic disease and whose risk factors place them at high risk of CHD death is recommended. Older adults in their late 70s and beyond generally need not be screened or treated for high blood cholesterol.

Diabetes: Diabetes is one of the top ten leading causes of mortality in the United States for older adults. Non-insulin dependent diabetes mellitus, the more common form of diabetes in the elderly, affects 10% of subjects over 65 years of age and 25% of adults over 85 years of age. The prevalence is 60 to 100% higher among African-Americans. For a firm diagnosis of diabetes, an individual must have a fasting plasma glucose of 140 mg/dL or greater on 2 occasions. However, no specific glucose level discriminates completely between persons with impaired glucose tolerance or diabetes in the normal population. There is no evidence regarding age-, gender- and race-adjusted guidelines for the diagnosis of diabetes. Nor is there evidence demonstrating reduction in disease-specific outcomes as a result of screening asymptomatic older adults. Current recommendations are for periodic/annual fasting plasma glucose measurements in persons over the age of 65 years, especially those who are at high-risk for diabetes mellitus such as marked obesity, persons with a family history of diabetes mellitus, or women with a history of gestational diabetes mellitus.

Electrocardiography: The electrocardiogram (ECG) is the principal test for early detection of coronary atherosclerotic disease (CAD). However, there are important limitations to the sensitivity and specificity of electrocardiography when used as a screening test. A normal resting ECG does not rule out CAD. Conversely, an abnormal ECG does not reliably predict the presence of CAD. Some advocate obtaining a "baseline" ECG to assist in interpreting subsequent ECG, but studies indicate that in actual practice, most baseline tracings are either unavailable, or do not provide information that effects treatment decisions. There are no recommendations for routine or baseline electrocardiography in asymptomatic elderly patients.

When considering screening tests for the older adult, the following questions may be helpful in determining the necessity of the test:

* Is the target disease an important clinical problem?

* Does the burden of disability warrant early detection?

* Is the natural history of the target disease understood?

* Is there a latent or early symptomatic period?

* Is the screening diagnostic strategy effective?

* Is the accuracy of testing (sensitivity and specificity) established?

* Is the test acceptable to patients with low discomfort or risk?

* If the screening test is positive, will patients accept subsequent diagnostic evaluation?

* Is there a known treatment for the target disease?

* Is the treatment effective and available?

* Are there risks of treatment, such as adverse drug effects or adverse outcomes of surgical treatment?

* Is the cost of testing balanced by the benefit of treatment?

- Does the patient have insurance that covers the cost?

REHABILITATION

Rehabilitation is defined as any intervention designed to restore physical, emotional, or cognitive functioning. The main goal of rehabilitation is to increase or preserve the autonomy and well-being of the older adult elderly by providing treatments that are designed to improve functional abilities to the highest level possible. Principles of rehabilitation are of major importance in working with elderly patients in all settings. The first principle is that rehabilitation should start as soon as the disability is evident. Another is that treatment should be in the interdisciplinary manner. This could include nursing, physical, speech, recreational and occupational therapy, social work, and dietary in addition to the physician or physiatrist. A physiatrist is a physician who specializes in medicine and rehabilitation. The goals of rehabilitation are to

- promote the patient's functional independence.

- prevent secondary disabilities.

- control underlying disease or impairment.

- preserve the dignity of the individual.

- improve level of independence and live in a preferred and less costly community setting.

Rehabilitation can occur in many settings. Often the determining factor is the patient's medical insurance and what it will cover. Medicare will allow rehabilitative therapies in the acute care setting if there is an appropriate diagnosis and significant deficit. Often patients are discharged before they regain function and must seek further rehabilitation in other settings such as rehabilitation units of hospitals, nursing facilities, or through home health care. Medicare will pay for acute needs, but not for maintenance or chronic needs. There must be documentation of daily progress for Medicare reimbursement. Patients who are poorly motivated are quickly dropped from rehabilitation programs. There is research efficacy to support rehabilitative efforts for cardiovascular accidents, numerous neurological disorders, traumatic brain injury, hip fracture, arthritis, dementia, deconditioning, and post-amputation.

Successful rehabilitation is dependent on the positive outlook and the mutually agreeable goals of both staff and patient. Three frequently encountered attitudinal stumbling blocks in geriatric rehabilitation are ageism or negative attitudes toward the elderly, feelings that dependency is a right that elders have earned by virtue of their longevity, and apathy towards therapy that results from fatigue, pain, or depression. Negative attitudes toward aging and the elderly lead to a defeatist attitude with respect to rehabilitation. Elderly patients, their families, and sometimes even healthcare staff may feel that being old is synonymous with functional decline, and thus little effort will be made to promote independence. There may be little faith in what rehabilitation can accomplish. This attitude also interferes with rehabilitation efforts. Finally, some patients may not have the energy, either physical and emotional, to cooperate with a strenuous program. For these patients, setting small, limited goals may be helpful.

THE THERAPIES

Physical Therapy

A physical therapist (PT) is a licensed professional with at least a 4-year degree. Although the profession is relatively new, physical therapy initially began during World War I with the work done by restorative aides. Physical therapists (PT) today work in a variety of settings: hospitals, nursing homes, senior centers, outpatient clinics, fitness facilities, and home environment. The physical therapist may use massage, exercise, manual therapy, joint mobilization, myofascial release, and neurodevelopmental (NDT) techniques to treat patients to help decrease disability and pain, and improve overall function and quality of life. Therapists use various treatment modalities such as electrical stimulation, hot or cold packs, infrared, and ultrasound to help the healing and recovery of an injury. As part of the treatment and the rehabilitation process, a PT will often stretch, strengthen, facilitate muscles, challenge balance, test coordination abilities, teach home exercise programs, and enhance basic mobility skills. The PT also evaluates need for assistive and other seating and mobility devices such as walkers and wheelchairs. To obtain services of physical therapy a physician order is required for reimbursement purposes in many settings. A PT is often used after a hip fracture or stroke.

Speech Therapy

The speech therapist (ST) has similar educational requirements as the PT and works with problems in human communication and swallowing. The most common cause of communication disorders in the older adult is stroke; however, ST may also be needed for older adults with head injuries, after cancer surgery involving the mouth or throat, and other neurological disorders such as supranuclear palsy. Speech therapy includes assessment and evaluation of communication and swallowing abilities, training and repetitive exercises, and use of devices that can make it easier for some people to speak, communicate, or swallow safely. They may also recommend types of diet or thickening of fluids to prevent aspiration when swallowing. STs also work closely with the family members and other care providers, who will help care for the person upon discharge from the hospital or treatment center. This may include positioning and other tips for safe eating or use of specific communication devices.

Occupational Therapy

Occupational therapists (OT) are licensed rehabilitation care professionals who work to restore or improve physical abilities, promote behavioral

changes, adapt surroundings, and teach new skills; the goal is to have the individual achieve her or his best physical and/or mental functioning in daily life tasks. OTs provide these services on the referral or prescription of a physician, physician assistant, or nurse practitioner. The OT may work with older adults who have had stokes or injuries, neurological problems, psychosocial disorders, chemical dependency, or age-related disorders. An OT has a minimum of a bachelor's degree in occupational therapy, had supervised experience, and has passed a national licensing examination. OTs help people lead more productive, active and independent lives through a variety of methods, including the use of adaptive equipment. An OT's main objective is to improve people's ability to perform tasks associated with activities of daily living (ADLs). OTs instruct in the use of adaptive equipment such as wheelchairs, splints, and aids for eating and dressing. OTs help to create a treatment plan that may improve basic motor skills, increase reasoning abilities, and compensate for permanent loss of function. For the older adult, the OT assists mostly in regaining ADLs functions, such as dressing, bathing, and self-feeding. OT's also evaluate the environment for safety and perform driving evaluations.

Recreational Therapy

Certified therapeutic recreational specialists (CTRS) are care professionals who work to restore, remediate, or rehabilitate to improve function and independence, as well as reduce or eliminate the effects of illness or disability. The CTRS has a 4-year degree and is often mistakenly confused with activity directors and others working in recreation. Recreation therapy is not Bingo, large entertainment programs, or birthday parties. These, although an important part of long-term care facilities, are diversional, entertainment programs without individual goals. The difference is that the CRTS may take physicians' orders for their service that may be reimbursable, and provide individualized outcome-based interventions. Unlike PT or OT, the CRTS in a long-term care facility may be a staff member working with patients based on nursing and other referrals, regardless of reimbursement status. They often work or co-treat with PTs and OTs. The CRTS works with older adults in a variety of care settings such as in-home, senior centers, long-term care, psychiatric, rehabilitation, and acute settings. The CRTS may work on preventative programs such as falls prevention or on improving function, mood, anxiety, maintaining weight, improved sleep, or for behavior management for older adults with dementia to name a few. Interventions may include various exercise programs, psychosocial groups, community re-integration, music, dance, or relaxation programs, wheelchair biking, and Somatron Air mattress for relaxation and tactile defensiveness.

As recreational therapy has always been a strong component of psychiatric services, the CRTS is often a vital team member on special care units. See Chapter 6 on dementia for how the CRTS works with wandering, repetitive vocalization, weight loss, physical aggression, bathing, anxiety, and other problems. Programs are offered that are outcome-based in small groups (4:1) or one-on-one. The CRTS assesses the patients, then formulates goals based on strengths and weaknesses. Interventions to achieve these goals are selected based on past leisure interest and current cognitive and physical functioning levels. Oftentimes the CRTS adapts or modifies the intervention to the patient's functioning level. The use of recreational interventions to reach goals can have multiple outcomes. An example is the older adult who is post stroke but with no motivation to exercise his weak side who was discharged from PT services. The CTRS uses a dog, as the patient always had dogs in the past. Placing the dog on the patient's weak side, the patient is encouraged to brush the dog's coat and play fetch, using the weak side. Not only does the patient benefit from exercising the weak side,

but also his or her mood elevates and motivation improves. CRTSs provide these services on the referral or prescription of a physician, physician assistant, or nurse practitioner. The CTRS also educates patients, formal and informal staff members on leisure education and choices for the older adult.

Nursing advocating for recreational interventions started over 150 years ago with Florence Nightingale during the Crimean War. While there she organized and reformed the nursing profession. At that time the physician's administration of drugs or performance of surgery was basically the beginning and end of the treatment process. Nightingale (1859) wrote of the benefits to patients from caring for pets, listening to and performing music, doing needlework, and writing. She chastised healthcare administrators to be more inclusive in their provision of services to patients: "Bearing in mind that you have all these varieties of employment which the sick cannot have, bear also in mind to obtain them all the varieties which they can enjoy." She then established a large recreation room and coffeehouse and developed various programs based on the patients functioning level (Nightingale, 1859).

PHYSICAL ACTIVITIES

Physical activity is an effective strategy for promoting wellness in people of all ages. Exercise levels decline with age for many reasons, most commonly because chronic conditions and current illnesses in the older adult limit physical activity. About 35 to 45% of older adults participate in minimal exercise, while only 20 to 25% participate in regular exercise > 30 minutes 5 times/week. Women are less active than men. Low income and educational level are stronger predictors of inactivity than older age and female sex. Physical inactivity is the second leading cause (after tobacco use) of premature death in the United States.

Direct correlations between fitness and specific health benefits have been scientifically supported.

Fortunately, significant attention has been focused on the effects of exercise on older adults. A growing body of literature supports increased physical activity in the older population as a means of counteracting the negative physiological effects of normal aging. Physical activity in older patients has also been shown to be a powerful prevention and treatment strategy for many medical conditions. Even activities such as gardening, housework, and other everyday tasks can have similar benefit as a formal exercise program. Exercise programs may include any combination of four types of therapeutic exercise — endurance, muscle-strengthening exercises, balance training, and flexibility exercises. The activities must be appropriate for a patient's level of fitness and medical condition. Exercise may employ stretching, range-of-motion, isometric, isotonic techniques, endurance, aerobic, strength training, balance, resistance, weight bearing, and/or fat burning. Exercise has shown to be beneficial for cardiovascular health, diabetes, osteoporosis, arthritis, insomnia, high blood pressure, chronic lung disease, constipation, obesity, neurological disorders such as dementia, Parkinson's, and cardiovascular accidents. In the older adult, regular exercise increases insulin sensitivity and glucose tolerance, reduces resting systolic and diastolic blood pressure, normalizes blood lipid levels (including a reduction in circulating triglycerides and an increase in high-density lipoprotein cholesterol), and reduces visceral fat content. Thus, regular exercise can help prevent cardiovascular disease (e.g., CAD, hypertension), diabetes, osteoporosis, obesity-related disorders, colon cancer, and psychiatric disorders (especially mood disorders such as depression). Regular exercise can preserve skeletal muscle strength, aerobic capacity and bone density, contributing to mobility and independence. Indirect benefits include opportunities for social interaction, a sense of well-being, and improved sleep, mood, coping, depression, anxiety, and cognition. Exercise is one of the few interventions that can restore physiologic capacity once it has been lost. Exercise may be used to increase ADL function such as self-feeding, dressing, and toileting and appears to improve quality of life by improving physical functioning (Lazowski, Ecclestone, & Myers, 1999). Exercise can help skin integrity such as maintaining the ability to turn and position self.

Regular exercise can help prevent falls and fall-related injuries by improving several risk factors for falls related to poor mobility, including strength, balance, neuromuscular coordination, joint function, and endurance. Exercise provides an overall benefit, despite a modest increased risk of falls during the exercise. Many cohort studies report that regularly active elderly persons have 20 to 50% lower mortality rates, despite a slight temporary increase in the risk of sudden death during exercise. The most common health risks of exercising are musculoskeletal injuries such as torn ligaments and pulled muscles. Falls and fall-related injuries can occur during exercise.

To determine if a patient is safe to exercise, screening by interview or questionnaire is recommended for all elderly patients starting an exercise program. It is useful to note that there are few older adults for whom exercise is inappropriate. Conditions such as recent cardiac events, pulmonary or systemic embolus, severe hypertension, arrhythmias, angina, or thrombophlebitis should be stabilized prior to beginning an exercise program. For these patients and frail older adults with multiple chronic conditions, the physician should make the exercise recommendations. For community-dwelling older adults, most community exercise classes and fitness centers commonly screen new participants to identify those with chronic disorders or symptoms of chronic disorders. They will also determine if the participant needs to see their physician prior to starting to exercise.

TABLE 11-1: EXERCISE TIPS FOR THE OLDER ADULT

Is It Safe for Me to Exercise?

- It is safe for most adults older than 65 years to exercise. Usually patients with chronic illnesses such as heart disease, high blood pressure, diabetes, and arthritis, can exercise safely. Many of these conditions are improved with exercise. If you are not sure if exercise is safe for you or if you are currently inactive, ask your doctor.

Getting Started

- Select an activity you know you will enjoy or one that you would like to try. Exercising with friends or family members can increase your enjoyment. If you are afraid of getting hurt try aquatic exercise.

- It is important to wear loose, comfortable clothing, and well-fitting, sturdy shoes. Your shoes should have a good arch support and a cushioned heel to absorb shock.

- If you are not already active, begin slowly. Start with exercises that you are already comfortable doing. Starting slowly makes it less likely that you will injure yourself and also helps prevent you from getting sore. The saying "no pain, no gain" is not true for older adults. You do not have to exercise at a high intensity to get most health benefits. Walking is an excellent beginning activity.

- Avoid exercising outdoors in extreme heat or cold. Drink extra fluids to prevent dehydration.

Exercise

- Do some type of aerobic activity for at least 30 minutes on most, and preferably, all days of the week. Examples are walking, swimming, dancing, and bicycling. You should also do resistance, or strength training two days per week. Exercises for balance are important to prevent falls. These types of exercises are good to try at a senior center or exercise center.

- Warm up for five minutes before each exercise session. Walking slowly and stretching are good warm-up activities. You should also cool down with more stretching for five minutes when you finish exercising. Cool down longer in warmer weather.

- Exercise is only good when you are feeling well. Wait to exercise until you feel better, if you have a cold, flu, or other illness. If you miss exercises for more than two weeks, be sure to start slowly again.

When Should I Call My Doctor?

- If your muscles or joints are sore the day after exercising, you may have done too much. Next time exercise at a lower intensity. If the pain or discomfort persists, you should talk to your doctor. You should also talk to your doctor, before resuming exercising, if you have any of the following symptoms while exercising: chest pain or pressure, trouble breathing or excessive shortness of breath, light-headedness or dizziness, difficulty with balance, or nausea.

To encourage exercise participation, assist the patient to select the activities they enjoy. Older adults do maintain interest in activities they enjoyed in the past (Strain, Grabusic, Searle, & Dunn, 2002). Some patients may want to do the same activity every day while others may want variety. Many patients prefer to exercise alone; some prefer exercise classes. Some want to exercise outdoors or at an exercise center while others prefer or have to exercise at home indoors. Exercises should be started at a low intensity for a short time, then gradually increased to the recommended intensity level. Urge all patients to exercise in the presence of another person, at least during the first few weeks of their program. Maintaining contact with the patient over time in regard to their exercise program is a simple method of maintaining adherence (Dubbert, Cooper, Kirchner, Meydrech, & Bilbrew, 2002). Patients whose exercise program is interrupted for more than a few weeks should resume exercising at about half the intensity level, then gradually increase to previous levels. Prolonged inactivity, especially bed rest, is not usually advised during recovery from illness. Each day of strict bed rest causes an incremental loss of muscle mass of about 1.5% and substantial losses in muscular performance and in cardiorespiratory fitness. See Table 11-1 for Exercise Tips for Older Adults.

Of all types of exercise, endurance exercises (walking, cycling, dancing, swimming and low-impact aerobics) provide the most well-documented health benefits for the elderly. Walking is the most common exercise among the elderly in the United States (about 50% of the elderly walk for exercise) and is recommended clinically. Jogging is generally inappropriate for elderly persons not already accustomed to it. Yoga, tai chi, and various types of aquatics programs are good for balance and flexibility and are generally safe.

SUMMARY

Due to the complexities of needs of the older adult, illness prevention and methods of maintaining or regaining function are best delivered in an interdisciplinary manner. Advocating for the use of the specialized skills and training of other disciplines increases opportunities for improved function, independence, and quality of life. Nurses are more capable of reaching their patients' goals while working as a part of a strong team.

EXAM QUESTIONS

CHAPTER 11

Questions 76-80

76. Which of the following is an example of a primary preventative health program?

    a. Exercise group for older adults with diabetes

    b. Walking program for post-hip fracture

    c. Aquatic therapy for post-stroke

    d. Falls prevention exercise program

77. Mr. Smith is a 70-year-old male in for a yearly physical. The screenings he should receive, assuming he has never had any of screenings in the past, are

    a. a chest x-ray for lung cancer, although he is asymptomatic.

    b. a cognitive screening, though his family reports no symptoms.

    c. a sigmoidoscopy, although he has no GI symptoms.

    d. a bone density examination, although he has had no fractures.

78. Rehabilitation is best described as

    a. assisting the older adult to live comfortably in his or her environment.

    b. using interventions to restore physical, emotional, or cognitive function.

    c. teaching an older adult how to use assistive devices.

    d. assisting an older adult to use a communication board.

79. A nursing home activity that is considered to be recreational therapy is a/an

    a. Halloween costume parade of a local pre-k class that walks through all units.

    b. after lunch music hour for all who are interested in the main hall.

    c. ice cream social: Sundaes for all, scooped and served by the activity staff.

    d. a cooking group of 4 residents, 3 times per week, with measurable, individual goals.

80. Regular physical activity in the older adult

    a. increases their mortality rate by 50%.

    b. should always be avoided if they have heart disease.

    c. can counteract the negative physiological effects of normal aging.

    d. should be done at a high intensity to get the most health benefits.

CHAPTER 12

SPECIAL ISSUES

CHAPTER OBJECTIVE

After studying this chapter, the reader will be able to discuss how select special issues including sexual orientation, driving, and smoking impacts the rights and quality of life of older adults.

LEARNING OBJECTIVES

After studying this chapter, the reader will be able to

1. discuss the unique problems facing older adults who are homosexual.

2. describe strategies to reduce discrimination for older adults with alternative lifestyles.

3. list reasons why AIDS may not be diagnosed in the older adult.

4. recognize the difficulties in determining when an older adult is at risk for accidents while driving.

5. indicate possible health benefits for older adults who quit smoking.

6. discuss the concerns associated with residents' rights and smoking in a long-term care facility.

INTRODUCTION

Nurses, like many in our society, have strong opinions concerning homosexuals. Nursing is based on doing what is in the best interest of the patient, not what is best for the nurse. This may be dif-

ficult for some when it means having to advocate for a right in which you morally do not believe. Many people in society today, look down on smokers, acting as if they are secondhand citizens. Keep in mind that they are not doing anything illegal and once again you might find yourself in the position of advocating for a right in which you do not believe. Many older adults are no longer safe drivers and determining when someone is no longer safe is a difficult issue. Do not assume a diagnosis of Alzheimer's disease or another dementing illness means an unsafe driver. Giving up the freedom to drive, smoking, or a partner after 50 or so years is a tremendous loss and should not be given away lightly.

HOMOSEXUALITY AND OLDER ADULTS

In our society older adults who consider themselves homosexuals have been invisible for much of their lives. Estimation as to numbers of older adults who are gay is difficult to determine because of its invisibility. However, it is generally agreed on that between 1 and 3 million older adults are homosexuals in the United States. In 1942 the American Psychiatric Association (APA) classified homosexuality as a disease; however, states did not start decriminalizing it until 1961. In 1973 it was declassified and no longer considered a disease. However, discrimination based on sexual orientation for employment, housing, and other rights still exists in many states. It is a certainty that a nurse working with older adults will encounter and give care to patients who are openly gay or in the closet. As nurses, it is paramount not to allow personal morals to influence the type of care we provide to any older adult.

As gay people grow older they, like their heterosexual counterparts, rely more and more on public programs and social services for care and assistance. This exposes the gay older adult to depend upon strangers for care and to feel fear of experiencing discrimination. Gay elders may be more dependent on strangers as they are less likely to have children and may even be estranged from their families due to homophobia or fear of rejection.

When an older adult enters independent elderly housing, retirement communities, assisted living, or nursing homes, they are most often presumed to be heterosexual. Thus, for gay older adults, their identities are immediately challenged. Many have lived their lives openly as a gay person and don't want to go back in the closet. There is significant prevalence of homophobic attitudes on the part of staff, an assumption that every resident is heterosexual, and a general, negative attitude concerning sex and any older adult. For the gay older adult, their long-term relationships are often devalued and not recognized. The lack of sensitivity to any type sexual activity, and particularly a homosexual orientation, often puts gay elders in vulnerable and uncomfortable circumstances, reinforcing social isolation, placing them at higher risk for self-neglect, and decreased quality of life. Consider this actual incident: A nursing assistant enters a room without knocking to find two elderly male residents engaged in sex. The two are separated immediately after the assistant notifies her supervisor. Within a day, one man is transferred to a psychiatric unit and placed in four-point restraints. A community health board, holds that the transfer was a warranted response to "deviant behavior" (Kaplan, 2002).

Homophobia and neglect appear widespread in nursing homes. In a recent survey of nursing home social workers, more than half said their coworkers were intolerant or condemning of homosexuality among residents (Cahill, South, Spade, 2000). Other studies report staff refusing to bathe a resident because they did not want to touch "the lesbian," and a homecare assistant threatened to "out" a gay patient if he reported her negligent care. Many state Area Agencies on Aging (AAA), the regional entities that distribute federal funds for senior services, report that openly gay and lesbian seniors would not be welcome at senior centers in their areas. A survey of physicians and medical students found that half reported witnessing colleagues providing reduced care or denying care to patients because of their sexual orientation, and 88 percent reported hearing colleagues make disparaging remarks about gay and lesbian patients (Raphael, 1997).

Same sex couples are treated unfairly by Social Security and Medicaid systems, and in the taxation of pensions and 401(k) plans. This costs homosexual seniors hundreds of millions of dollars each year in lost benefits that heterosexuals take for granted, such as Social Security survivor and spousal benefits, and the pension income of a deceased partner. This is particularly unfair since, without legal recognition of same-sex marriages, gay workers pay higher income taxes, on average, than straight people. Medicaid regulations offer no protections to the home or other assets when a same-sex spouse must enter a long-term care facility. Then there is the regulation involving the Medicaid spend-down. Same-sexed couples are not protected against seizure of their home by the government in the same way married couples are. If one of the couple enters long-term care and dies there, the government takes the survivors' house to pay the bill. There are no rights if there was no specifically stated share in the mortgage. The policies protect married couples, even if the house is in one person's name. Those policies are not in place for same sex couples. Even federal programs designed to help elder Americans are often either ineffective or irrelevant to the lives of gay elders.

Homosexuals are allowed to be discriminated against in long-term care settings, and the Patients' Bill of Rights does not apply to every older adult in the same way. Established policies in many long-term care institutions don't allow same sex partners to visit let alone allow a gay couple, who enter a nursing home together, to share a room. Homosexual older adults face particular health risks, and may be less likely to have the insurance benefits that their heterosexual counterparts have. Nurses in all settings are responsible for caring for a range of populations. People have mixed feelings about homosexuality depending on their experience, whether anyone is gay in their family, what generation they represent, and from where they come. No matter what one's religious or moral basis is, the nurse whose job is caring for people will – knowingly or unknowingly – provide care to homosexuals.

Nursing Intervention for Homosexual Older Adults

- Treat all patients with basic dignity and respect, and with no tolerance for bigotry or harassment.

- Educate other staff members when discrimination or disrespect is noticed.

- Advocate for the rights of all older adults.

- Assess your patient to determine who is the important person in his or her life.

- Provide privacy for all consenting couples.

- Help arrange power-of-attorney or other legal rights for same sex couples.

- Keep partner informed of status of same sex couple, as you would any other family member.

HIV/AIDS AND OLDER ADULTS

Disease prevention strategies often ignore gay and lesbian older adults or the possibility of HIV/AIDS in heterosexual older adults. As treatments for HIV/AIDS have improved, persons afflicted with the condition are living longer. As a result, the number of persons with HIV/AIDS over age 65 is increasing. Minorities comprise 50 – 70% of people over the age of 50 with HIV/AIDS and the number of HIV/AIDS cases continues to rise especially in communities of color. Educators, healthcare workers, and community leaders need to inform and warn people about HIV — the dangers of having sex without a condom, injecting drugs, using infected needles, and the importance of getting tested.

Many older adults believe that because they are beyond childbearing years, sex is no longer risky. Many healthcare professionals assume their older patients are no longer interested in sex and therefore do not consider sexually transmitted disease (STD) prevention or diagnoses. Of the AIDS-infected population, 15% are over 50 years old, yet health care professionals may not consider an HIV/AIDS diagnosis when examining an older patient (McLennon, Smith, & Orrick, 2003). It may be difficult to determine if dementia is HIV-related or a sign of Alzheimer's disease (AD) and to discern that an infection is an opportunistic one linked to HIV, not an unrelated condition such as pneumonia or herpes zoster. Experts believe AIDS might be misdiagnosed or under-diagnosed in elderly patients for many reasons (Willard & Dean, 2000):

- Stereotypical thinking perpetuates the myth that seniors are not sexually active.

- Older adults don't get tested for HIV/AIDS on a regular basis; thus, there may be even more cases than realized.

- Older adults know less about HIV/AIDS than younger age groups: how it is spread; the importance of using condoms and not sharing needles; the importance of getting tested; the importance of talking to their doctor.

- Healthcare workers and educators have neglected the middle age and older population in terms of HIV/AIDS education and prevention.

- Older adults are less likely than younger people to talk about their sex lives or drug use with their doctors.

- Doctors don't tend to ask older patients about sex or drug use.

- It is more difficult to recognize symptoms of HIV/AIDS in older adults. Doctors need to talk to their patients about the specific behaviors that put them at risk for HIV/AIDS.

- Older adults often mistake HIV/AIDS symptoms for the aches and pains of normal aging so they are less likely than younger people to get tested for HIV/AIDS. They may be embarrassed, ashamed, and fearful of being tested for HIV/AIDS, a disease connected with having sex and injecting drugs.

- People age 50 and over may have had the virus for years before being tested. By the time they are diagnosed with HIV/AIDS, the virus may be in its most advanced stages.

As older patients contract HIV, they experience a shorter disease free interval and a more rapid progression (Baldwin, 2001). Possible explanations for the apparent acceleration of HIV progression in older patients include the theory that the virus replicates more rapidly in older patients, the immune system of the older patient may be less competent, and cells may be destroyed more rapidly. The immune system of the older patient, unlike the younger patient, suffers from declining regenerative powers (Goodroad, 2003). Age-related declines in thymic function and replacement of CD4 cells occurs after 6 years and 40 years,

respectively. Patients require expensive treatment including multiple hospitalizations with stressed finances and dwindling resources as their disease progresses and they are no longer able to work. Therapeutic goals are similar to the goals in geriatric patients that include maximizing function, independence and quality of life while minimizing hospitalization.

Nursing Assessment for HIV/AIDS

- Assess the need for STD prevention education. Ask if they are sexually active.

- Assess patients for risky sexual activity. How many partners?, Condom usage?, HIV tested?

- Assess risky activity such as IV drug usage.

- For patients with risky behaviors:
  - If having sex, make sure your partner is HIV negative.
  - Use male or female condoms (latex or polyurethane) during sex.
  - Do not share needles or any other drug use paraphernalia.

- If the patient or partner had a blood transfusion between 1978 and 1985 or an operation or blood transfusion in a developing country at any time, get tested.

Nursing Interventions For HIV/AIDS Patients

- Many older people who have HIV/AIDS live in isolation because they are afraid to tell family and friends about their illness. Assist them with telling someone they can trust.

- They may have more severe depression than younger people. Screen for depression if suspected.

- Older people are less likely to join support groups. They may need to find other types of support such as one-on-one, Internet, spiritual, etc.

- Older people with HIV/AIDS need help coping both emotionally and physically with the disease. Assess need frequently.

- As the infection progresses, they will need help getting around and caring for themselves. Older people with AIDS need support and understanding from their doctors, family, friends, and community. Establish needs and set services in place.

DRIVING AND TRANSPORTATION

Driving is a complex task that demands quick reactions, alert senses, and split-second decisions. Psychomotor skills, good visual health, and intact cognitive functioning are needed, as the ability to accomplish the task safely requires highly complex interactions between the eyes, brain, and muscles. For many in our society, driving a car is the only available form of transportation. The ability and freedom to slide behind the wheel of a vehicle and drive away is important for the maintenance of a person's independence, convenience, self-esteem, and quality of life. In our culture driving is synonymous with adulthood and autonomy, and giving up this privilege and freedom is particularly difficult, especially after 50 or more years of driving. It is understandable that older adults want to be able to drive for as long as possible.

Advanced age brings a decrease in vision and hearing, and a slowing of reflexes. The majority of older adults learn to compensate for such diminished abilities by driving slower, avoiding night driving, and congested driving times and places. Though it is not an easy choice, most older adults determine for themselves when it is time to stop driving. For a person with Alzheimer's disease (AD), or other dementing disorders, the decision to stop driving is often not voluntary and compensation techniques may be forgotten. Unfortunately, for these older adults, the struggle to drive is particularly challenging since memory, information processing, visual spatial skills, and rapid decision-making are impaired and are critical components of

driving. Just how long a person with AD, or another compromising condition, should be permitted to drive is an issue that stirs the emotions of many families, healthcare providers, and the public, in general. Most states do not require healthcare providers to report the older adult with dementia to the Department of Motor Vehicles. In the majority of the states, it is up to the healthcare provider and the family to determine when and how to stop the older adult from driving. Unfortunately, there is no consensus on how this should be accomplished.

For families, determining when driving is unsafe is a very stressful event. Everyone simply hopes that the older adult will voluntarily stop driving on his or her own. But frequently older adults with dementia lack the insight and foresight to do so. Because the disease progresses differently in each person, it is hard to generalize about when older adults with dementia lose their ability to safely handle a motor vehicle.

There are conflicting opinions about whether someone with AD should drive because this diagnosis does not mean a person has lost the required abilities. This is particularly true when someone is diagnosed in the very early stages of the disease. Driving relies on visual and spatial sensitivity, which is not immediately impaired in all persons with AD. More people are being diagnosed earlier in the course of the disease due to increased public and healthcare provider's awareness. Research has not yet been able to identify, with 100% accuracy, which individuals with early AD are unsafe to drive. But, it is agreed that eventually all persons with AD will eventually lose the ability to drive safely. Studies have suggested that 50% of older adults with AD disease stop driving within 3 years of the onset of the disease and the risk for a motor vehicle accident increases with the duration of driving after disease onset (Carr, 1997).

Many studies have researched the association between driving and cognitive ability in attempts to help determine if a dementia diagnoses actually increases traffic accidents and fatalities. Some studies find that older adults with dementia do have a higher traffic crash rate but so do older adults without dementia but with other types of diagnoses and impairments. This signifies that further studies are required to determine the characteristics of "high risk" drivers.

In one study of 121 participants, 58 without dementia and 63 with dementia were compared for crash rates and roadway exposure. Results found the greater the cognitive impairment, the less actual miles were driven each year. They also found no statistically significant difference in crash frequency between groups, even when adjusting for exposure (Carr, Duchek, & Morris, 2000).

A national probability sample of 467 geriatricians examined knowledge and attitudes regarding the restriction of patients with dementia from driving (Cable, Reisner, Gerges, & Thirumavalavan, 2000). More than 75% of the responding geriatricians agreed that it was their responsibility for reporting patients; however, only 28% knew how to go about reporting such patients and less than 10% knew the actual steps involved. Unfortunately, this survey did not ask how many of these physicians actually ever reported a patient; one would think this number to be small based on the admitted lack of knowledge on how to report such patients. A discrepancy may exist between what these physicians state is their responsibility, and what they actually do in practice.

Older drivers do have more accidents and due to frailty have more serious injuries and fatalities than younger drivers do. The decision to end driving however, should be done on an individual basis, because during the 2–4 years after a dementia diagnosis, the risk of crashes is considerably lower than that for young men between the ages of 16 and 24 (Freund & Szinovacz, 2002). Table 12-1 lists education for safe driving points to use with patients that continue to drive. The following are general guidelines to follow when discussing driving with the patient and their families.

Addressing Driving with the Older Adult

Let the patient know that nurses realize that the ability and freedom to slide behind the wheel of a vehicle and drive away is important for the maintenance of a person's independence, convenience, self-esteem, and quality of life. Acknowledge that giving up driving is particularly difficult and determining when driving is unsafe is a very stressful event for everyone. Inform the patient that he/she should consider giving up driving for the following reasons:

- If feeling anxious about driving
- If unable to see well despite corrective lens
- If forgetting where you are going
- If getting lost in familiar surroundings
- If having near misses or crashes
- If getting traffic violation tickets

For patients who seem to be at risk for driving but are unwilling to voluntarily give up driving there are still other suggestions. Determine if the Department of Motor Vehicles will do a road test, if the patient is willing. Refer to an occupational therapist for a road test, again if patient is willing. Request for the physician to write a "Do not drive" prescription" as many in this generation pay strict adherence to the physician. Education for family members and the older adult sometimes helps the patient make a decision. These are some educational points to use:

- Driving is a complex task that demands quick reactions, alert senses, and split-second decisions.
- As people age, reaction time slows.
- Most traffic violations in older adults are due to failure to observe rules of the road, such as yielding or obeying traffic signs.
- The majority of traffic violations in older adults occur at lower speeds and more often at intersections.

TABLE 12-1: EDUCATION FOR INCREASING DRIVING SAFETY

- Exercise regularly: This increases flexibility, maintains range-of-motion in your joints and muscle strength. Always include neck exercises for good range-of-motion.

- Have your eyes checked annually: You may need glasses, or to update your prescription.

- Don't drink and drive.

- Keep your automobile in good condition.

- Ask you doctor or pharmacist if your medications may affect driving

- Take "At risk" defensive driving classes such as:
    American Association of Retired Persons (AARP) 55 Alive Driver Safety Program
    (8 hour course) 1-888-227-7669
    Coaching the Mature Driver offered by the U.S. National Safety Council 1-630-285-1121

- Use Compensation Methods:
    Drive slower, but remain within posted limits.
    Avoid night driving.
    Avoid congested driving times.
    Avoid congested areas or highways.
    Drive fewer miles.
    Limit driving to familiar roads.
    Only drive in good weather conditions.

- Safe Driving Checklist:
    Adjust seat and rear-view mirrors.
    Make sure seat belt is buckled.
    Wear glasses if prescribed and keep sunglasses in the car.
    Make sure someone knows where you are going.
    Make certain windshield is clear before starting.
    Pull off the road to use the cell phone, eat, apply make-up, or read a map.
    Keep the radio off or on low volume.
    Get directions for your destination and leave a copy with a friend or family member.
    Keep keys in the same place all the time so they are easy to find.
    Leave an extra set of keys with a friend or family member.

- Driving with Grandchildren in the Car:
    Make sure safety seats are correctly strapped into the seat.
    Make sure child is buckled correctly.
    If in doubt ask a police officer, they have been trained in safe use of child car seats.
    Bring another adult along for the ride. Another hand is always helpful with children.

- Safety When Out Shopping:
    Park near a light pole, a particular entrance to the store or in the same aisle each time.
    Get a handicap-parking permit if you need one.
    Put a ribbon on your car antenna to easily identify your car.
    Keep keys in your hand, ready to unlock your car when you leave the store.
    Hold purse with shoulder straps over shoulder and tucked under your arm.
    Always be aware of who is around you.

- Advanced age brings a decrease in vision and hearing.

- Many older adults take medication that may cause drowsiness, increase the slowing of reflexes, or reduce blood pressure.

- Many older adults have chronic physical conditions that may affect driving such as: arthritis, mobility impairment, angina, seizures, Parkinson's, tremors and strokes.

- Many older adults have AD and other dementias which may affect ability to remember how to get to familiar places. Visual spatial skills and slowing of rapid decision-making are impaired and critical components of driving.

- Because dementia progresses differently in each person, it is hard to generalize about when the older adults loses the ability to safely handle a motor vehicle. All persons with AD will eventually lose this ability.

Keep in mind that mandated reporting may compromise physician-patient confidentiality. Fear of losing one's license may delay a diagnostic workup for dementia in some older adults. Families and caregivers of older adults deemed unfit to drive should be responsible for making the vehicle less accessible by changing the locks, hiding the keys, disabling the vehicle or simply removing or selling it, if necessary. In addition, arrangements for consistent, reliable, alternative forms of transportation for the older adult who has lost driving privileges must be made. This could be a ride from friends or family, community senior ride programs, public transportation, taxis, or alternative forms of transportation.

Older adults frequently use other forms of transportation to get around their communities, especially in places with year-round warm climates. This could be a bicycle or a motorized cart, scooter, or wheelchair. These types of transportation enable the older adult to maintain independence and provide short-distance mobility. These forms of transportation are often unregulated, offer little protection from the weather, and have limited distances they can travel. Many towns and areas do not have designated biking pathways and often a traffic light walk sign is not on long enough for the older adult to get across safely. When assessing transportation and alternative forms of transportation:

- Determine alternative transportation mode

- Who maintains the vehicle? How often? How reliable?

- Do you wear a helmet?

- Do you have lights and a horn for safety?

- Does it have a means of carrying items such as a basket?

- How far do you go in it?

- Do you let others know where you are going?

- Do you bring identification with you?

These questions will help nurses assess if the older adult is in need of any repairs, or equipment or education for safety.

SMOKING AND OLDER ADULTS

Older adults began smoking before its harmful effects were well understood. They are significantly less likely than younger smokers to believe that smoking harms their health. This generation of older adults is now experiencing the health consequences of an average of 40 years of smoking. An estimated 3.5 million adults over the age 65 smoke, accounting for over 10% of all smokers. Each year 440,000 Americans die from diseases caused by smoking. Smoking is responsible for an estimated 1 in 5 U.S. deaths and costs the U.S. at least $150 billion each year in health care costs and lost productivity (MMWR, 2001). All the major causes of death among the elderly are associated with smoking and secondhand smoke. One of every 3 deaths among older men who smoke more than a pack of cigarettes a day is related to smoking. Smoking is estimated to be responsible for 87% of lung cancer cases, 21% of deaths from heart disease, 18% of deaths from stroke, and 82% of deaths from chronic obstructive pulmonary disease (emphysema and chronic bronchitis). Men 65 or older who smoke are twice as likely to die from a stroke, and women smokers are about 1.5 times as likely to die from a stroke than their non-smoking counterparts. The risk of dying from ischemic heart disease is 60% higher for smokers than nonsmokers 65 or older.

Older adult smokers are different from younger smokers in several ways. High nicotine brands of cigarettes are more popular with older smokers, with 58% smoking brands with estimated nicotine levels of 1.0 mg. Older smokers are highly nicotine dependent as measured by the need to smoke within 30 minutes of waking. Older smokers aged 50 to 74 are less likely to have tried to quit than smokers aged 21 to 49. Self-help and formal smoking cessation treatments for older adults must emphasize strategies to overcome high levels of nicotine dependence and lifelong psychological dependence on smoking.

Quitting smoking has supportive health benefits, even at a late age. When an older person quits smoking, circulation improves immediately, and the lungs begin to repair damage. In one year, the added risk of heart disease is cut almost in half, and risk of stroke, lung disease, and cancer diminishes. Of the older adults who have quit, more than 90% have done so on their own, citing these reasons for quitting: to maintain good health, take control of their lives, and/or avoid the unpleasant smell of cigarettes

Nurses will want to encourage smoking patients to quit. For many smokers, being nagged or pressured about their habit will be met with resistance and may harm the nurse/patient relationship. It is critical to have an approach that is non-

judgmental. Ask if they have considered quitting. If they have, probe deeper and determine if they have a specific plan in mind. Offer whatever assistance is needed. If they have not considered quitting, provide education material as to the benefits of quitting, or help them do the smoking quiz (Tables 12-2). When finished let them know what happens to them when they quit (Table 12-3) and if they decide they wish to stop smoking, offer to either assist them or find the help they need. Table 12-4 provides tips to stop smoking. Review the Stages of Change Theory in Chapter 1 for more detail on targeting interventions to modify behaviors.

Reasons for Not Quitting, and How to Respond:

"I am under a lot of stress and smoking relaxes me." The human body can become accustomed to nicotine, so smokers naturally feel more relaxed when they obtain the nicotine on which they have come to depend. However, nicotine is actually a stimulant that temporarily raises heart rate, blood pressure, and adrenaline levels. After a few weeks of not smoking, most ex-smokers feel less nervous.

"I have already cut down to a safe level." Cutting down is a good first step toward quitting, but smoking at any level increases the risks of illness. In fact, some smokers who believe they have cut back actually inhale more often and more deeply, thus maintaining the nicotine dependence. It is best to quit smoking completely.

"I don't have the willpower to give up smoking." It can be difficult for some people to give up smoking, but for others it is much easier than they expect. More than 3 million Americans quit every year. It might take more than one attempt and people might need to try different methods of quitting. Good programs help quitters analyze when and why they smoke, and help them tailor new routines to replace smoking, while teaching good nutrition and exercise.

Quitting smoking may cause short-term after-effects, especially for those who have been heavy

TABLE 12-2: SMOKING QUIZ — TRUE OR FALSE

____ 1. If you have smoked for most of your life, it's not worth stopping now.

____ 2. Older smokers who try to quit are more likely to stay off cigarettes.

____ 3. Smokers get tired and short of breath more easily than non-smokers the same age.

____ 4. Smoking is a major risk factor for heart attack and stroke among adults 60 years of age and older.

____ 5. Quitting smoking can help those who have already had a heart attack.

____ 6. Most older smokers don't want to stop smoking.

____ 7. An older smoker is more likely to smoke more cigarettes than a younger smoker.

____ 8. Someone who has smoked for 30 to 40 years probably won't be able to quit smoking.

____ 9. Very few older adults smoke cigarettes.

____ 10. Lifelong smokers are more likely to die of diseases like emphysema and bronchitis than nonsmokers.

ANSWERS

1. FALSE: Stopping now will help you live longer and feel better. You will reduce your risk of heart attack, stroke and cancer; improve blood flow and lung function; and help stop diseases like emphysema and bronchitis from getting worse.

2. TRUE: Once they quit, older smokers are far more likely than younger smokers to stay away from cigarettes.

3. TRUE: Smokers, especially over age 50, are much more likely to get tired, feel short of breath, and cough more. These symptoms can signal the start of bronchitis or emphysema, both of which are suffered more often by older smokers. Stopping will help reduce these symptoms.

4. TRUE: Smoking is a major risk factor for 4 of the 5 leading causes of death (heart disease, stroke, cancer, and lung diseases, emphysema, and bronchitis). For adults 60 +, smoking is a major risk factor for 6 of the top 14 causes of death. Older male smokers are nearly 2x as likely to die from stroke than older men who do not smoke, and the odds are nearly as high for older females. Cigarette smokers of any age have a 70% greater heart disease death rate than do non-smokers.

5. TRUE: The good news is that stopping smoking does help people who have suffered a heart attack. In some cases, ex-smokers can cut their risk of another heart attack by half or more.

6. FALSE: Most smokers prefer to quit. In fact 65 % of older smokers said that they would like to stop. What keeps them from quitting? Fears of being irritable, nervous, and tense, concerns about cravings for cigarettes, and not wanting to gain weight. Many think it's too late to quit, that quitting after so many years will not help but this is not true.

7. TRUE: Older smokers usually smoke more cigarettes than younger people. Plus, older smokers are more likely to smoke high nicotine brands.

8. FALSE: Older smokers are more likely to succeed at quitting smoking. Older smokers who stop want to avoid further health problems, take control of their life, get rid of the smell of cigarettes, and save money.

9. FALSE: One out of 5 adults aged 50+ smoke cigarettes. This is more than 11 million smokers, 1/4 of the US 43 million smokers! About 25% of the general population still smoke.

10. TRUE: Smoking greatly increases the risk of dying from diseases like emphysema and bronchitis. In fact, over 80 percent of all deaths from these two diseases are directly due to smoking. The risk of dying from lung cancer is also a lot higher for smokers than nonsmokers: 22 times higher for males, 12 times higher for females.

Note. From National Heart, Lung and Blood Institute, (2000). You Can Quit Smoking. Consumer Guide No. 91-3031. Bethesda, MD: U.S. Public Health Services. National Institute of Health.

TABLE 12-3: WHAT HAPPENS WHEN YOU STOP SMOKING

- 20 minutes after you quit—your blood pressure, pulse rates, and body temperature of your hands and feet drop to normal.

- 8 hours after you quit—the carbon monoxide level in your blood drops and the oxygen level in your blood increases to normal.

- 24 hours after you quit—your chance of heart attack decreases.

- 2 days after you quit—your nerve endings start regrowing and your ability to smell and taste is enhanced.

- After 15 years of not smoking—your risk of heart disease is that of a non-smoker!

Note. From U.S. Department of Health and Human Services. (1990). The Health Benefits of Smoking Cessation. Public Health Service, Center for Disease Control, Center for Disease Prevention and Health Promotion, Office on Smoking Health. DHHS Publicatin No (CDC), 90-846.

smokers for a long period of time. People who quit smoking initially are likely to feel anxious, irritable hungry, more tired, and have difficulty sleeping. They may also have difficulty concentrating. Many tobacco users gain weight when they quit, but usually less than 10 pounds. These changes do subside. It is important to tell patients ahead of time what they are up against. Many smokers find it difficult to quit smoking, and it may take 2 or 3 attempts before they are finally able to quit. Although relapse rates are most common in the first few weeks or months after quitting, people who stop smoking for 3 months are often able to remain cigarette-free for the rest of their lives.

Smoking and Care Settings

It is impossible to generalize about the policy of smoking and long-term care units as facility, local, state, and federal ordinances apply differently to different facilities. Some facilities have no policies prohibiting smoking and there are no city/county ordinances that prohibit smoking. It is generally agreed upon that although everyone in the healthcare community is keenly aware of the dangers of smoking, it is also recognized that many older adults have smoked for years and depriving them of the opportunity to smoke could be counterproductive to their welfare. Consideration must be given for residents' rights issues and accommodations for those who wish to smoke before a facility

changes policy and becomes smoke-free. Aside from safety issues, smoking in nursing homes can be problematic. A resident running out of cigarettes can experience the unpleasant physical symptoms of nicotine deprivation which is a reasonable concern for caregivers. Additionally, if residents are reduced to begging for cigarettes or stealing cigarettes when they run out, it is an affront to their dignity. This raises the issue of caregivers rationing cigarettes for residents. In light of the limited financial resources of some residents, it does make sense for staff to control cigarette use in order to stretch the resident's resources as far as possible. This should be done with the resident's permission. It would be a violation of a resident's rights to ration tobacco use when money is not a concern. A provider does not have the right to restrict a resident's access to his or her own property, money, or tobacco. Limiting smoking areas is reasonable. Segregating smokers from non-smokers in recreation areas and requiring all smoking to take place in a common area is appropriate. It is appropriate to forbid smoking in resident rooms. Caregivers may need to keep cigarettes and/or lighters at the nurse's station in order to assure that smoking policies are followed. Providers have the right, and indeed the duty, to assure safety in the facility. Smoking rules need to be tempered with genuine concern for the resident's welfare.

TABLE 12-4: TIPS TO STOP SMOKING

1. Set a quit date.

    My quit date:_____

2. Change the things around you.
    Get rid of all cigarettes and ashtrays in your home, car and place of work.
    Do not let people smoke in your home.

3. After you quit, don't smoke—not even a puff!

Get Medicine to Help You Quit
* You can buy nicotine gum or the nicotine patch at a drug store. You can ask your pharmacist for more information.
* Ask your doctor about other medicines that can help you.
    Nicotine nasal spray.
    Nicotine inhaler.
    Bupropion SR (pill).

Get Help
* Tell your family, friends and people you work with that you are going to quit. Ask for their support.
* Talk to your doctor, nurse, or other health care worker. They can help you quit.
* Get together with other people who are trying to quit, or join a smoking cessation program.
* To find out where to get help in your area, call the American Cancer Society toll-free: 1-800-ACS-2345.

Helpful Hints to Stay Quit
* If you "slip" and smoke, don't give up. Set a new date to get back on track.
* Avoid alcohol.
* Avoid being around smoking.
* Eat healthy food and get exercise.
* Keep a positive attitude. You can do it!

Note. From U.S. Department of Health and Human Services (2002). Tobacco Intervention Prevention. Tips To Stop Smoking. Washington, DC: National Center for Chronic Diseases and Health Promotion.

Offering assistance to quit smoking should be provided but according to research, smokers in these settings have little desire to quit, advice is rarely offered by either physicians or nurses, and smoking cessation programs are even scarcer (Capezuti, Brush, & Lawson, 1997). Provide educational material to smokers on safety factors, such as safe disposal of matches and cigarette butts, and the dangers of flames and oxygen. For older adult smokers in acute settings where smoking is strictly prohibited, determine if nicotine replacement is a viable option.

SUMMARY

This chapter was intended to bring to light these special issues that cause controversy. Older adults facing these issues need the kindness and understanding of the nurse caring for them. The nurse may not approve of all behaviors but advocates for the needs of all patients regardless.

EXAM QUESTIONS

CHAPTER 12
Questions 81-86

81. An older adult who is homosexual and living in a nursing home

    a. experiences all the rights that heterosexual residents have.

    b. is no longer interested in homosexuality.

    c. may encounter homophobic reactions by staff.

    d. has the right to share a room with their partner.

82. A nurse can best reduce discrimination against homosexual residents in a nursing home by

    a. encouraging the residents to be heterosexual.

    b. keeping sexual orientation in the closet.

    c. educating other staff member on rights of all residents.

    d. assist in having resident transferred to a more tolerant facility.

83. A major reason why older adults are not being screened or diagnosed with HIV/AIDS is that they

    a. have symptoms that are difficult to recognize.

    b. are no longer interested in sex, and therefore, are not at risk.

    c. engage in monogamous heterosexual activities only.

    d. use proper prevention, and therefore, are not at risk.

84. To help promote safe driving for a patient that drives, a nurse might encourage him/her to

    a. never drive anywhere alone.

    b. take a "55 Alive" driver safety class.

    c. encourage buying a large car.

    d. never exceed 40 mph, even on highways.

85. Your 76-year-old patient has smoked one pack of cigarettes per day for the past 60 years. He does not feel there is any benefit in stopping now. To help educate and encourage him to quit you tell him that if he stops, after one year he will have

    a. reduction in depression.

    b. reduction in cholesterol levels.

    c. reduced risk of heart attack, stroke, and cancer.

    d. reduced health insurance rate.

86. Mr. Jones is a 90-year-old nursing home resident who is cognitively intact and smokes cigarettes on a daily basis. In order to best preserve the rights of all of the residents in the nursing home you would allow Mr. Jones to smoke

    a. 2 times a shift, with staff members.

    b. anytime and anyplace.

    c. only when out of facility with family.

    d. only in the facility's designated areas.

CHAPTER 13

CARE SETTINGS

CHAPTER OBJECTIVE

After studying this chapter, the reader will be able to discuss the various aspects of different care settings of the older adult.

LEARNING OBJECTIVES

After studying this chapter, the reader will be able to

1. discuss the importance of aging in place to older adults.

2. detail the various assessments required for at-home dwelling older adults.

3. describe the problems associated with older adults as caregivers to their grandchildren.

4. identify common complications that occur in acute care settings.

5. explain the demographic make-up of the assisted living population.

6. describe the difficulties older adults may face when moving into nursing home settings.

7. explain the philosophy of hospice care.

8. indicate some of the physical changes associated with the dying process.

INTRODUCTION

A community should offer older adults a wide variety of living and care options, enabling them to remain as independent as possible in the least restrictive living environment of their choice. It also means seamless care from one setting or agency to another. This type of care is not only in the best interest of the older adult, but it also is cost effective as services are not duplicated, more older adults are able to remain in their homes, and emergency room visits decline. A true community-based Continuum of Care incorporates the collaboration of the healthcare system with the myriad of community-based services for the aging population. Typical of these service agencies are Meals-on-Wheels, lifelines, senior centers, congregate living facilities, home health, hospice, skilled nursing, adult day care, rehabilitation services, and many others. Frequently these agencies view one another as competitors (at least for funding), and they do very little collaborating.

Nursing practice can improve the outcomes for older adults when the expectation is to collaborate with multidisciplinary services and multiple sites of care (Tichawa, 2002). Supporting different living options for clients requires a comprehensive needs assessment taking into consideration chronic conditions, co-morbidities, disability, cognitive impairments, availability of informal caregivers and most of all, the wishes of the older adult.

Knowing what is available, and where, will help achieve the goals for the clients.

AGING IN PLACE

Aging in place is growing older without having to move from one's present residence in order to secure necessary healthcare services in response to changing needs. It means living where you have lived for many years, or living in a non-healthcare environment, and using products, services, and conveniences to allow, or enable one, to not have to move as circumstances change.

It is also a term used in marketing by those in the rapidly evolving senior housing industry. Continuing Care Retirement Communities (CCRCs) by definition offer the chance to age in place, but first one must move to the community to "start aging." Multi-level campuses market independent living, assisted living and perhaps Alzheimer's care and skilled nursing in one location, and claim to offer the opportunity to "age in place," but again, the adult must move there first. In many cases one must also move from one wing of the campus to another to receive the increased services. Some older adults prefer the security of a CCRC, knowing that their needs, and perhaps that of their spouses, will be met no matter what problems arise. One study found that 40% of the participants who moved to a CCRC did so with the intention of dying with dignity on the CCRC campus rather than in an acute care setting (Hays, Galamos, Palmer, McQuoid, and Flint, 2001). Generally these communities require considerable financial investment to initially move in. Care to older adults living in CCRCs is provided by both facility and community services and the concerns for nursing are similar to the ones for the community and residential dwelling elder.

OLDER ADULTS LIVING AT HOME

The value of remaining in one's home varies significantly with each individual. For many, home provides a sense of identity, security, and belonging that transcends any rational calculation of benefits. Living in one's home provides the older adult with a locus of control and a familiar environment that does not change rapidly. It may be the only substantial remaining symbol of independence and autonomy. Taking into account the psychological meaning of home for each patient is imperative in setting realistic and achievable goals and will assist in determining what interventions are necessary to keep the older adult in the home. The nurse working with older adults living at home has the unique advantage of assessing the client in their natural environment, of building a strong, trusting relationship with the client, and having a significant impact on the health and welfare of the client. The following areas of assessment should be considered for the home-dwelling client in addition to the routine physical assessment. These assessment areas will help determine the services needed by the older adult. The services will vary depending upon the specific state and community. A few examples are:

Accessibility and Safety: Inside and outside safety of home, need for adaptations, accessibility of equipment such as hospital bed or wheelchair in home, outdoors, and in the community. May need physical or occupational therapist (PT/OT) referral to do extensive assessments and interventions.

Activities of Daily Living (ADL): Ability to bathe, toilet, feed, and move about. May need assistive devices, home modifications, in-home meal program, home health aide, PT, or OT.

Instrumental Activities of Daily Living (IADL): Ability to shop for food and clothing, get to doctors' appointments, transportation, handle medications, phone calls, laundry, housekeeping, and manage finances. May need in-home care services, community-based programs, legal services, or home delivered meals.

Nutritional Needs: Assess weight history; hydration; ability to afford, purchase, and prepare food; special nutritional needs and diets; eating habits; and oral health. May need speech therapist, nutritionist or dietitian, in-home services, or meal program.

Social Function: Assess social history, support and network. Assess for any possible abuse. May need referral to social worker, volunteer visiting program, recreational therapist, or outreach programs.

Financial: Assess ability to afford housing cost, food, medications, and other expenses. Determine ability to handle insurance claims. May need referral to case management, social services, social worker, or county or local agencies.

Mood and Memory: Assess for depression, anxiety, grief and memory impairment. Refer to a memory clinic for diagnoses of memory loss or to a psychologist or psychiatrist for depression and/or other emotional disturbances.

OLDER ADULTS AS CAREGIVERS TO OLDER ADULTS

Caregivers are family members who find themselves in the role of providing unpaid assistance to see that the physical, psychological, and/or social needs of an aging loved one are met. In 2000, 54 million people were involved in some level of caregiving and spent, on average, more than 20 hours per week in this capacity. Older adults make up 20–40% of all caregivers with 76% of them being female. Those caring for older adults with Alzheimer's, stroke and Parkinson's report an average of 87 hours of care a week. About one-half of primary caregivers provide care with no formal or informal assistance whatsoever and contrary to popular belief, only an estimated 10% to 20% of family caregivers use formal services through public or private agencies (Family Caregiver Alliance, 2001). As many caregivers are older adults, it is vital to include an assessment of their needs. This should include their physical, psychological, emotional, social and financial burden, and stresses. Often times the health of the caregivers are overlooked. Research has demonstrated that over 23% of family caregivers met the requirements for home health services for themselves and that 50% report their own health to be fair or poor (Bradley, 2003). This study showed that the older caregivers have numerous unmet needs and that caregiver assessment, not just initial but rather periodically, becomes routine for at-home clients. The most common self-reported health problem of caregivers is depression (66%) followed by hypertension (34%), and arthritis (30%).

Providing care for someone who is no longer able to take care of him or herself can produce a wide range of emotions. It's natural for the caregiver to feel sadness and grief for the care receiver and for the loss of their own previous life. Retirement dreams of travel, leisure pursuit, and other plans are no longer viable options. The caregiver may feel angry and resentful toward the care receiver, guilty and impatient, ashamed and lonely, pity for himself or herself, anger towards other family members, and/or fearful of the future. Nurses should respond to these expressed emotions as a cry for help as the caregiver may be near the end of his or her ability to cope. Research indicates that caregivers are more likely to have stress-related physical problems than others in their age group. Be aware that chronic muscle tension, insomnia, indigestion, trembling, teeth grinding, jaw clenching, sweaty hands, changes in appetite, dizziness, stomachache, headache, and back pain are signs of stress. These signs warn of depression, exhaustion, and other illnesses and they won't go away by themselves. Various methods of assisting the caregiver are in Table 13-1 with Table 13-2 listing several resource

TABLE 13-1: ASSISTING CAREGIVERS TO COPE

- Provide information for local caregiver support group.
- Provide respite options so social needs of caregiver are met, such as adult daycare or in home respite.
- Provide in-home health care and other services from housekeeping, and home modification to nursing needs of carereciever.
- Provide listing of state, regional, and other resources.
- Provide information on outreach and community programs: referral programs, telephone reassurance, Internet support, friendly visitor programs, peer counseling, transportation, meal and social programs, senior centers, and university programs.
- Provide information on financial assistance programs such as legal services, income assistance, medication programs, Supplemental Security Income (SSI).
- Educate caregivers on care receivers condition.
- Encourage caregivers to maintain own health.
- Teach relaxation techniques such as guided imagery, meditation, or relaxation-breathing techniques.
- Encourage the caregiver to ask for help and to be very specific about what is needed and when. When offered help, say "yes."
- Encourage the caregiver to take time to do enjoyable activities.
- Avoid destructive coping behaviors such as alcohol, overeating, and smoking.
- Encourage caregivers to express their feelings.
- Caregiver should establish daily routines. Having a routine will help to minimize stress.
- Have a plan in the event of you being unable to care for the care receiver.
- Provide assistance into other care options when caregiver has reached emotional overload or maximal stress levels.
- Keep organized. Keep all of your important information in one easily accessible place. Be sure to include insurance, legal, and financial information (i.e. insurance cards, advance directives, social security, etc.).

contacts. The goals of nursing care for the home-dwelling older adult is maintaining and improving health and quality of life along with preventing need for acute care and transfer to higher level of care, and assisting the caregiver to cope.

Keeping clients in their homes not only has a psychological advantage, but also a financial advantage. Assisting the client to remain in the home is much more cost effective than long term placement. If the services provided by informal caregivers had to be replaced with paid services, it would cost an estimated $196 billion (Arno, Levine, & Memmott, 1999).

Many older adults, unable to live independently and not able to afford assisted living, enter nursing homes but really do not need the extensive care that nursing facilities offer. An example of this is in Tennessee where 2,900 low-income older adults were waiting for nursing home placement. A program called Options for Community Living allows the state to coordinate the services needed for low-income older adults to remain in their homes. Although the program cost the state $27 million dollars, it saves the state $2000 per month per participant, or the equivalent of almost $70 million dollars (Gearon, 2003).

TABLE 13-2: CAREGIVER RESOURCES

American Bar Association: Referrals and listings of legal aid offices where older people can get free or low-cost legal assistance. 1-202-662-1000
Website: http://www.abanet.org/elderly

American Parkinson's Disease Association: 1-888-400-2732
Website: http://www.apdaparkinson.org

Alzheimer's Association: 1-800-272-3900
Website: www.alz.org

Alzheimer's Disease Education and Referral Center: 1-800-438-4380
Website: http://www.alzheimers.org

Eldercare Locator: A nationwide toll-free service, helps older adults and their caregivers find local services for seniors. Information Specialist: 1-800-677-1116
Website : http://www.eldercare.gov/

Eldercare On-line: Includes information, chat rooms, forums, state directories of services.
Website: http://www.ec-online.net/

Elderweb: A website for older people, professionals and families seeking information on elder care and long-term care. 1-309-451-3319
Website: http://www.elderweb.com

National Adult Day Services Association: 1-866-890-7357
Website: http://www.nadsa.org

National Institute on Aging and Administration on Aging: Extensive Resource Directory for older adults. 1-202-619-0724
Website: http://www.aoa.gov

National Organization For Empowering Caregivers has a tremendous amount of resources links for national and state organizations covering a multitude of economic, legal and various care issues. 1-212-807-1204
Website: http://www.nofec.org

Oftentimes it is a difficult decision for the older caregiver to give up providing care due to emotional, physical, or other reasons. Assisting the caregiver emotionally through this is important for a smooth transition for all. The need for long-term care is different for each client and situation. The following are some reasons why long-term care may be needed:

- Around the clock care is required.
- Frequent falls.
- Limited mobility.
- Patient wanders from home.
- Patient displays behaviors that are of danger to self or others.
- Caregiver health is adversely affected: exhaustion, stress, or medical deterioration.
- Incontinence of bowel or bladder.
- Patient no longer able to cooperate significantly with care.
- Patient needs services unobtainable at home.
- No caregiver available.

For those older adults who are no longer capable or who no longer want the responsibility of living in their own home, finding the appropriate set-

TABLE 13-3: ASSISTING WITH TRANSITION TO NURSING HOME

How to Make the Transition Successful for Everyone
- Speak with staff ahead of time residents needs, likes, and dislikes.
- Make the room as personalized as possible: own furniture, bedspread, or picture.
- Orient family and resident to the "culture" of the unit. If a special care unit, provide philosophy concerning freedom and behaviors.

Encourage Communication with Staff
- Share information with staff about resident's life, work, family, leisure history etc.
- Provide staff with daytime, nighttime, and alternative phone numbers.
- Introduce resident and family to staff and provide name and numbers to call for concerns
- Participate in care planning meetings.

How Family Members Can Be an Advocate or Involved in Care
- Staff and families are partners in care and should share information.
- Families may take on meaningful roles to the extent desired. Inform families what they can do with their family member if they wish (help with activities, provide direct care: feeding, bathing, toileting, or grooming).

Suggestions for Family Visits
- Bring newspapers, magazines to discuss together.
- Engage in cards or games with no rules.
- Take resident for walk or exercise.
- Take resident to out-of-facility appointments such as doctor, dental, or hairdresser.
- Share meal with resident either in facility or out.
- Bring children or pets. Check facility rules.
- Limit number of visitors at one time.
- Make visits brief, one hour or less, unless tolerated.
- Plan visit around unit schedule.
- Participate in activities with resident.
- Share your skills, piano, sewing etc.
- Help decorate the resident's room.
- Help resident with calls or correspondence.
- Take for ride in car.
- Make videotape or cassette tape for resident to enjoy when your gone.

ting, with the required level of care is important. Assisting the older adult to visit the various setting options, providing choices and ensuring that the older adult has a voice is important for a smooth transition. See Table 13-3 for Assisting with Transition to Nursing Home.

OLDER ADULTS AS CAREGIVERS TO GRANDCHILDREN

Many older adults find themselves caring for and raising their grandchildren. Nurses may come in contact with these situations when working with older adults. The grandparent stepping in to raise grandchildren or other relatives is not a new development, but the dramatic increase in it is new. There are grandparent-headed households in every socioeconomic and ethnic group. According to the U.S. Census Bureau, in 2000 4.5 million children were living in homes maintained by their grandparents, which is 6.3% of all children under 18. This is an increase from 2.2 million in 1970. In one-third of the cases, grandparents are the only caregivers. Researchers report that at some point, more than 1 in 10 grandparents raise a grandchild for at least 6 months. Typically, grandparents are caregivers for periods that are far longer. Older adults who raise grandchildren tend to be women and are younger than age 65, but between 20 and 25% are over the age 65 (AOA, 2000).

There are many reasons why grandparents step in to care for their grandchildren. The older adult is responding to a problem in the middle (parent) generation, such as death of the parent, illness, divorce, immaturity, incarceration of the parent, parental substance abuse, child abuse, neglect, unemployment, and HIV/AIDS.

The grandparents are motivated by the love they feel for their grandchildren and step in to fill a gap created by the problem. Grandparent caregivers face a myriad of challenges in nearly all aspects of their lives when they assume the role of parent. They are prone to psychological and emotional strain as well as feelings of helplessness and isolation. Many grandparents raising grandchildren face financial difficulties and are 60% more likely to live in poverty than are grandparents not raising grandchildren. Grandparent caregivers often neglect their own physical and emotional health because they give priority to the needs of their grandchildren. Often the grandchildren in their care have unmet physical, emotional, and developmental needs that require special assistance.

Grandparents raising grandchildren encounter problems that can require them to seek legal authority in order to make decisions on behalf of their grandchildren. Grandparents may need legal authority to get their grandchildren medical care,

enroll them in school, enable them to receive immunizations and vaccinations, public assistance, and supportive services. Grandparents can find themselves in need of respite services, affordable housing and access to medical care. State and area agencies on aging across the country have instituted programs and services to assist grandparent caregivers. Many have published information guides and have established resource centers to assist grandparent caregivers to identify and access available services. Other important interventions offered around the country include respite services and support groups. An area agency on aging can also be located by contacting the Eldercare Locator at 1-800-677-1116.

For the nurse working with older adults who are raising grandchildren, the goals are to insure the older adult has all the available resources from the community for child raising. The other, equally important goal is to insure the needs of the older adult are assessed and met.

OLDER ADULTS IN THE ACUTE CARE SETTING

People over age 65 constitute the greatest consumers of acute hospital services in the United States (Kozak, Hall, and Owings, 2002). More than 5 million persons over age 65 are hospitalized yearly. Admission to the hospital often results in complications and adjustment problems not seen in younger persons as hospitalized individuals with functional disabilities often regress to a state of helplessness rapidly (Khasraghi, Lee, Christmas, & Wenz, 2003). Older adults tend to have chronic problems that hospitals are poorly equipped to handle and have complications that extend their hospital stay. Hospitalization is often followed by an irreversible decline in functional status and quality of life. At its worst, hospitalization can result in permanent institutionalization or death, the so-called cascade of disasters. For example, an elderly woman experiences hypotension and falls as a result of too vigorous treatment for hypertension. Having broken a hip, she is admitted to the hospital for surgical repair. Following surgery, she initially does well for a day or two. Fever then develops, and it is determined she has pneumonia. She becomes disoriented and, as a result, cannot participate in rehabilitation. Her hospital discharge is delayed, and she eventually needs to go to a nursing facility until she is able to independently care for herself.

A systematic assessment of elderly patients soon after admission is critical to promote timely interventions for minimizing disability and maximizing independence. Nurses should play a major part in the screening, assessment, and management of delirium in older people in acute settings (Schofield & Dewing, 2001). The assessment should include determining the older adult's normal cognitive and physical functioning. That is functioning prior to the illness, accident, or reason for current admission. This is important for discharge goals, which should be to return to those normal functioning levels. Also assess for social functioning, including family systems, significant relationships and support, depression, prosthetic aids used, and availability of community resources that could provide assistance after discharge and the patient's goals.

Care should be taken not to put elderly patients into a passive role while they are hospitalized. Though it can be more time-consuming for staff, elderly patients should be allowed to do as much of their ADLs as possible. This is of particular importance for patients who were independent before their hospitalization. Common problems that arise due to hospitalization include immobility, cognitive impairment, incontinence, skin breakdown, and falls.

Immobility is a problem for older adults in the acute setting (Inouye, et al, 2000). Other than hypotension, an acute neurological or cardiovascu-

lar event, recent surgery and unstable fractures, there are very few reasons for immobilizing hospitalized older patients. Factors that cause immobilization in the hospital without legitimate reasons include environmental barriers such as bedrails, restraints, high beds, lack of staff to help with mobility, cognitive impairment, pain with movement, affective disorders, sensory changes, terminal illness, overuse of sedative and psychoactive drugs, and acute episodes of illness. Immobility or bedrest can result in severe deconditioning because the rate of recovery for lost strength is much slower than the speed of the loss. A person at bedrest can lose 1–3% of his or her muscle strength per day. It may take 6 weeks to recover from 3 weeks of immobilization. In addition, the immobilized patients are at risk for the development of other complications, including stiffness or contractures of joints, pressure sores, pneumonia, constipation, fecal impaction, and deep-vein thromboses. Prevention involves mobilizing patients as soon as possible and doing daily range of motion exercises.

Cognitive Impairment may be seen in a delirium or acute confusional state and occurs in up to 50% of older adult patients at some point in their hospitalization, placing them at risk for complications. Delirium is a disturbance of cerebral function with global cognitive impairment that has an abrupt onset; is brief in duration; and is characterized by evident concurrent disturbances in attention, sleep-wake cycle, and psychomotor behavior. Post-surgical, medication, strange environment, unfamiliar staff, pain, and discomfort are some of the reasons why delirium is so common in hospitalized patients. See Chapter 9 for additional information on delirium. One effective intervention is the continuous presence of a reliable family member or friend who can reassure the individual that the terrifying experience is temporary. Signs of delirium seen in hospitalized clients:

• Behavioral disturbances such as pulling dressings or tubes, or physical combativeness.

- Inappropriate communication such as incoherent speech, or verbal combativeness.

- Visual or auditory hallucinations.

Whenever possible, one should try to prevent the occurrence of delirium. Nursing measures that may be helpful in preventing delirium include the following:

- Visit the patient frequently, especially in the beginning of the hospitalization. Provide a supportive environment.

- Orient the patient to hospital routines.

- Explain diagnostic tests and treatments. Explain rationale for various steps.

- Use physical and chemical restraints as a very last resort for the treatment of anxiety, agitation, and insomnia.

- Anticipate common problems, such as nocturnal falls, incontinence, missed meals, and lack of sleep.

- Place the patient in a quiet, well-lighted room in which a clock, a calendar, and a few familiar objects are clearly visible.

Incontinence is a leading cause of social isolation and institutionalization of the elderly. Incontinence should not be ignored or viewed as an inevitable consequence of aging. The major causes of incontinence in the acute care setting are medications, mental status changes, fecal impaction, immobility, restraints, indwelling catheters, and psychological regression. Catheters tend to promote urinary tract infections and immobility. Once incontinence begins, it tends to persist. Therefore, prevention during hospital stay is critical. The simplest method is for nursing to offer assistance in toileting every 2 hours.

Skin Breakdown and pressure sores are predictable, preventable problems in most hospitalized older patients. The best intervention is prevention. Elderly patients who are at risk for skin problems should be placed on appropriate pressure-relieving devices early in their hospitalization, and a regular turning schedule should be implemented. Preventing incontinence and promoting mobility are important preventive measures.

Falls are a common problem among hospitalized elderly patients. Patients are considered as being at risk for falls if one or more of the following conditions are present:

- Polypharmacy

- A known fall before or after admission

- Confusion, disorientation, uncontrolled restlessness, sedation, or post-operative

- Unsteady gait

- Muscle weakness or interference with sense of balance

- Inability to call for help when walking

- An interruption of cerebral oxygenation with dizziness, syncope or vertigo

- A history of crawling out of bed

- Incontinence of bowel and/or bladder

Interventions such as providing bedside commodes, nonskid footwear, night-lights, low bed positions, and frequent checks can result in a greatly reduced prevalence of falls. Devices such as bed alarms may be useful. Encourage family members to remain with the patient both day and night. Another preventive measure is to move the patient's room near to nursing station and/or allow the patient to sit by the nursing station.

Physical Restraint usage may result in incontinence, skin breakdown, behavioral problems, constipation, depression, loss of function, and negative clinical outcomes (Gallinagh, et al, 2001). Rather than make patients safer from falls in the hospital or other care settings, physical restraints have been found to increase risks for patients (Dunn, 2001). Typically, nursing staff initiates the use of physical restraints to manage patients' problem behaviors and to protect patients from hurting themselves. Rate of restraint usage in hospitalized hip fracture patients was found to be 33.2%. Nurses in acute care settings have reported increased use of physical restraints when they felt that they were working short-staffed. OBRA and the Joint Commission for the Accreditation of Hospitals (JCAHO) have taken stands recognizing the potential negative outcomes associated with the use of physical restraints. Assessment for the underlying cause of the restlessness or other behaviors often results in a basic unmet need such as pain, itching, thirst, need for toilet, hunger, or boredom. Alternatives to restraints include orientation, active listening, therapeutic touch, beds closer to the floor, electronic alarms for beds and wheelchairs, accessible call lights, and — most important — adequate supervision by staff. Reducing the use of restraints in the acute care setting is a priority for gerontological nurses.

Avoiding Complications

Low-tech interventions with little if any side effects are extremely beneficial for preventing the numerous complications of hospitalization. Providing activities to fill idle and "anxious time" such as reading materials and television are found to reduce the stress of hospitalization (Huckstadt, 2002). Request that the hospital recreational therapist evaluates and works with the patient on remaining active, maintaining function, maintaining mood, and preventing falls. See Chapter 12 for additional information on recreation therapy.

Discharge Planning

Shortened hospital stays due to the implementation of the Medicare prospective payment plan based on diagnosis-related groups (DRGs) has resulted in the earlier discharge of patients, many of whom still have significant health problems. Discharge planning is essential and should begin when the patient is first hospitalized. Older patients, the patients' families and all members of the healthcare team should be involved. Discharge planning involves assessing the needs and limitations of patients and their caregivers during hospitalization, planning for continuity of health care on discharge, and coordinating needed individual, family, and hospital and community resources to implement the discharge plan. Some patients are likely to resume their lives as before, but others will require community supports or institutionalization. Comprehensive discharge planning is especially important for patients being discharged to the community. Discharge planning sessions with the family and patient are invaluable in giving information, clarifying understanding of the illness, and answering questions. Information can be shared regarding community agencies and other available resources.

Discharge planning includes assessing the amount of support a patient will need in the community, taking into consideration the following: mobility, ADL functioning (ability to dress, toilet, bathe, feed, and transfer), ability to take medications, fix meals, shop, get to medical appointments, and type of support available with family and friends. Other important factors to consider are environmental factors such as stairs; distance from bedroom to bathroom; and needed medical equipment and safety hazards, particularly with respect to risk of falling. The weeks following hospitalization are crucial. The patient and the patient's family will need as much support as possible. Patients without a primary caregiver who are not capable of caring for themselves or those who are in need of special rehabilitation services may need to be discharged to a nursing facility or rehabilitation facility for a period of time prior to returning to their home. See Chapter 12 for a discussion on rehabilitation.

OLDER ADULTS IN EXTENDED CARE FACILITIES

Assisted living and other forms of supportive housing are specifically designed for those who need extra help in their day-to-day lives but who do not require the 24-hour skilled nursing care found in traditional nursing homes. The trend over the past 2 decades has fortunately been to create a wider variety of living options that are much more homelike than the institutional facilities of the past. The multiple terms used to describe assisted living makes it difficult to pinpoint the exact number of assisted living facilities in the United States. A study conducted by the National Academy for State Health Policy in 2000 reported 32,886 licensed assisted living residences with 795,391 units or beds nationwide (NCAL, 2000). The "typical" assisted living resident is a woman (69%) between 75 and 85 years of age and is self-ambulatory, but needs assistance with approximately two activities of daily living. The survey found that 19% of all residents require no help with ADLs, and on average, assisted living residents need help with 2.25 ADLs, compared to 3.75 ADLs for nursing. Sixty percent require significant help with medications, 26% some help, and 14% need no assistance. Just under half of the residents (46%) came from their home, while 20% from another ALS, 14% from a hospital, and 10% from a nursing home. The most common destination for residents moving out was nursing homes (33%) or died (28%). Costs for assisted living residences vary greatly and depend on the size of units, services provided, and location. The NCAL survey found that 48% of surveyed assisted living centers (ALC) charge between $1,000 and $2,000 in average monthly rent and fees, 23% charge between $2,000 and $3,000, 9% charge more than $3,000 each month, and 16% charge less than $1,000. About two-thirds of ALC residents pay with their own funds, 8% rely on family funding, and 14% pay with Supplemental Security Income (SSI). Assisted living is covered in a growing number of long-term care insurance policies. Medicare does not cover assisted living costs, but certain services are paid under Supplementary Security Income and Social Services Block Grant programs. Thirty-eight

states reimburse or plan to reimburse for assisted living services as a Medicaid service. In addition, states have the option to pay for assisted living under Medicaid by including services in the state's Medicaid plan or petitioning the U.S. Department of Health and Human Services (DHHS) for a waiver. For the nurse working with older adults in assisted living, the overall goal is to maintain function and prevent the need for acute or skilled nursing care transfer.

Nursing Home Settings

While a relatively small number (1.56 million) and percentage (4.5%) of the 65+ population lived in nursing homes in 2000, the percentage increases dramatically with age, ranging from 1.1% for persons 65–74 years to 4.7% for persons 75–84 years and 18.2% for persons 85+.

Early discharge from acute settings often requires a temporary stay in a nursing facility before returning to their own home. When the nursing home admission is expected to be a permanent placement the older adult should be encouraged to visit nursing facilities they are considering before they make a decision. If the patient is too ill, family members or friends should be encouraged to do so. National data is now available to the public on nursing home quality by the DHHS. The data shows how individual facilities compare with others, both nationally and in their region. This may be accessed on-line under Nursing Homes Quality Initiatives www.cms.hhs.gov or by calling 1-800-Medicare. There are 10 quality indicators listed, divided into 2 groups, one for long-term stay and the other for short-term stays. For each facility a percentage is listed for long-term residents with: loss of ADL ability, infection, pain, pressure sores, pressure sores after risk adjustment, and physical restraints. For short-term stay residents the incidents are: delirium, delirium with risk adjustment, improvement in walking, and pain (Pettey, 2003).

These indicators should assist in to some extent in choosing a nursing home.

The nursing facility industry has suffered from a poor public image. The reality is that nursing facilities, as a whole, try to provide good services to a very frail and ill population with limited resources. When patients enter a nursing facility, they must adapt to a totally different environment from their own home. Privacy is diminished, and personal effects are minimal and may be lost or stolen. There is a need to conform to the schedules for bathing, eating, sleeping, and activities as determined by the nursing facility staff. Staff is often overwhelmed with paperwork and following state regulations, making individualized care difficult to provide. A patient may be forced to spend time in the company of persons with whom he or she has little in common. It is important that family members maintain close contact with family members in a nursing facility, to help alleviate feelings of depression and loss of self-esteem. Although placement in a nursing facility can be difficult, with proper and adequate preparation, patients and their families may find the quality of family relationships really improved, to the benefit of all.

It may be useful for nurses working in long-term care to understand what quality of life features are important as defined by residents and their families and attempt to provide the residents with them. For cognitively intact residents the following were important: staff behavior, freedom of choice, quality of food, ambiance at mealtimes, compatible roommate or private room, getting outdoors in good weather, maintaining contact with friends and family, getting a good night's sleep, and infrequent contact with residents with behavioral disturbances. For those with cognitive impairments, features important to quality of life included pleasurable interactions such as meaningful appropriate activities and avoidance of discomfort as identified by forced bathing and restraints (Wunderlich and Kohler, 2001).

END OF LIFE CARE

At present, the only existing alternative to aging is, of course, dying. Eventually, everyone will die. Currently, most persons in Western industrialized cultures have difficulty accepting this simple but inescapable truth. Uncounted millions have been spent on medical research in an attempt to prevent illness and postpone death. The process of dying has been removed from common experience by the practice of putting sick persons in hospitals and nursing homes.

Consequently, many persons today reach the time of their own death without ever having participated in helping anyone through the dying process. This unfamiliarity with death contributes to fear and anxiety surrounding the idea of dying.

Another reason for difficulties in dealing with death and dying in today's culture is the development of medical technology to the point that we often have the ability to keep a person's organs functioning after normally he or she would have died. This capability creates a whole array of ethical dilemmas surrounding the care of those who can no longer care for themselves or even breathe or maintain a heartbeat without the intervention of medical machines.

Many different federal agencies are interested in improving the care given to persons approaching the end of life. Over the past few years an explosion of funding for end-of-life issues has occurred. These range from complimentary pain methods, education, spirituality, death settings mood, and many other end of life support measures (Knebel, 2002). The results of this interest will show promising improvements in the end of life care in the next several years.

Hospice Care

Dying patients often need specific types of care to make them comfortable and to assist them in the process of dying with dignity. Nurses sometimes provide this care directly, and sometimes they teach, counsel, or assist the patients' family members in the provision of this care. The hospice movement in the United States arose to offer this kind of nursing care, and to differentiate it from the cure-oriented care provided by most healthcare institutions. Hospice care originated as a philosophy of care, based on the British model of hospice care developed by Dr. Cicely Saunders, a nurse and physician and founder of St. Christopher's Hospice in London. The U.S. government now forbids an organization from calling itself a hospice unless it is a Medicare-certified hospice. Consequently, the term in this country has come to have a fairly specific meaning. The term palliative care is used to describe the type of care given to provide comfort and support, rather than diagnosis and cure (HFA, 2003).

Hospices in the United States are primarily home care organizations, but some inpatient hospice facilities do exist. Hospices can contract with hospitals and nursing facilities to provide inpatient services, but it can be difficult to retain the hospice philosophy of care in these settings. The long-term care facility and the hospice must have an agreement spelling out the care to be given by both providers to the individual. The care of the resident must reflect the hospice philosophy that is palliative rather than curative. The care given in long term care to a hospice resident is directed at symptoms and circumstances surrounding the physical, psychosocial, and spiritual needs of the individual and their family. A hospice can supply routine or continuous home care to a Medicare beneficiary who lives in a long-term care facility. The Hospice has the responsibility to provide professional case management that a registered nurse must coordinate as well as all core services given routinely by hospice employees. Core services include medical care by a physician, and nursing care such as personal care, social services, and bereavement counseling. Both the long-term care staff and the hos-

pice staff are responsible for delineating and performing their respective services. Coordination and planning of care are imperative according to Medicare guidelines. Long-term care facilities often become the "home" for many elderly individuals. The atmosphere is often more flexible than an acute care setting. Because of these differences, families and residents can disclose and carry out their wishes regarding death in a relaxed manner. Death can occur in a calm and empathic setting.

The hospice philosophy involves recognition that a person has a terminal illness and no longer seeks treatment aimed at providing a cure for that illness. The care is family oriented, and family members usually provide the bulk of hands-on care. An interdisciplinary team that includes the patient and the patient's family, primary physician and/or hospice physician, nurses, social workers, clergy, volunteers, dietitians, and physical therapists provides care. Team members start with a common purpose: to provide care to the dying patient and the patient's family, with the understanding that death does not represent failure, but rather a natural stage of life. Through working together, team members ideally develop mutual respect, open communication, and shared decision making. The focus of hospice care is on symptom management and on coping with anticipatory grief and bereavement. Symptom management is aimed primarily at controlling symptoms before they become distressing rather than only trying to relieve them after they become a problem. It also deals with such issues as pain, hypoxia, nausea and anorexia, incontinence, constipation, and emotional reactions such as depression and anxiety.

Pain Control At End Of Life

One of cancer patient's greatest fears is the fear of uncontrollable pain. One of the major sources of pain in cancer is from bone cancer or from metastases to the bones. Swelling at a tumor site can also cause pain when pressure is put on nerve cells or when organs are blocked. Compassionate, terminal care involves the utmost effort to control pain while keeping the patient as alert as possible. Controlling pain is different from alleviating pain. Control implies that the pain is never allowed to get to the point of causing distress to the patient. Nurses need to remember that a patient may have more than one source of pain. When a patient requests medication for pain, the nurse must understand which pain and how severe it is. A patient with cancer, whose pain is from a long-standing arthritis normally controlled with aspirin, does not need a narcotic to control that pain. In attempting to choose the correct medication and dosage to relieve pain, nurses are usually involved in assessing the effectiveness and side effects of the medicine. If the medicine does not relieve the pain, a different medicine or a stronger dose may be needed. If the medication relieves the pain but does not last until the next dose, then the interval between doses needs to be adjusted. Many medication regimens are available to achieve the optimum effect. Some types of pain medication allow the patient to be in control of the dosing. Patient-controlled analgesia (PCA) can be provided as a "pain cocktail" liquid that the patient can sip as needed or via a subcutaneous pump that allows the patient to determine the dosage needed. One type of schedule that can work well is to have a long-acting pain medication used on a schedule, with a shorter-acting drug available, as needed. Frequently, additional medicines will be added to an analgesic to potentiate the pain-relieving effect.

Historically, physicians and nurses have not been comfortable allowing patients to take adequate pain medicine to control the patients' symptoms. With hospice as a model, nurses in most settings are becoming more aware of the techniques for providing adequate pain control. Nurses used to be afraid that patients might become addicted, or, of more significance in the terminally ill, that they might become tolerant and no longer get adequate relief from available medications. Obviously the problem of addiction is irrelevant for anyone who is in the process of dying. With the development of many different kinds of synthetic narcotics, tolerance is also not usually a problem. Although tolerance does develop, the reduced respiratory depression of newer drugs means that the dose can be increased when more medicine is needed, without causing respiratory arrest. Eventually, high doses of pain medications may, in fact, cause impaired respirations. Many patients choose to receive adequate pain medicine even if this regimen would shorten their lives.

End of Life in a Nursing Home

Research into death experiences within a nursing home is limited. However, some interesting studies have taken place. A summary compilation article reported a lack of attention to cultural needs, with 35% of dying residents unable to speak English, unable to request help, unable to ask for pain relief, and socially isolated (Kayser-Jones, 2002). Some of the residents basically starved to death due to not being accustomed to Western foods served. Dying residents without family members and with cognitive impairment are often neglected under the assumption that they are comfortable. Less than adequate staffing resulted in lack of oral hygiene and lack of bathing dying residents. Poor pain control, poor staff to resident communication, disrespectful and insensitive communication, lack of meaningful activities, psychosocial care, and meeting spiritual needs were a few of the issues mentioned. Another study found that failure to recognize treatment futility was a major obstacle to palliative and end-of-life care (Travis, et al., 2002). In the defense of the nursing home staff, much of the problems are due to inadequate staffing to provide quality end-of-life care.

PHYSICAL CHANGES ASSOCIATED WITH APPROACHING DEATH

Several physical changes can signal the approach of death. Although the last stage of dying can occasionally take several days, it is usually over within a day or two unless medical intervention leads to further delays. Nurses can help patients and families by providing counseling on what to expect and how to cope with problems that develop. Recognizing these signs can also help nurses' plan for a more intensive period of support for patients and the patients' families.

Persons stop eating and drinking when they have no energy or desire to force themselves to eat, or when their disease stops them from digesting food. Providing food and fluid is a basic caregiving process in our society, and persons often react to a patient's cessation of oral intake with an impulse to give food and fluids by enteral or parenteral tubes. Such feeding and hydration are actually more of a treatment for the living than for the dying. Dehydration actually seems to provide a natural anesthesia with lessening edema, less vomiting, fewer lung secretions and even less need to void (Lynn, & Harrold, 1999). The U.S. Supreme Court, in the case of Nancy Cruzan, recognized that giving food and fluid to a patient who is unable to eat or drink is a medical treatment and patients may refuse such a treatment.

Changes in breathing usually occur as death approaches, with breaths becoming shallow, noisy and labored. Breathing patterns can become irregular, with longer and longer periods of apnea. Slowing circulation will occur as the heart pumps blood less strongly. Feet and hands, then arms and legs will cool and become cyanotic. Vital signs change with approaching death, but when death is expected, it is not appropriate to continually disturb a patient just to get accurate readings of temperature and blood pressure. Pulse and respirations can

be measured without disturbing the patient and typically will show tachycardia and tachypnea that become irregular in pattern. Level of consciousness can decrease, but this is very unpredictable, and a person can regain full consciousness when least expected to do so. Nurses should always remember that hearing is the last sense to disappear. Always speak as if the dying person can hear what is being said. Restlessness can occur, and effort should be made to ensure that it is not a sign of a specific physical discomfort such as pain or a need to void.

One of the most difficult occurrences for families to tolerate is bleeding. Although it is not a usual occurrence, it can be an extremely frightening one. If the bleeding is accessible, pressure on the bleeding site can reduce it. Internal bleeding can cause painful swelling that can sometimes be alleviated with ice packs. Frequent changes of towels can reduce the frightening impact of the bleeding. One hospice is reported to calmly bring out red blankets to absorb the bleeding. Families may find themselves unable to cope with significant bleeding in the home.

Finally, when a person dies, there may be an exhalation of air through collected bronchial secretions that produces a gurgle or rattle. Eyes may remain open, and family members may feel more comfortable if the eyes are gently closed. A damp gauze placed on the eyelids is usually sufficient to close them. The body should be placed in a physiologically neutral position, but tying of the hands and feet is an archaic custom that should be abandoned. When combined with the edema that occurs with the collapse of the circulatory system, this practice can result in marking the body unnecessarily. Frequently, the bowel and bladder empty, and for patients dying at home, the family may want to have a plastic sheet on the mattress to prevent soaking the mattress. Some family members want to stay with the body for a period, and this should always be accepted. For a patient dying in a hospital or nursing home, the body should not be moved until the patient's family has had a chance to see and sit with the body if they desire.

A nurse can help a patient and the patient's family prepare for the experience of death by explaining what to expect. Knowing what may happen helps patients and their families cope without panic, especially when an emotional acceptance of the impending death has been reached. A nurse may also suggest that patients and their families make arrangements in advance for funerals, memorial services, and organ donations. When death is expected, autopsies are not generally required, and a physician's presence is not required to complete a death certificate. In some locations, calls to an emergency medical system will result in compulsory cardiopulmonary resuscitation (CPR) and transport to a hospital. When this is not the desired outcome, families need to be warned not to call an emergency number. One of the advantages of hospice involvement is that many of these arrangements are made more easily in a system where the providers have had much experience in coping with death.

SUMMARY

Care provided to older adults may occur in a variety of settings and may be anything from a healthy well visit to the care of the dying. The environment that the older adult is in can have a significant impact on quality of life and perception of care. Assisting the older adult to be in an environment that he or she is comfortable in is an important function of nursing.

EXAM QUESTIONS

CHAPTER 13

Questions 87-94

87. The concept of aging in place is best illustrated by an older adult who

    a. moves in with his/her daughter and her family.

    b. enters an assisted living center.

    c. obtains care services to remain at home.

    d. transfers into a CCRC.

88. An assessment of instrumental activities of daily living (IADL) include

    a. the social support available to the patient.

    b. the ability to obtain groceries and do shopping on a regular basis.

    c. how well the patient is able to bathe.

    d. how a patient feeds him or herself.

89. One of the common challenges of raising grandchildren is

    a. not having enough bedrooms for the grandchildren.

    b. avoiding resentment towards both the children and the parents.

    c. obtaining legal authority to make decisions on the child's behalf.

    d. providing a loving, warm environment for the grandchildren.

90. The older adult in an acute care setting is likely to

    a. have more visitors than younger people.

    b. not require as much pain mediation than a younger person.

    c. have a shorter length of stay than a younger adult.

    d. have more complications than younger adults.

91. The older adult in an assistive living center is likely to need

    a. little assistance with ADLs.

    b. assistance with 2 ADLs.

    c. help with all ADLs.

    d. assistance with 3 ADLs.

92. Transition into a nursing home can be made easier for the older adult by

    a. moving familiar items and furniture into the room ahead of time.

    b. requesting that family does not visit for the first 24 hours.

    c. provide one-on-one care for the first 24 hours.

    d. have admissions occur in the early evening.

93. Hospice care is best described as

    a. assisting nursing home staff members to provide end of life care.

    b. providing specific care to assist in a comfortable death with dignity.

    c. providing end of life care to dying patients with no family.

    d. providing end of life care to persons wishing to remain at home.

94. The best way to prevent family members from being frightened over the physical changes that occur with approaching death is to

    a. prevent the family from seeing the patient during the death process.

    b. keep the room dark and cover the patient with many blankets.

    c. educate the family as to what they might witness ahead of time.

    d. darken the room, play soft music, and burn incense.

CHAPTER 14

LEGAL ISSUES

CHAPTER OBJECTIVE

After studying this chapter, the reader will be able to discuss legal issues that are pertinent to the older adult.

LEARNING OBJECTIVES

After studying this chapter, the learner will be able to

1. describe the concept of autonomy and how it applies to healthcare decisions of older adults.

2. identify the components of informed consent.

3. discuss different types of surrogate-decision making.

4. recognize why older adults are not likely to have advanced directives.

5. describe estate-planning issues for the older adult.

6. identify how older adults become victims of illegal and legal methods of spending down their life savings.

INTRODUCTION

In this country every competent person has the freedom to determine and carry out his or her own decisions. Autonomy comes from the Greek word for "self rule," and is the ability or capacity to make informed choices, free of coercion, based on one's own personal beliefs and values. All adults are presumed to have decision-making capacity and are therefore afforded the right to self-determination, that is, the freedom to make decisions for themselves in all areas of their lives. The concept of autonomy reinforces this right to be free from unwanted interference, which means that there must be legal justification for any curtailment of autonomy. Nurses have a responsibility to respect a patient's right to self-determination. This right is more important than the nurse's values, beliefs or what the nurse may perceive is most beneficial to the patient. All healthcare organizations that receive Medicare or Medicaid reimbursement are required to adhere to regulations of the Patient Self-Determination Act. This act, passed in 1990, requires that all adult patients be informed of their rights under state laws to make their own medical care decisions. Issues surrounding competency, capacity, and decision-making are common with this population and frequently are not addressed until a crisis occurs.

INFORMED CONSENT, COMPETENCY AND CAPACITY

The law presumes all adults are competent to make their own medical care decisions. Generally there are 3 areas concerning medical decisions: informed consent, the patient's competency, and the role of surrogate decision-makers. Informed consent is the process by which a fully informed patient can participate in choices about his/her health care. It originates from the legal and ethical right the patient has to direct what happens to his or her body and from the ethical duty of the physician to involve the patient in his/her health care. The most important goal of informed consent is that the patient has an opportunity to be an informed participant in his healthcare decisions. It is generally accepted that complete informed consent includes a discussion of the following elements:

- The nature of the decision/procedure.

- Reasonable alternatives to the proposed intervention.

- The relevant risks, benefits, and uncertainties related to each alternative.

- Assessment of patient's understanding.

- The acceptance of the intervention by the patient.

In order for the patient's consent to be valid, he or she must be considered competent to make the decision at hand and his/her consent must be voluntary. It is easy for coercive situations to arise when dealing with older adults who often feel powerless and vulnerable. Comprehension on the part of the patient is equally as important as the information provided. Consequently, the discussion should be carried on in layperson's terms and the patient's understanding should be assessed along the way. In some cases, it is unclear whether or not the older adult is competent to make their own decisions. Patients are under an unusual amount of stress during illness and can experience anxiety, fear, and depression. The stress associated with illness should not necessarily preclude one from participating in one's own care. However, precautions should be taken to ensure the patient does have the capacity to make good decisions. There are several different standards of decision-making capacity. Generally the nurse should assess the patient's abil-

ity to understand his or her situation, understand the risks associated with the decision at hand, and communicate a decision based on that understanding. Mental incompetency is not limited to those who legally have been declared incompetent. It includes those who, in the opinion of the attending physician, are either permanently (e.g., cognitive impairment, dementia) or temporarily (e.g., head injury, coma, alcohol, sedated) incapable of giving consent. In some cases, it is necessary to have a psychiatric consultation to evaluate the person to determine competency. Use of forms for documenting the required legal aspects of informed consent can reduce the paperwork and avoid litigation and other problems associated with the documentation of consent (Starr, 2002).

SURROGATE DECISION-MAKER

A surrogate decision-maker is a person designated by the patient, a court-appointed person, or the patient's closest available relative. The surrogate should be guided by the patient's own desires and feelings to the extent that they were expressed before the patient became incompetent or by the patient's best interest. Granting durable power of attorney for healthcare is the preferred method for patients to establish their wishes in advance. A power of attorney enables patients to grant decision-making authority about health-related matters to someone trustworthy in the event they become incompetent.

ADVANCED DIRECTIVES (AD)

Encourage older adult patients to complete advanced directives (AD) to document their preferences regarding treatment and care, including end-of-life wishes. Historically, patients are not given choices or information pertaining to AD and

TABLE 14-1: WHAT TO DO WITH YOUR ADVANCE DIRECTIVES
Make sure your doctor, lawyer, and/or family member knows that you have an advance directive and where it is located.
• If you have designated a health care surrogate, give a copy of the written designation form or the original to the person.
• Give a copy of your advance directive to your doctor for your medical file.
• Keep a copy of your advance directive in a place where it can be found easily.
• Keep a card or note in your purse or wallet which states that you have an advance directive and where it is located.
• If you change your advance directive, make sure your doctor, lawyer, and/or family member has the latest copy.

of those with AD only one-third had them documented in their medical chart (Douglass & Brown, 2002). Research shows that up to 95% of older adults felt they had someone they trusted to make medical decisions for them, but less than half, had talked to that person about preferences for care (Hopp, 2000). Older adults give several reasons for not having discussed AD wishes: " It's too depressing," "Can't cope with the thought of it," "Haven't gotten around to it." Reasons for not completing a formal document were "I intend to," "Don't have a copy of one to use," "Do not want to." When asked to define the best time to be educated about AD the overwhelming number of older adults (80%) said "When you are well" (Inman, 2002). Encourage patients to talk with their family, doctor, and anyone else that they trust, such as a minister, about their preferences for end of life care. Do this when they are well, or at least stable and not in a crisis situation. Inform them that if they do not decide now, their family may have to make decisions for them at some point without knowing their preferences.

Two common forms of AD are a *living will* and the *durable power of attorney for healthcare.* A living will states choices for future medical care decisions, including the use of artificial life support systems. A person has the legal right to limit or forgo medical or life-sustaining treatment, including the use of mechanical ventilators, cardiopulmonary resuscitation, antibiotics, feeding tubes, and artificial hydration. In a living will, a person describes the kind of treatment desired in certain situations. A living will does not allow selection of someone to make decisions for another person. A durable power of attorney for health care allows the patient to appoint an agent (usually a trusted family member) to make all decisions regarding health care. These decisions may be about healthcare providers, medical treatment, and end-of-life decisions. The term durable means that this agent can act on a person's behalf after they are unable to make decisions for themselves. Laws about advance directives are different in each state and vary in terms of content. These can create confusion and a possible failure to honor healthcare wishes of persons who execute healthcare documents in one state and receive treatment in another (Gunter-Hunt, Mahoney, & Sieger, 2002). Nurses need to be aware of the laws in their states when advising patients. Patients who spend the summer or winter in another part of the country ("Snowbirds") should have AD for each state.

Patients may change or cancel AD at any time, as long as they are considered of sound mind to do so. Being of sound mind means that they are still able to think rationally and communicate their wishes in a clear manner. Again, the changes must be made, signed and notarized according to the laws in your state. Make certain the patients' primary physician and any family members who knew about the directives are also aware if they have changed them (see Table 14-1). A durable power of attorney is generally more useful than a living will but may not be a good choice for those who do not have another person they trust to make these decisions for them.

DO NOT RESUSCITATE

A do not resuscitate (DNR) order is another kind of advance directive (AD). A DNR is a request not to have cardiopulmonary resuscitation (CPR) if a patient's heart stops or if the patient stops breathing. (Unless given other instructions, staff will try to help all patients whose heart has stopped or who have stopped breathing.) The patient can use an AD form or tell his or her doctor that they don't want to be resuscitated. In this case, the doctor puts a DNR order in the medical chart. Doctors and hospitals in all states accept DNR orders.

For patients with cognitive impairment it is important that these decisions be executed while the patient is in the early stages of dementia; he or she must be awake, alert, oriented, and legally competent to sign the document. The extent of the durable power of attorney is limited to 7 years unless the patient has become incapacitated at the end of 7 years, during which time the power of attorney continues to be valid or durable.

CONSERVATORSHIP

Conservatorship of a person is a legal procedure that allows the conservator to assume control over a completely incapacitated individual. The conservator is responsible for making sure the conservatee is properly fed, clothed, and housed. A court hearing is required before a conservator can be appointed. Conservatorship provides an incapacitated person with as much legal protection, through court involvement, as possible. On the other hand, conservatorship can incur high and continuous legal fees, increase demands on the judicial system, and offer no guarantee that decisions always will be made in the best interests of the incompetent person or in keeping with that person's desires.

LEGAL ISSUES

Covered in this section are legal issues that may require the use of legal services to resolve. In most states legal services for older adults, who do not have the financial means to obtain a lawyer, are provided by a network of law schools, federal, state, and local grants and the courts. Many of these programs have eligibility standards. However, some programs have special grants that allow them to serve special populations regardless of income. Obtain the resources for your state so they can be made available for any patient who needs them.

Estate planning involves the legal and financial strategies to transfer property from one generation to another. A person's estate is the assets and liabilities remaining after death. Many older adults think that estate planning is just for "wealthy" people. Older adults who do not develop a plan, run the risk of not having their wishes fulfilled. Without a will or trust instrument, upon death the deceased assets will be probated in courts. Probate is a legal process required when transferring assets from a deceased person to beneficiaries in a will, or in the absence of a will, to those entitled to inherit under state intestacy laws. Probate process, in the absence of a will, can be expensive and drawn out, lasting anywhere from several months to several years. All older adults are to be encouraged to do estate planning in advance of health crisis. A *will* is a document that directs how property will be disposed upon death and designates a person to be responsible for assembling the property, paying debts and taxes, and distributing what is left. There are two types of trusts, revocable and irrevocable. A *revocable trust* allows control over assets and unrestricted access to the assets. It provides no protection for assets when it comes to paying for long-erm care. The older adult has no control over assets with an *irrevocable trust* as that is left to the designated trustee. These are often used to get around Medicaid eligibility rules. Medicaid has regulations that severely restrict the use of trusts to hide assets. Medicaid is able to look back 60 months and disqualify an applicant who has hidden assets in a trust. In addition, every state has laws that permit them to place liens on the estate of individuals receiving benefits for long-term care, including funds held in trusts. Older adults are the objects of marketing by large companies that hold free seminars with meals with the goal of encouraging the attendees to open up trust accounts through them. The best method for older adults to protect their assets yet not violate laws or rules, is for them to seek assistance of a trusted local attorney who specialized in estate planning.

LEGAL ISSUES INVOLVING FINANCES

Older adults are vulnerable to various types of legal and illegal methods of spending down their life savings. The isolated, lonely adult who lives alone is particularly at risk as they are often starving for someone to talk to, some mail to arrive, or for the thrill of winning something. The older adult who is poorly educated, has limited income, or has cognitive impairment is often defenseless against fast-talking, convincing scam artists. The older adult is manipulated using fear tactics, promises of prizes or money, or simply by smooth-talking. The results are often financial losses, despair, anxiety, anguish, and emotional distress. Nurses working in home health care are frequently

the ones to uncover these situations and need to direct the patient to the legal services needed to resolve these issues. As various states have specific regulations over these types of problems a general overview follows.

Home repair fraud may occur in many forms and older adults are frequent victims. The most common is the worker who shows up at a homeowner's door offering to do work at what seems to be a good deal. The homeowner is pressured into deciding on the spot as the worker "can only make this offer because he has left over materials from another local job." Generally the homeowner has no opportunity to get a second estimate and is scared into thinking the repairs are needed immediately before more damage occurs. Work is often done quickly and poorly and the final price is much higher than the estimate. Afterwards the homeowner feels he/she is left with faulty repairs and little likelihood of getting their money back. The second form of home repair fraud is the provision of brochures that offer to do an expensive repair for little money. The homeowner signs a contract and pays the money and never hears from the firm again. A third method is the repairman or utility worker showing up in the neighborhood to do a free inspection. These inspections always turn up repairs that most people do not need. Homeowners who have been scammed should contact their states Department of Consumer Repairs and local sheriff's office. To file a complaint they may also contact their state attorney's office or local Better Business Bureau.

Identity theft does happen to older adults, even to those who do not use a computer. It is ranked as one of the top consumer fraud complaints in the nation according to the Federal Trade Commission. This occurs when an impostor uses someone else's name, social security number, or other personal information. Many people do not know their identities have been stolen until they receive bills for credit accounts they never opened, their credit report include debts they did not know they had, or they see charges on their bill they did not authorize. Identity theft can cause a great amount of emotional distress to the older adult. To assist patients in prevention of identity theft, or the steps to take if theft has occurred see the information in Table 14-2.

Sweepstakes companies make millions of dollars each year from misguided and uninformed consumers. Many sweepstakes are legitimate, but large percentages are deceptive promotions designed to rob older adults of their money. The mailings often mislead consumers into believing they have won a valuable prize or that their chances of winning will increase if they purchase certain merchandise. They often appear to announce that "you are the winner," but reading further, the older adult must send in money to receive their prize. Even large well-known major sweepstakes companies have legal actions filed against them.

Telemarketing fraud has become a multi-billion dollar business in this country with thousands of older adults losing a few dollars to their entire life saving as a result of telephone scams (Department of Elder Affairs, 2003). This may be an offer for merchandise, which never arrives, requests from charities that do not exist, or services that are never received. Services scams often occur when consumers are given an 800 number to call, thinking that it is a toll free call when it actually has high phone charges. Cramming is when companies add charges to phone bills for optional services never agreed to such as voice mail or club memberships. These monthly charges, added to the phone bill, may not be noticed as they are relatively small charges ($5–$30) and look like regular phone charges. To prevent these types of frauds instruct patients to:

- Never buy items over the phone from companies they are not familiar.

- If offered an unsolicited rebate or check it is probably a scam.

- Ask for written materials for any offer or charity.

- Call the local Better Business Bureau to determine if a company or offer is legitimate.

- Take time to make a decision.

- Never give out bank account or credit card information.

- The Telephone Consumer Protection Act gives consumers the right to ask companies to place them on their "do not call list" and sue if they do not comply.

- Further information on telemarketing scams: contact the state attorney's office or call Federal Trade Commission 1-877-438-4338.

- If a call is received asking if you are the telephone account holder you may be receiving a slamming pitch. This is the illegal act of switching long distance, local toll, or local telephone company without permission. For information or to file a complaint: Federal Communications Commission 1-888-225-5322.

Television Shopping Channels, Mail Order Catalogs, and Health Product Marketing are another problem for the older adult. Many older adults with mild cognitive impairments spend large amounts of money, their entire savings, on unnecessary items. Family and professional caregivers become aware of this when they either receive expensive gifts or notice many unneeded new items around the older adult's home. The older adult, with or without dementia, may spend large amounts of money on needless "cures" or "anti-aging" products that in fact have no legitimate basis. Generally these are bought by legitimate businesses with attractive advertising methods. The older adult may require the nurse's assistance in determining if these items actually have a positive impact on their health. Older adults with dementia may need assistance in returning unneeded items and require legal assistance to allow a named person to take over the finances of the older adult.

TABLE 14-2: IDENTITY THEFT ISSUES

Prevention of Identity Theft

- Do not leave name and address on discarded mail.
- Use a shedder to destroy papers with personal information.
- Store important papers in a secure location.
- Never leave mail in your box overnight.
- Don't divulge personal information to strangers.
- Report lost or stolen items immediately.
- Keep a list of your credit cards and their phone numbers in a secure place in the event of your wallet or purse being stolen.
- Avoid giving personal information at registrations for door prizes, discounts and coupons.
- Check your credit report frequently.

Steps to take if identity has been stolen

- Contact the fraud department of each of the major credit bureaus. Ask them to flag your file with a fraud alert and include a statement that creditors should get your permission before opening any new accounts. Number to call to report fraud:

Equifax	1-800-525-6285
Experian	1-888-397-3742
Trans Union	1-800-680-7289

- Ask the credit bureaus for copies of your credit. Review these carefully for fraudulent account or unauthorized charges made to existing accounts. Number to call for copies:

Equifax	1-800-685-1111
Experian	1-888-397-3742
Trans Union	1-800-916-8800

- Speak to creditor for any accounts that have been tampered with or opened without your permission. This should be someone in the security or fraud department.
- Follow up with a written account of what was said. (This is one of the procedures spelled out in the Fair Credit Billing Act for resolving errors on credit billing statements).
- File a report with your local police and keep a copy of the police report.
- You will be asked to provide creditors with notarized affidavits identifying all fraudulent accounts and requesting that they be closed. The consumer information center has a form that can be downloaded and used: www.consumer.gov.idtheft/affidavit.htm.
- Additional information: Federal Trade Commission 1-877-438-4338.

SUMMARY

Decisions about life-sustaining treatment are frequent during end-of-life care and become difficult when patient wishes have not been documented or discussed with either the healthcare providers or the family. Nurses must facilitate discussion about AD with their patients in order to allow them to maintain control over healthcare decisions. Prevention of financial losses on unnecessary items or fraudulent schemes helps the older adult afford basic needs, medical care, and treatment and avoid emotional distress. The older adult who fraudulently loses their life savings must depend upon public healthcare dollars for their needs. Therefore it is a responsibility of nurses to help prevent this from happening.

EXAM QUESTIONS

CHAPTER 14
Questions 95-100

95. The Patient Self-Determination Act protects a patients right to

   a. beneficence.

   b. justice.

   c. self-deliverance.

   d. autonomy.

96. In order for a patient's informed consent to be valid a patient must be

   a. given a 2-hour training and pass an exam.

   b. considered competent and give consent voluntarily.

   c. considered near end of life with chance of recovery.

   d. a patient in a hospital or extended care facility.

97. An older adult who wants to name a family member to make healthcare decisions for him/her in the event that he/she is unable needs

   a. to request the doctor to give a Do Not Resuscitate order.

   b. a durable power of attorney for health care decisions.

   c. to complete a Living Will for his/her state.

   d. to see an attorney for a Conservatorship.

98. When would be the best time to initially discuss advanced directives with your client?

   a. During a routine well visit.

   b. During admission to a nursing home.

   c. During a hospitalization for pneumonia.

   d. During an emergency room visit.

99. The best method for an older adult to protect their assets yet not violate laws or rules is to

   a. attend a free seminar for advice.

   b. develop a living will.

   c. seek assistance of a trusted local attorney.

   d. hide their money.

100. An older adult realized that a company has added charges to his/her phone bill for optional services he/she never agreed to. This practice is called

   a. cramming.

   b. identity theft.

   c. repair fraud.

   d. bait-and-switch.

GLOSSARY

absorption: The movement and uptake of substances (liquids and solutes) into cells or across tissues such as skin, intestine, and kidney tubules, by way of diffusion or osmosis.

acetylcholine: A neurotransmitter released at autonomic synapses and neuromuscular junctions, active in the transmission of nerve impulses, and formed enzymatically in the tissues from choline.

Activities of Daily Living (ADL): The basic activities of daily living including bathing, dressing, toileting, transferring, feeding, and continence.

advanced directive: A document that a competent adult can complete and share with a healthcare provider that tells what the person would want to happen in case he or she becomes unable to make his or her wishes known.

aerobic: Living, active, or occurring only in the presence of oxygen, (aerobic respiration); involving, utilizing, or resulting from aerobics (aerobic exercise or fitness).

agnosia: The inability to recognize a familiar stimulus (visual, auditory, or tactile) although primary sensory receptors are intact.

agoraphobic: Abnormal fear of being helpless in a situation from which escape may be difficult or embarrassing that is characterized initially often by panic or anticipatory anxiety and finally by avoidance of open or public places.

akinesia: An agitated motor restlessness that is one of the extrapyramidal side effects of neuroleptic medications.

albumin: The main protein in human blood and the key to the regulation of the osmotic pressure of blood. Chemically, albumin is soluble in water, precipitated by acid, and coagulated by heat.

anhedonia: A psychological condition characterized by inability to experience pleasure in acts which normally produce it.

anaerobic: Living, active, or occurring in the absence of free oxygen. During heavy exercise anaerobic respiration occurs, pyruvic acid acts as a hydrogen acceptor, and lactic acid builds up in the tissues.

anosmic: The absence of the sense of smell, also called anosphrasia and olfactory anesthesia.

antropometrics: The use of body measurements for estimating subcutaneous fat and skeletal muscle stores as well as overall body composition. Examples include weight for height, triceps skin fold, and mid-arm muscle circumference.

anticholinergic: Opposing or blocking the physiological action of acetylcholine.

apraxia: The inability to perform previously learned motor activities in the presence of intact motor and sensory systems (e.g. inability to tie a shoe).

ataxia: The failure of muscular coordination, irregularity of muscular action.

autonomic dysfunction: Also termed dysautonomia refers to a disorder of autonomic nervous system (ANS) function which are involuntary such as blood pressure. Most view dysautonomia in terms of failure of the sympathetic or parasympathetic components of the ANS, but can involve excessive ANS activities.

avitaminosis: A disease resulting from or caused by a vitamin deficiency.

azotemia tube feeding syndrome: An abnormally high level of nitrogen-type wastes in the bloodstream, (elevated blood urea nitrogen or BUN) caused by excessive protein intake or protein catabolism with dehydration (inadequate fluid intake).

bereavement: Refers to the whole process of grieving and mourning and is associated with a deep sense of loss and sadness.

bibliotherapy: A discussion process guided by a facilitator that uses literature as the catalyst to promote insight, normal development or rehabilitation.

bioavailability: The degree and rate at which a substance (as a drug) is absorbed into a living system or is made available at the site of physiological activity.

bradykinesia: Extreme slowness of movements and reflexes (as in catatonic schizophrenia or in weightless space flight).

cogwheeling: A type of rigidity seen in Parkinsonism in which the muscles respond with cogwheel-like jerks to the use of constant force in bending the limb.

conservatorship: A legal procedure that allows the conservator to assume control over a completely incapacitated person.

creatinine clearance: A measurement of the clearance of endogenous creatinine, used for evaluating the glomerular filtration rate (GFR).

discrimination: Unfair treatment or denial of privileges because of an individual's membership in a protected group such as age, race, and gender.

durable power of attorney for healthcare: A legal procedure that enables one person to give another person the legal authority to make health care decisions on behalf of the first person.

dyspareunia: Difficult or painful sexual intercourse.

emotional lability: Excessive emotional reactivity associated with frequent changes. Being emotionally unstable.

failure to thrive: A clinical syndrome encompassing a number of biologic and psychosocial problems associated with increased morbidity and mortality that occurs near the end of life. It may be defined as an unexplained decrease in function, structure, or metabolic process occurring in excess of that expected for age. The easiest measurement to define this syndrome is "unexplained weight loss", though loss of function and loss of lean body mass may also be seen.

free radicals: Highly reactive molecules with an unsatisfied electron valence pair. Free radicals are produced in both normal and pathological processes. They are proven or suspected agents of tissue damage in a wide variety of circumstances including radiation, damage from environment chemicals, and aging.

gastrostomy: The operation of making a permanent opening into the stomach, for the introduction of food.

glaucoma: A group of eye diseases characterized by an increase in intraocular pressure, which causes pathological changes in the optic disk and typical defects in the field of vision.

guided imagery: The use of relaxation and mental visualization to improve mood and/or physical well-being.

Hayflick phenomenon: A theory of aging that proposes that cells loose the ability to reproduce themselves after 50 divisions.

homophobia: The irrational fear and hatred of gays and lesbians.

hyperchloremia: The presence of an excessive amount of chloride. This electrolyte helps to control blood pressure.

hyperkalemia: The presence of an abnormally high concentration of potassium in the blood — called also hyperpotassemia.

hypernatremia: The presence of an abnormally high concentration of sodium in the blood.

hypokalemia: A deficiency of potassium in the blood — called also hypopotassemia.

hyponatremia: Deficiency of sodium in the blood

hypophosphatemia: Deficiency of phosphates in the blood that is due to inadequate intake, excessive excretion, or defective absorption and that results in various abnormalities (as defects of bone).

informed consent: Means that a physician (or other medical provider) must tell a patient all of the potential benefits, risks, and alternatives involved in any surgical or medical procedure, or other course of treatment, and must obtain the patient's written consent to proceed. The concept is based on the principle that a physician has a duty to disclose information to the patient so he or she can make a reasonable decision regarding treatment.

Kegel exercises: Repetitive contractions by a woman of the muscles that are used to stop the urinary flow in urination in order to increase the tone of the pubococcygeal muscle especially to control incontinence or to enhance sexual responsiveness during intercourse. (Kegel, Arnold Henry (b 1894), American gynecologist).

lipophilic: Having an affinity for lipids (as fats).

living will: A form of advance medical directive which preserve the person's right to accept or reject a course of medical treatment even after that person becomes mentally or physically incapacitated to the point of being unable to communicate those wishes. With a living will the person outlines specific treatment guidelines that are to be followed by healthcare providers.

locus of control: A theoretical construct designed to assess a person's perceived control over his/her own behavior; classified as internal if the person feels in control of events, external if others are perceived to have that control.

macular degeneration: The physical disturbance of the center of the retina called the macula. The macula the part of the retina which is capable of our most acute and detailed vision. The macula is used for reading, driving, recognizing faces, watching television, and fine work. Macular degeneration is the leading cause of legal blindness in people over age 55 causing a loss of central vision, however, color vision and peripheral vision may remain clear. Vision loss usually occurs gradually and typically affects both eyes at different rates.

memory tea: A recreational program that utilizes a peer social setting to promote socialization, belonging and an opportunity to express emotions.

myocardial infarction: A term used to describe irreversible injury to heart muscle.

myocardial ischemia: A disorder of cardiac function caused by insufficient blood flow to the muscle tissue of the heart. The decreased blood flow may be due to narrowing of the coronary arteries (coronary arteriosclerosis), to obstruction by a thrombus (coronary thrombosis) or less commonly, to diffuse narrowing of arterioles and other small vessels within the heart. Severe interruption of the blood supply to the myocardial tissue may result in necrosis of cardiac muscle (myocardial infarction).

myofascial release: A stretching technique used by physical therapists to treat patients with a variety of soft tissue problems.

myopia: A condition in which the visual images come to a focus in front of the retina of the eye because of defects in the refractive media of the eye or of abnormal length of the eyeball resulting especially in defective vision of distant objects — called also nearsightedness.

neuralgia: Acute paroxysmal pain radiating along the course of one or more nerves usually without demonstrable changes in the nerve structure.

neurodevelopmental techniques: A therapy method used to inhibit spasticity and synergy using inhibitory posture and movements, and to facilitate normal autonomic responses that are involved in voluntary movement.

pill-rolling: A circular movement of the opposed tips of the thumb and the index finger appearing as a form of tremor in paralysis agitans.

pneumothorax: An abnormal state characterized by the presence of gas (as air) in the pleural cavity.

positive affirmations: Repeatedly speaking or thinking a positive thought about oneself, or others, as a method of motivating, being optimistic and having a positive attitude.

prompted voiding: A technique applicable in which frequent (1 to 2 hourly) checks for dryness are made, reminding the patient to void and praising success.

osteoblastic bone formation: Osteoblast cells arise from fibroblasts and which, as they mature, are associated with the production of bone.

osteoclastic bone resorption: Osteoclasts cells resorb calcified bone or cartilage by secreting acids. When osteoblastic activity no longer balances osteoclastic activity this leads to a great absorption of bone than creation of bone resulting in decreased bone mass.

paraesthesia: A sensation of pricking, tingling, or creeping on the skin having no objective cause and usually associated with injury or irritation of a sensory nerve or nerve root.

paralysis: Complete or partial loss of function especially when involving the power of motion or of sensation in any part of the body.

perseveration: Continual involuntary repetition of a mental act usually exhibited by speech or by some other form of overt behavior.

physiatrist: A physician specializing in physical medicine and rehabilitation.

pica: An abnormal craving for and/or eating of substances (as chalk, ashes, or bones) not normally eaten that occurs in nutritional deficiency states, some forms of mental illness or neurological conditions.

presbyopia: A visual condition that becomes apparent especially in middle age. Loss of elasticity of the lens of the eye occurs causing defective accommodation and inability to focus sharply for near vision.

primary prevention: Prevention of disease or mental disorders in susceptible individuals or populations through promotion of health, including mental health, and specific protection, as in immunization, as distinguished from the prevention of complications or after-effects of existing disease.

secondary prevention: Measures as those that identify and treat asymptomatic persons who have already developed risk factors or preclinical disease but in whom the condition is not clinically apparent.

self determination: Provision of information relating to the individual's rights to make decisions concerning medical care, including the right to accept or refuse medical or surgical treatment and the right to formulate advance directives.

somatization: Conversion of an emotional, mental, or psychosocial problem to a physical complaint.

tertiary prevention: Involve the care of established disease, with attempts made to restore to highest function, minimize the negative effects of disease, and prevent disease-related complications.

visual spatial skills: The ability to localize objects or to appreciate distance, motion, and spatial relationships.

BIBLIOGRAPHY

Advisory (2002). Too many seniors, not enough doctors: Lack of geriatricians is creating a health care crisis. *Senior Market Advisor,* May. Retrieved on January 9, 2003, from http://www.seniormarketadvisor.com/Archives/may02/advisory3.cfm

Administration on Aging (AOA) (2000). Statistical Information on Older Persons. Retrieved on January 9, 2003, from http://www.aoa.gov/prof/Statistics/statistics.asp

Agency for Health Care Policy and Research (1997). In: Medical Expenditure Panel Survey (MEPS) NHC-00P: Round 1 Sampled Facility and Person Characteristics, March [CD-ROM]. Rockville (MD), 1997. AHRQ Pub. No. 97–DP21.

Algase, D., Beck, C., Kolanowski, A., Whall, A., Berent, S., Richards, K., et al. (1996). Need-driven dementia-compromised behavior: An alternative view of disruptive behavior. *American Journal of Alzheimer's Disease, 11*(6), 10–19.

Allen, L.A. (1999). Treating agitation without drugs. *American Journal of Nursing, 99*(4), 36–41, quiz 42.

Alzheimer's Association (n.d.). Ten Warning Signs of Alzheimer's. Retrieved on December 10, 2003, from http://www.alz.org/AboutAD/10Signs.htm

Alzheimer's Association (2002). Alzheimer's Disease Costs Business $61 Billion a Year in Caregiver Time, Productivity Loss and Medical Expenses, Study Shows. Retrieved on January 9, 2003, from http://www.alz.org/Media/news releases/current/062702cost.html

American Medical Directors Association (AMDA). (1999). *Chronic pain management in the long-term care setting.* Columbia (MD): American Medical Directors Association.

American Geriatrics Society. (1998). The management of chronic pain in older persons: AGS panel on chronic pain in older persons. *Journal of American Geriatric Society, 46*(5), 635–651.

American Geriatric Society/British Geriatric Society and American Academy of Orthopedic Surgeons Panel on Falls Prevention. (2001). Guideline for the prevention of fall in older persons. *Journal of Amerian Geriatric Society, 49*(5), 664–672.

American Hospital Association (1992). A Patient's Bill of Rights. Retrieved on May 20,2003, from: http://www.injuredworker.org/Library/Patient_Bill_of_Rights.htm

American Psychiatric Association (APA). (1994). *Practice guidelines for the treatment of patients with Alzheimer's disease & other dementias of late life.* Retrieved on March 7, 2003 from: http://www.psych.org/clin_res/pg_dementia_32701.cfm

Andersen, U., Andersen, M., Rosholm, J., & Gram, L. (2000). Contacts to the health care system prior to suicide: a comprehensive analysis using registers for general and psychiatric hospital admissions, contacts to general practitioners and practicing specialists and drug prescriptions. *Acta psychiatrica Scandinavica.Acta, 102*(2), 126–134.

Andrews, W. (2002). Advances in prevention and treatment of osteoporosis. *Patient Care for the Nurse Practitioner*, Special Edition, December, 21–28.

Antai-Otong, (2000). D. Schizophrenia in the elderly: Managing acute and chronic symptoms. *Advance for Nurse Practitioners, 8*(3), 38–40,46.

Aravanis, S. C., Adelman, R. D., Breckman, R., Fulmer, T. T., Holder, E., Lachs, M., et al. (1993). Diagnosis and treatment guidelines on elder abuse and neglect. *Archives of Family Medicine, 2*, 371–388.

Arno, P., Levine, C., & Memmott, M. (1999). The economic value of informal caregiving. *Health Affairs, 18*(2), 182–188.

Arthur, A., Matthews, R., Jagger, C., & Lindesay, J. (2002). Factors associated with antidepressant treatment in residential care: Changes between 1990 and 1997. *International Journal of Geriatric Psychiatry, 17*(1), 54–60.

Aubert, J., Brochu, C., Vezina, J., Landreville, P., Primeau. G., Imbeault, S., et al. (2001). Environmental conditions associated with agitated behavior among demented patients. Vancouver, British Columbia. *The XVII World Congress of the International Alzheimer's Association of Gerontology*, July 1–6, 7–11.

Ayello, E. A. (1999). Predicting pressure ulcer sore risk. *The Hartford Institute for Geriatric Nursing: Best Practice in Nursing Care to Older Adults*, (5). Retrieved on January 9, 2003 from: http://www.hartfordign.org/publications/trythis/issue05.pdf

Baldwin, J. (2001). AIDS may escape diagnosis in older people. *Geriatric Times, 2*(1). Retreived on July 11, 2003 from http://www.geriatrictimes.com/g010106.html

Barenbrock, M., Kosch, M. & Hausberg, M. (2003). Sodium intake and vessel wall properties of large arteries. *Journal of Hypertension, 21*(1), 33–35.

Baltes, P., & Baltes, M. (1990). Psychological perspectives on successful aging: The model of selective optimization with compensation. In P. B. Baltes & M. M. Baltes (Eds.), *Successful Aging* (pp. 1–27). Cambridge, Mass: Cambridge University Press.

Barash, R. A. (1991). How Aging Effects Sexual Functioning. California Nursing. May-June, pp. 25–28.

Beers, M. H. (2000). The medication list-a portrait of a patient's health. *Journal of Gerontology, Biological Sciences and Medical Sciences*, SS(20), M549.

Beers, M., Ouslander, J., Rollingher, I., Reuben, D., Brooks, J., & Beck, J. (1991). Explicit criteria for determining medication use in nursing home residents. *Archives of Internal Medicine, 151*(9), 1825–1832.

Bell, J. (1978). Disengagement versus engagement – a need for greater expectations. *Journal of American Geriatric Society, 26*(2),89–95.

Beullens, J. (2001). Sleep and intellectual functioning in the elderly: The role of sleep quality and apnea. *Tijdschr Gerontology & Geriatrics, 32*(4), 165–173.

Biggs, A. & Freed, P. (2000). Nutrition and older adults: What do family caregivers know and do? *Journal of Gerontological Nursing, 26*(8), 6–14.

Blum, H. (1980). Social perspective on risk reduction, family and community health. *The Journal of Health Promotion and Maintenance, 3*(1), 41–61.

Bowles, S. (1991). In F. F. Rogers-Seide, (ed.)., *Geriatric nursing care Plans*. St. Louis: Mosby-YearBook.

Braden, B., & Bergstrom, N. (1988). Clinical utility of the Braden scale for predicting pressure sore risk. *Nursing Times, 84*(25), 69–70.

Bradley, P. J. (2003). Family caregiver assessment: Essential for effective home health care. *Journal of Gerontological Nursing, 29*(2), 29–36

Brunk, U., & Terman, A. (2002). Lipofuscin: mechanisms of age-related accumulation and influence on cell function. *Free Radical Biology Medicine, 33*(5), 611–619.

Bryant-McKenney, H. (2000). Clinical management of the geriatric stroke patient. *Advance for Nurse Practitioners, 8*(7), 36–38, 43,84.

Buettner, L. (2002). Tips for older adults with Alzheimer's Disease and other dementias. *Health Promotions for the Body, Mind and Spirit.* Fort Myers, FL: Florida Gulf Coast.

Buettner, L. (1997). *The art of dementia care: A training manual.* Binghamton, NY: Binghamton University.

Buettner, L., & Fitzsimmons, S. (2003). *Dementia practice guidelines for recreational therapy: Treatment of disturbing behaviors.* Alexandria,VA: American Therapeutic Recreation Association.

Burgio, L., Butler, F., Roth, D., Hardin, J., Hsu, C., & Ung, K. (2000). Agitation in nursing home residents: The role of gender and social context. *International Psychologeriatrics, 12*(4), 495–511.

Burgess, M., McCrea, J., & Hedrick, H. (2001). Age-associated changes in cardiac matrix and integrins. *Mechanisms of Aging and Development, 122*(15):1739–1756.

Buysse, D. J., Reynolds, C. F., Monk, T. H., Berman, S.R., & Kupfer, D. J. (1989). The Pittsburgh sleep quality index: A new instrument for psychiatric practice and research. *Journal of Psychiatric Research, 28*(2), 193–213.

Cable, G., Reisner, M., Gerges, S., & Thirumavalavan, V. (2000). Knowledge, attitudes, and practices of geriatricians regarding patients with dementia who are potentially dangerous automobile drivers: A national survey. *Journal of American Geriatric Society, 48*(1), 14–17.

Cadieux, R. (2002). Legal and ethical issues in treating the elderly. *Penn State*, July. Retrieved on January 9, 2003, from http://www.parc.xerox.com/solutions/enhancedthumbnails/demo-enh/Demo-Halcion/497/www.mhsource.com/gericongress/423s.html

Cahill, S., South, K., Spade, J. (2000). *Outing Age*: Public Policy Issues Affecting Gay, Lesbian, Bisexual, and Transexual Elders. New York, NY: Policy Institute of NGLTF Foundation, http://www.ngltf.org/downloads/outingage.pdf

Capezuti, E., Brush, B., & Lawson, W. (1997). Reporting elder mistreatment. *Journal of Gerontological Nursing, 23*(7), 24–32.

Carosella, A., Ossip-Klein, D., Watt, C,. & Podgorski, C. (2002). Smoking history, knowledge, and attitudes among older residents of a long-term care facility. *Nicotine Tobacco, 4*(2), 161–169.

Carr, D. (1997). Motor vehicle crashes and drivers with dementia of the Alzheimer's type. *Alzheimer's Disease Association Disorder, S-1*, 38–41.

Carr. D., Duchek, J. & Morris, J.C. (2000). Characteristics of motor vehicle crashes of drivers with dementia of the Alzheimer's type. *Journal of American Geriatric Society, 48*(1), 18–22.

Carstensen, L. (2002). *Difficult dialogues program: Aging in the 21st century: Consensus report.* Stanford CT: Institute on Research on Women and Gender.

Center for Drug Evaluation and Research. (2002). *Preventable Adverse Drug Reactions: A Focus on Drug Interactions.* Retrieved on May 20,2003, from http://www.fda.gov/cder/drug/drugReactions/default.htm

Centers for Medicare & Medicaid Services, (n.d.). *Psychotropic drug use in skilled nursing facilities (SNF).* Retrieved December 10, 2003, from http://www.cms.hhs.gov/medlearn/articleSNF1002.pdf

Cesari, M., Landi, F., Torre, S., Onder, G., Lattanzio, F., & Bernabei, R. (2002). Prevalence and risk factors for falls in an older community-dwelling population. The Journals of Gerontology: Medical Science, 57(11), M722–M726.

Chaudhry, K. (2003). Cardiovascular system. Synopsis of pathology and microbiology. Retrieved on May 20, 2003, from http://medicalbooks.a2zfree.net/pathsynopsis/

Cheitlin, M. (2003). Cardiovascular physiology-changes with aging. *American Journal of Geriatric Cardiology, 12*(1),9–13.

Chin, J., Sahadevan, S., Tan, C., Ho, S. & Choo, P. (2001). Critical role of functional decline in delayed discharge from an acute geriatric unit. *Annals of Academic Medicine Singapore, 30*(6), 593–599.

Closs, S. (1996). Pain and elderly patients: A survey of nurses' knowledge and experiences. *Journal of Advanced Nursing, 23*(2),237–242.

Cobb, E., Duthie, E., Jr., & Murphy, J.B. (2002). Geriatrics review syllabus: a core curriculum in geriatric medicine. New York: *American Geriatric Society.*

Cockcroft, D. & Gault, M. (1976). Prediction of creatinine clearance from serum creatinine. *Nephron, 16*(1), 31–41.

Conwell, Y. (1994). Suicide, religion, and the elderly. *Crisis, 15*(1), 9–10.

Corbin, J., & Strauss, A. (1991). A nursing model for chronic illness management based upon the trajectory framework. *Scholarly Inquiry Nursing Practice, 5*(31), 155–174.

Coyne, A. C. (2001). The relationship between dementia and elder abuse. *Geriatric Times, 2*(45). Retreived on July 11, 2003, from http://www.geriatrictimes.com/g010715.html

Crutchfield, D. (2002). Medication review: Don't forget the OTCs. *Geriatric Times, 3*(2), 13–15.

Crutchfield, D. (2002). Managing weight loss in the elderly: An interdisciplinary approach. *Geriatric Times, 3*(4), 18–20.

Day, L., Fildes, B., Gordon, I., Fitzharris, M., Flamer, H., & Lord, S. (2002). Randomized factorial trial of falls prevention among older people living in their own homes. *British Medical Journal, 325*(7356), 128.

Davis, G., Hiemenz, M., & White, T. (2002). Barriers to managing chronic pain of older adults with arthritis. *Journal of Nursing Scholarship, 34*(2), 121–126.

Dechant, K., & Clissold, S. (1991). Paroxetine: A review of its pharmacodynamic and pharmaco-kinetic properties, and therapeutic potential in depressive illness. *Drugs,* 41(2), 225–235.

Department of Elder Affairs. (2003). *Consumer resource guide.* Tallahassee, Fl: Florida Department of Elder Affairs.

Dellasega, C., Klinefelter, J., & Halas, C. (2000). Psychoactive medications and the elderly patient. *Clinician Reviews, 10*(6), 53–74.

Demirci, S., & Savas, S. (2002). The auditory event related potentials in episodic and chronic pain sufferers. *European Journal of Pain, 6*(3), 239–44.

Derouesne, C., Piquard, A., Thibault, S., Baudouin-Madec, V., et al. (2001). Non-cognitive symptoms in Alzheimer's disease: A study of 150 community-dwelling patients using a questionnaire completed by caregivers. *Reviews of Neurology, 157*(2), 162–177.

Derouesne, C., Thibault, S., Lozeron, P., Baudouin-Madec, V., Piquard, A., & Lacomblez, L. (2002). Perturbation of activities of daily living in Alzheimer's disease. A study of 172 patients using a questionnaire completed by caregivers. *Reviews of Neurology, 158*(6–7), 684–700.

Dhalla, I., Anderson, G., Mamdani, M., Bronskill, S., Sykora, K. & Rochon, P. (2002). Inappropriate prescribing before and after nursing home admission. *Journal of American Geriatric Society, 50*(6), 995–1000.

Douglas, R. & Brown, H. (2002). Patients' attitude toward advance directives. *Journal of Nursing Scholarship, 34*(1), 61–65.

Dowd, J. (1975). Aging as exchange: A preface to theory. *Journal of Gerontology, 30*(5),584–594.

Dowling-Castronovo, A. (2001). Urinary incontinence assessment. *Journal of Gerontological Nursing, 27*(5), 6–7.

DrugIntel. (2003). Adverse drug reactions, adverse drug events, and medication errors are a leading cause of death in USA: Retrieved on January 9, 2003, from http://www.drugintel.com/pharma/cause_of_death.htm

Droge, W. (2002). Free radicals in the physiological control of cell function. *Physiological Review, 82*(1), 47–95.

Dubbert, P., Cooper, K., Kirchner, K., Meydrech, E., & Bilbrew, D. (2002). Effects of nurse counseling on walking for exercise in elderly primary care patients. *Journal of Gerontology: Medical Sciences, 57A*(11), 733–740.

Dunn, K. (2001). The effects of physical restraints on fall rates in older adults who are institutionalized. *Journal of Gerontological Nursing, 27*(10), 40–48.

Durso, S. (2001). Helping patients adhere to medical instructions. *Lifeline Connections for the Healthcare Professional.* Summer. Farrington, MA. Retrieved on January 9, 2003, from http://www.lifelinecanada.com/english/publications/index.shtmlc

Ebersole, P., & Hess, P. (1998). *Toward healthy aging: Human needs and nursing response,* (5th ed). St. Louis: Mosby.

Elliott, B. (2000). Diagnosing and treating hypothyroidism. *The Nurse Practitioner, 25*(3), 92–94, 99–105.

Engelman, K., Mathews, R., & Altus, D. (2002). Restoring dressing independence in persons with Alzheimer's disease: A pilot study. *American Journal of Alzheimer's Disease and Othe Dementias, 17*(1), 37–43.

Erkinjuntti, T., & Rockwood, K. (2003). Vascular dementia. *Seminar in Clinical Neuropsychiatry, 8*(1), 37–45.

Erikson, E. (1963). *Childhood and society.* (2nd Ed.), New York: W. W. Norton & Co.

Family Caregiver Alliance. (2001). Fact Sheet: Selected Caregiver Statistics. Retrieved on March 9, 2003, from http://www.caregiver.org/factsheets/selected_caregiver_statistics.html

Farmer, B. (2000). Fall risk assessment. *Journal of Gerontological Nursing, 26*(7), 6–7.

Farrell, J. (1990). *Nursing care of the older person.* Philadelphia: Lippincott.

Farrell, M., Gibson, S., & Helme, R. (1996). Chronic nonmalignant pain in older people. In: B. A. Ferrell, & B.R. Ferrell, (eds). Pain in the Elderly: *A report of the task force on pain in the elderly.* Seattle, WA: International Association for the Study of Pain.

Feil, N. (1992 & 1994). *V/F Validation: The Feil Method, how to help disoriented old-old.* Cleveland, OH: Edward Feil Press.

Feil, N., & Klerk-Rubin, V. de, (2002). *The validation breakthrough: simple techniques for communicating with people with Alzheimer's-type dementia (2nd edition).* Baltimore, MD: Health Professions Press.

Field, D., & Gueldner, S. (1999). The oldest-old: How do they differ from the old-old? *Journal of Gerontological Nursing, 27*(8), 20–7.

Fitzsimmons, S., & Buettner, L. (2003). Therapeutic recreation interventions for need-driven dementia-compromised behaviors in community-dwelling elders. *American Journal of Alzheimer's Disease and Other Dementias, 17*(6), 367–381.

Flannelly, L., Flannelly, K., & Weaver, A. (2001). Religious and spiritual variables in three major oncology nursing journals: 1990-1999. *Oncology Nursing Forum, 29*(4), 679–85.

Flint, A. J. (2001). Anxiety disorders. *Clinical Geriatrics, 9*(11), 21–30.

Folkins, J. (1992). Resource on person-first language: The language used to describe individuals with disabilities. American Speech, Language and Hearing Publication Board. December.

Folstein, M., Folstein, S., & McHugh, P. (1975). 'Mini-Mental State': A practical method for grading the cognitive status of patients for the clinician. *Journal of Psychiatric Research, 12*(3), 189–198.

Foreman, M., Wakefield, B., Culp, K,. & Milisen, K. (2001). Delirium in elderly patients: An overview of the state of the science. *Journal of Gerontological Nursing, 27*(4), 12–20.

Foster, D., Phillips, R., Hamel, M., & Eisenberg, D. (2000). Alternative medicine use in older Americans. *Journal of American Geriatric Society, 48(12).* 1560–1565.

Freedman, M. (1999), Assessment and treatment of erectile dysfunction in late life. Presented at the *American Association for Geriatric Psychiatry Annual meeting.* New Orleans; March 13.

Freund, B., & Szinovacz, M. (2002). Effects of cognition on driving involvement among the oldest old: Variations by gender and alternative transportation opportunities. *Gerontologist, 42(5),* 621–633.

Friedland, R., & Summer, L. (1999). *Demography is not Destiny.* Washington D.C.: National Academy on an Aging Society.

Fry, P. S. (2001). The unique contribution of key existential factors to the prediction of psychological well-being of older adults following spousal loss. *The Gerontologist, 41*(1), 69–81.

Frenchman, I. B. (2001). Cost of urinary incontinence in two skilled nursing facilities: A prospective study. *Clinical Geriatrics, 9*(1), 49–52.

Fugh-Berman, A. (1996). *Alternative medicine what works.* Philadelphia: Williams Wikins.

Fugh-Berman, A. (2002). Herbal supplements: Indications, clinical concerns, and safety. *Nutrition Today, 37*(3), 122–124.

Funk, S.G., Tornquist, E.M., Champagne, M.T., & Wiese, R.A. (Eds.). (1992). Key Aspects of Elder Care: Managing Falls, Incontinence, and Cognitive Impairment. In L. Hollinger & R. Patterson, *A Fall Prevention Program for the Acute Care Setting.* New York, NY: Springer Publishing Company.

Furlanetto, L., von Ammon Cavanaugh, S., Bueno, J., Creech, S., & Powell, L. (2000). Association between depressive symptoms and mortality in medical inpatients. *Psychosomatics, 41*(5), 426–432.

Gallinagh, R., Nevin, R., McAleese, L., & Campbell, L. (2001a). Perceptions of older people who have experienced physical restraint. *British Journal of Nursing, 10*(13), 852–858.

Gallinagh, R., Nevin, R., McIlroy, D., Mitchell, F., Campbell, L., et al. (2001b). The use of physical restraints as a safety measure in the care of older people in four rehabilitation wards: Findings from an exploratory study. *International Journal of Nursing Studies, 39(2),* 147–156.

Gallo, J., & Rabins, P. (1999). Depression without sadness: alternative presentations of depression in late life. *American Family Physician, 60*(3), 820–826.

Gaston-Johansson, F., Johansson, F., & Johansson, N. (1999). Undertreatment of pain in the elderly: Causes and prevention. *Annals of Long-Term Care, 7*(5), 190–196.

Gatz, M., Kasl-Godley, & Karel, M. (1996). *Aging and mental disorders: Handbook of psychology of aging,* (4th ed.) (pp. 367–382), J. Birren & K.W. Schaie, (eds). San Diego, CA: Academic Press, pp. 367–382.

Gearon, C. (2003). Southeast region report: Tennessee: Nursing home care alternative launched. *American Association of Retired Persons (AARP) Bulletin, 44*(2), 13.

Gibbs-Brown, J. (1997). Prescription drug use in nursing homes. *Department of Health & Human Services,* Nov. OEI-06-96-00080.

Glaser, V. (2000). Effective approaches to depression in older adults. *Patient Care for Nurse Practitioners, 3*(9), 53–69.

Goodroad, B. K. (2003). HIV and AIDS in people older than 50. A continuing concern. *Journal of Gerontological Nursing, 29*(4), 18–24.

Graeber, M. B., & Mehraein, P. (1999). Reanalysis of the first case of Alzheimer's disease. *European Archives of Psychiatry Clinical Neuroscience, 249 Suppl* 3, 10–13.

Grandjean, C. K., & Gibbons, S. W. (2000). Assessing ambulatory geriatric sleep complaints. *The Nurse Practitioner, 25*(9), 25–32, 35, 40–41.

Guigoz, Y., Lauque, S., & Vellas, B. J. (2002). Identifying the elderly at risk for malnutrition the Mini Nutritional Assessment. *Clinical Geriatric Medicine, 18*(4), 737–757.

Gunter-Hunt, G., Mahoney, J. E. & Sieger, C. (2002). A Comparison of state advance directive documents. *The Gerontologist, 42*(1), 51–60.

Gurvich, T., & Cunningham, J. A. (2000). Appropriate use of psychotropic drugs in nursing homes. *American Family Physician, 61*(5), 1437–1446.

Gurwitz, J. H., Field, T. S., Avorn, J., McCormick, D., Jain, S., Eckler, M. (2000). Incidence and preventability of adverse drug events in nursing homes. *American Journal of Medicine, 109*(2), 87–94.

Guy, W. (1976). *ECDEU assessment manual for psychopharmacology.* (rev. ed.) Washington, DC: US Department of Health, Education, and Welfare.

Hall, G., & Buckwalter, K. (1987). Progressively lowered stress threshold: A conceptual model for care of adults with Alzheimer's disease. *Archives of Psychiatric Nursing, 1*(6), 399–406.

Hall, G. (1991). *Altered thought processes: Dementia.* In M. Maas, K. C. Buckwalter, & M. Hardy, (eds). Nursing diagnosis and interventions for the elderly. Redwood City, CA: Addison-Wesley, Nursing, 322–347.

Hall, G., & Buckwalter, K., Stolley, J., Gerdner, L., Garland, L., et al. (1995) Standardized care plan: Managing Alzheimer's patients at home. *Journal of Gerontological Nursing, 21*(1), 43–44.

Hampton, J. L. (1991). *The Biology of Human Aging.* Dubuque, IA: W. C. Brown.

Hanlon, J., Shimp, L., & Semla, T. (2000). Recent advances in geriatrics: Drug-related problems in the elderly. *Annals of Pharmacotherapy, 34*(3), 360–365.

Hardten, D. (2003). Condition: Cataract. Retrieved on May 20, 2003, from: http://drhardten.eye mdlink.com/Condition.asp?ConditionID=4

Hayflick, L. (1984). Intracellular determinants of cell aging. *Mechanics of Aging Development, 28*(2–3),177–185.

Hays, J. C.,Galanos, A. N., Palmer, T., McQuoid, D. R., & Flint, E. P. (2001). Preference for place of death in a continuing care retirement community. *The Gerontologist, 41*(1), 123–128.

Health Care Financing Administration. (1992). *State operations manual.* Baltimore: U.S. Department of Health and Human Services.

Hegge, M., & Fischer, C. (2000). Grief responses of senior and elderly widows: Practice implications. *Journal of Gerontological Nursing, 26*(1), 35– 43.

Heinrich, J. (2001). Health products for seniors: "Anti-aging" products pose potential for physical and economic harm. Washington, DC: U.S. General Accounting Office.

Herr, K. (2002). Chronic pain in the older patient: Management strategies Part 2. *Journal of Gerontological Nursing, 28*(2), 28–34.

Herr, K. (2002). Chronic pain: Challenges and Assessment Strategies. Part 1. *Journal of Gerontological Nursing, 28*(1), 20–27.

Hicks, Jr., T. J. (2000). What is your life like now? Loneliness and elderly individuals residing in nursing homes. *Journal of Gerontological Nursing, 26*(8), 15–19.

Hill, L., & Smith, N. (1990). *Self-care nursing: Promotion of health (2nd ed.).* Norwalk, CT: Appleton & Lange.

Hinton, R., Moody, R., Davis, A. & Sean, T. (2002). Osteoarthritis: Diagnosis and therapeutic considerations. *American Academy of Family Physicians, 65*(S), 841–848.

Hobgood, G. (1997). On old age: A conversation wih Joan Erikson at 90. Produced by Frances Davidson. San Luis Obispo, CA: Davidson Films. Retrieved on July 19, 2003, from: http://www.davidsonfilms.com/age1revu.htm

Hopp, F. (2000). Preferences for surrogate decision makers, informal communication, and advance directives among community-dwelling elders: Results from a national study. *The Gerontologist, 40*(4), 449–457.

Horgas, A. L., & Dunn, K. (2001). Pain in nursing home residents. Comparison of residents' self-report and nursing assistants' perceptions. Incongruencies exist in resident and caregiver reports of pain; therefore, pain management education is needed to prevent suffering. *Journal of Gerontological Nursing, 27*(3), 44–53.

Hospice Foundation of America (HFA). (2003). What is hospice? *Hospice Foundation of America.* Retrieved on May 22, 2003, from: http://www.hospicefoundation.org/what_is/

Huckstadt, A. (2002). The experience of hospitalized elderly patients. *The Journal of Gerontological Nursing, 28*(9), 25–29.

Hurley, A., Volicer, B., & Hanrahan, P. (1992). Assessment of discomfort in advanced Alzheimer patients. *Research, Nursing Health, 15*(5), 369–377.

Huth, E. (1985). Source: *Hippocrates. The Book of Prognostics.* In F. Adams (ed). The genuine works of Hippocrates. London: C. and J. Adlard Printers; 1849. Reprinted in Birmingham, AL: *Classics of Medicine Library;* 1985, p. 238 (q.v.).

Hyman, S., & Rudorfer, M. (2000). Depressive and bipolar mood disorders. In: D. C. Dale, D. D. Federman, (eds.). *Scientific American® Medicine, 3,* (Sub-Section 11), 1 New York: Healtheon/Web MD Corp.

Ihara, E. (2002). *Challenges for the 21st century: Chronic and disabling conditions: Prescription drugs.* Center on an Aging Society. Retrieved on January 9, 2003 from: http://ihcrp.george town.edu/agingsociety/profiles.html

Inman, L. (2002). Advanced directives: Why community-based older adults do not discuss their wishes. *Journal of Gerontological Nursing, 28*(9), 40–46.

Inouye, S., van Dyck, C. H., Alessi, C. A., Balkin, S., Siegal, A. P., & Horwitz, R. (1990). Clarifying confusion: The confusion assessment method, a new method for detection of delirium. *Annals of Internal Medicine, 113*(12), 941–947.

Inouye, S. K., Bogardus, Jr., S. T., Baker, D. I., Leo-Summers, L., & Cooney, Jr., L. M. (2000). The hospital elder life program: A model of care to prevent cognitive and functional decline in older hospitalized patients. Hospital elder life program. *Journal of American Geriatric Society, 48*(12):1697–1706.

Jacelon, C. (1999). Preventing cascade iatrogenesis in hospitalized elders. An important role for nurses. *Journal of Gerontological Nursing, 25*(1), 27–33.

Janssen Pharmaceutica, Inc. (2003). Important drug information. WARNINGS: Cerebrovascular adverse events, including stroke, in elderly patients with dementia. Letter to Health Care Providers, April 16. Retrieved on May 20, 2003 from: http://www.fda.gov/medwatch/SAFETY/2003/risperdal.htm

Janz, N. K., & Becker, M. H. (1984). The health belief model: A decade later. *Health Education Quarterly, 11*(1),1–47.

Jenike, M. (1988). Alzheimer's disease: What the practicing clinician needs to know. *Journal of Geriatric Psychiatry and Neurology, 1*(1), 37–46.

Johne, A., Brockmoller, J., Bauer, S., Maurer, A., Langheinrich, & Roots, I. (1999). Pharmacokinetic interaction of digoxin with an herbal extract from St John's wort (hypericum perforatum). *Clinical Pharmacological Therapy, 66*(4), 338–345.

Joiner T., Jr., & Katz, J. (1999). Contagion of depressive symptoms and mood; Meta-analytic review and explanations from cognitive, behavioral, and interpersonal viewpoints. *Clinical Psychology: Science and Practice, 6*(2), 149–164.

Joint Commission on Accredition of Healthcare Organizations (JCAHO). (2002). *Healthcare at the crossroads: Strategies for addressing the evolving nursing shortage.* Joint Commission Public Policy Commission. Retrieved on January 9, 2003, from http://www.jcaho.com/

Joint Commission on Accreditation of Healthcare Organizations (2000). Sentinel Event Alert Issue 14 - July 12.

Joo, J., Y., Lenze, E. J., Mulsant, B. H., Begley, A., Weber, E. M., Stack, J., et al. (2002). Risk factors for falls during treatment of late-life depression. *Journal of Clinical Psychiatry, 63*(10), 936–941.

Kane, G. C., & Lipsky, J. J. (2000). Drug-grapefruit juice interactions. *Mayo Clinical Procedures, 75*(9), 933–942.

Kane, R., Ouslander, J., & Abrass, I. (1999). Drug therapy. In: R. L. Kane, J. G. Ouslander, & I. Abrass, (eds). *Essentials of clinical geriatrics.* (4th ed) (pp 379–411). New York: McGraw-Hill.

Kaplan, B. (2002). Gay elders face uncomfortable realities in LTC. *Caring for the Ages, 3*(11), 14–16.

Kasckow, J. W., Mulchahey, J. J., Aslam, M., Sobai, M., & Mohamed, S. (2003). When and how to use SSRI's to treat late-life depression. *Current Psychiatry, 2,* 43–47.

Katz, S., Ford, A., Moskowitz, R., Jackson, B. & Jaffe, M. (1963). Studies of illness in the aged. The index of ADL: A standar measure of biological psychosocial function. *Journal of American Medical Association, 185,* 914.

Katzman, R., & Terry, R. (1983). *The neurology of aging.* Philadelphia: F. A. Davis.

Katzman, R., Brown, T., Fuld, P., Peck, A., Schechter, R., & Schimmel, H. (1983). Validation of a short Orientation-Memory-Concentration Test of cognitive impairment. *Am J Psychiatry, 140*;734-739.

Kayser-Jones, J. (2002). The experience of dying: An ethnographic nursing home study. *The Gerontologist, 42*(Special Issue III), 11–19.

Kegel, A. (1948). Progressive exercise in the functional restoration of the perineal muscles. *American Journal of Obstetrics and Gynecology, 56,* 238–248.

Kennedy, K. (2002). Constipation in the elderly. Routine equals regularity. *Advance for Nurse Practitioners, 10*(7), 32–34, 37.

Kessler, D. (1993). Introducing MedWatch: a new approach to reporting medication and device adverse effects and product problems. *Journal of the American Medical Association (JAMA), 269*(25), 2765–2768.

Khasraghi, F. A., Lee, E. S., Christmas, C., & Wenz, J. F. (2003). The economic impact of medical complications in geriatric patients with hip fracture. *Orthopedics, 26*(1), 49–53.

Kilker, K. (2000). *Challenges for the 21st Century: Chronic & disabling conditions: Hypertension: A common condition for older Americans.* Washington DC: National Academy on Aging Society.

Kim, I. J., Stewart, R., Shin, I., Choi, S. K., & Yoon, J. S. (2003). Subjective memory impairment, cognitive function and depression — a community study in older Koreans. *Dementia, Geriatric, Cognitive Disorders, 15*(4), 218–225.

Klausner, E. J., & Alexopolous, G. S. (1999). The future of psychosocial treatments for the elderly. *Psychiatric Services, 50*(9):1198–1204.

Knebel, A. (2002). Pain & palliative care: Research initiatives to improve end-of-life care. *Geriatric Times, 3*(6), 23–26.

Kolanowski, A. M. (1999). An overview of the need-driven dementia-compromised behavior model. *Journal of Gerontological Nursing, 25*(9), 7–9.

Kozak, I. J., Hall, M. J., & Owings, M. F. (2002). National Hospital Discharge Survey: 2000 annual summary with detailed diagnosis and procedure data. *Vital Health Statistics, 13*(153), 1–194.

Kunzmann, U., Little, T,. & Smith, J. (2002). Perceiving control: A double-edged sword in old age. *Journal of Gerontology: Psychological Science, 57*(6), 484–491.

Lantz, M. (2002). Generalized anxiety in Anxious times. Helping older adults cope. *Clinical Geriatrics, 10*(1), 36–38.

Lazowski, D. A., Ecclestone, N. A., Myers, A. M., Peterson, D. H., Tudor-Locke, C., Fitzgerald, C., et al. (1999). A randomized outcome evaluation of group exercise programs in long-term care institutions. *Journal of Gerontology Association Biological Sciences and Medical Sciences, 54*(12), 621–628.

Lebowitz, B. D., Pearson, J. L., Schneider, L. S., Reynolds, III, C. F., Alexopoulos, G. S., Bruce, L., et al. (1997). Diagnosis and treatment of depression in late life. Consensus statement update. *Journal of the American Medical Association, 278*(14), 1186–1190.

Lebowitz, B. D., (1997). The future of clinical research in mental disorders of late life. *Schizophrenia Research, 27*(2–3), 261–267.

Lee, R. (1997). Intergenerational relations and the elderly: Between Zeus and the Salmon. *The Biodemography of Longevity.* W. Wachter & Caleb E. Finch. (eds) (pp. 212–233). Washington DC: National Academy of Sciences Press.

Lemon, B. W., Bengtson, V. S., & Peterson, J. A. (1972). An exploration of the activity theory of aging: Activity types and life satisfaction among in-movers to a retirement community. *Journal of Gerontology, 27*(4), 511–523.

Levy, M., Cummings, J., Fairbanks, L., Masterman, D., Miller, B., Craig, A., et al. (1998). Apathy is not depression. *Journal of Neuropsychiatry Clinical Neuroscience, 10*(3), 314–9.

Lieberman, A. (2002). *Changing views on dementia in Parkinson's disease.* Retrieved on December 17, 2002, from http://www.parkinson.org/dement.htm

Lifton, R. (1973). Twentieth Annual Karen Horney Lecture. The sense of immortality: On death and the continuity of life. *American Journal of Psychoanalysis, 33*(1),3–15.

Lighthouse International. (2002). *Prevalence of vision impairment: National estimates.* Retrieved on December 17, 2002, from http://www.lighthouse.org/vision_impairment_prevalence_older.htm

Liu, G., & Christensen, D. (2002). The continuing challenge of inappropriate prescribing in the elderly: an update of the evidence. *Journal of American Pharmacy Association, 42*(6), 847–857.

LoBuono, C. (2001). Managing problem behaviors in AD. *Patient Care, 35*(3), 34–53.

Loeb, S. J., O'Neill, J. & Gueldner, S. H. (2001). Health motivation: A determinant of older adults' attendance at health promotion programs. *Journal of Community Health Nursing; 18*(3):151–165.

Loera, J., Black, S., Markides, K., Espino, D. & Goodwin, J. (2001). The use of herbal medicine by older Mexican Americans. *Journal of Gerontology. Biological Sciences and Medical Sciences, 56*(11), 714–718.

Lord, S., Dayhew, J,. & Howland, A. (2002). Multifocal glasses impair edge-contrast sensitivity and depth perception and increase the risk of falls in older people. *Journal of American Geriatric Society, 50*(11), 1760–1766.

Lowe, J., & Struthers, R. (2001). A conceptual framework of nursing in native American culture. *Journal of Nursing Scholarship, 33*(3), 279–283.

Lowry, L., & Conco, D. (2002). Exploring the meaning of spirituality with aging adults in Appalachia. *Journal of Holistic Nursing, 20*(4), 388–402.

Luisi, A., Owens, N., & Hume, A. (1999). Drugs and the elderly. In: J. J. Gallo, & W. Reichel, (eds). *Reichel's care of the elderly: Clinical aspects of aging.* (5th ed.) (pp. 59–87). Philadelphia: Williams & Wilkins.

Lyketsos, C. G., Steinberg, M., Tschanz, J. T., Norton, M., Steffens, D. C., & Breitner, J. (2000). Mental and behavioral disturbances in dementia: Findings from the Cache County Study on Memory in Aging. *American Journal of Psychiatry, 157*(5), 708–714.

Lynch, S. H. (1997). Elder Abuse: What to look for, how to intervene. *American Journal of Nursing, 97*(1), 27–32, quiz 33.

Lynn, J., & Harrold, J. (1999). *Handbook for mortals: Guidance for people facing serious illness.* Oxford: Oxford University Press.

Manda, W. & Rennard, S. (2002). COPD in older adults, Part II: Treatment strategies. *Geriatric Times, 3*(4).

Mann, N. (2002). Management of smell and taste problems. *Cleveland Clinic Journal of Medicine, 69*(4), 329–336.

Manning, J. (2002). The Brain-body connection and the relationship between depression and pain. Medscape CME. Retrieved on Jan 30, 2003 from: http://www.medscape.com/viewprogram/2166

Manton, K., & Gu, X. (2001). Changes in the prevalence of chronic disability in the United States black and non-black population above age 65 from 1982 to 1999. *Proceedings of the National Academy of Sciences, 98*(11), 6354–6359.

Marik, P. (1997). Stroke patients in the ICU: Is there any benefit? *The Internet Journal of Emergency and Intensive Care Medicine, 11*(2). Retrieved on May 20, 2003 from: http://www.ispub.com/journals/IJEICM/Vol1N2/stroke.htm

Marin, R. (1991). Apathy: A neuropsychiatry syndrome. *Journal of Neuropsychiatry and Clinical Neurosciences, 3*, 243–254.

Maslow, A. (1954). *Motivation and personality.* New York: Harper & Row.

Mayo Clinic. (2001). Study, review and editorial focus on religion, spirituality and medicine. Retrieved on May 20, 2003 from: http://www.mayoclinic.org/news2001-rst/921.html

Mayo Clinic. (2003) Geriatric medicine: Topics in geriatrics. Retrieved on January 9, 2003 from: http://www.mayo.edu/geriatrics-rst/geriactrics.htm/

McElhaney, J. (2002). Influenza: A preventable lethal disease. *Journal of Gerontology: Medical Science, 57A*(10), 627–628.

McLennon, S. M., Smith, R.,& Orrick, J. T. (2003). Recognizing and preventing drug interactions in older adults with HIV. *Journal of Gerontological Nursing, 29*(4), 5–12.

McPherson, S., Fairbanks, L., Tiken, S., Cummings, J. L., & Back-Madruga, C. (2002). Apathy and executive function in Alzheimer's disease. *Journal of International Neuropsychology Society, 8*(3), 373–381.

Menon, A. S., Gruber-Baldini, A. L., Hebel, J. R., Kaup, B., Loreck, D., Itkin Zimmeran, S., et al. (2001). Relationship between aggressive behaviors and depression among nursing home residents with dementia. *International Journal of Geriatric Psychiatry, 16*(2), 139–146.

Mentes, J. C., Iowa: Veteran's Affairs Research Conservation. (2000). Hydration management program. *Journal of Gerontological Nursing, 26*(10), 6–15.

Mezey, M., Fulmer, T. & Fairchild, S. (2000). Enhancing geriatric nursing scholarship: specialization versus generalization. *Journal of Gerontological Nursing, 26*(7), 28–35.

Mezey, M., & Fulmer, T. (2002). The future history of gerontological nursing. *Journal of Gerontology: A biological science, 57*(7), M438–M441.

Michocki, R. (2001). Polypharmacy and principles of drug therapy. In: M. P. Daly, B. D. Weiss, & A. M. Adelman, (eds.). *20 common problems in geriatrics.* (pp. 69–81) New York: McGraw-Hill.

Milisen, K., Foreman, M. D., Wouters, B., Driesen, R., Godderis, J., Abraham, I., et al. (2002). Documentation of delirium in elderly patients with hip fractures. *Journal of Gerontological Nursing, 28*(11), 23–29.

Moore, S. (1998). Specific drug therapy. In R. Handy, J. Turnbull, J. Edwards, & M. Lancaster (eds.), *Encyclopedia of elder care: The comprehensive resource on geriatric & social care.* New York: Springer.

Morbidity and Mortality Weekly Report (MMWR). (2001). *State Medicaid Coverage for Tobacco-Dependence Treatments-U.S., 1998 and 2000.* 50, 40 & 44.

Mueller, P. J., Plevak, D. J., & Rummans, T. A. (2001). Religious involvement, spirituality, and medicine: implications for clinical practice. *Mayo Clinic Proc, 76*(12), 1225–1235.

Mulchahey, J. J., Malik, M. S., Sabai, M., & Kasckow, J. W. (1999). Serotonin selective reuptake inhibitors in the treatment of geriatric depression and related disorders. *International Journal of Neuropsychopharmacoly, 2*(2), 121–127.

Muller-Lissner S. (2002). General geriatrics and gastroenterology: constipation and faecal incontinence. Best of Practice in Resident *Clinical Gastroenterology, 16*(1), 115–133.

Murphy, C., Schubert, C. R., Cruickshanks, K. J., Klein, B. E., Klein, R., & Nondahl, D. (2002). Prevalence of olfactory impairment in older adults. *Journal of the American Medical Association (JAMA), 288*(18), 2307–2312.

National Center for Assisted Living (NCAL). (2000). *Survey of Assisted Living Facilities.* National Center for Assisted Living. Retrieved on March 9, 2003 from: http://www.ncal. org/about/facility.htm

National Center for Health Statistics. (1999). Health and aging chartbook. Hyattsville, Maryland: National Center for Health Statistics.

National Center on Elder Abuse. (2002). What are the major types of elder abuse? Retrieved on July 19, 2003 from: http://www.elderabuse center.org/default.cfm?p=basics.cfm

National Eye Institute. (2002). National Eye Institute report on blindness and visual impairment in the U.S. Retreived July 19, 2003. http://www.hospitalmanagement.net/informer/ breakthroughs/break126/

National Heart, Lung, and Blood Institute. (2000). You Can Quit Smoking. Consumer Guide No. 91-3031, U.S. Public Health Service, National Institutes of Health. Bethesda, MD.

National Institute of Diabetes and Digestive and Kidney Diseases. (2002). *National diabetes Statistics fact sheet: General information and national estimates on diabetes in the United States, 2000.* Bethesda, MD: U.S. Department of Health and Human Services, National Institutes of Health.

Neugroschl, J. (2002). Agitation. How to manage behaviour disturbance in the older patient with dementia. *Geriatrics, 57*(4), 33–37, quiz 40.

Neafsey, P. T., & Shellman, J. (2002). Knowledge and self-efficacy of community health nurses concerning interactions of prescription medicines with over-the-counter agents and alcohol. *Journal of Gerontological Nursing, 28*(9), 30–39.

Neff, N. (2002). Growing number of U.S.-Mexican border residents using herbs to treat ailments, creating potential problems. 28(14A). Austin: The University Of Texas At Austin.

Nightingale F. (1859). *Notes on Hospitals.* (3rd ed.). John London: W. Parker and Sons.

Noel, H. C., Saunters, E., & Smolensky, M. H. (2000). Hypertension, Chronotherapy, and Patient management. *The Nurse Practitioner, Special Report, 25*(3), 1–10.

Nutrition Screening Initiative (NSI). (1992). The Nutrition Screening Initiative: *Nutrition interventions manual for professionals caring for older Americans.* Washington, DC: Nutrition Screening Initiative.

Omnibus Budget Reconciliation Action (1987).

Onen, F. & Onen, S. (2003). Sleep rhythm disturbances in Alzheimer's disease. *Review of Medicine-Internal, 24*(3), 165–171.

Olive, J. (2002), Better Hearing Institute launches new physician referral development program. *Audiology Today, 14*(2), 23–24.

O'Neil, G. (2002). *The state of aging and health in America: Mental health and aging.* Washington, DC: Merck Institute of Aging & Mental Health & The Gerontological Society on Aging.

Payne, B., & Cikovic, R (1996). An empirical examination of the characteristics, consequences and causes of elder abuse in nursing homes. *Journal of Elder Abuse & Neglect, 7*(4): 61–74.

Perry, P., Alexander, B., & Liskow, B. (1991). *Psychotropic drug handbook* (6th ed). Cincinnati: Harvey Whitney.

Petersen, R. C., Smith, G. E., Waring, S. C., Ivnik, R. J., Tangalos, E., & Kokmen, E. (1999). Mild cognitive impairment: Clinical characterization and outcome. *Archives of Neurology, 56*(3), 303–308.

Pettey, S. (2003). National nursing home quality data release generally applauded. *Caring for the Ages, 4*(1), 29–30.

Petry, N. M. (2002). A comparison of young, middle-aged, and older adult treatment-seeking pathological gamblers. *The Gerontologist, 42*(1), 92–99.

Physician's Desk Reference (PDR). (2002). *Physicians' desk reference* (56th ed). Montvale, NJ: Medical Economics Co.

Potter, J. (2003). Bowel care in older people. *Clinical Medicine, 3*(1), 48–51.

Prigerson, H. G., Maciejewski, P. K., & Rosenheck, R. A. (2000). Preliminary explorations of the harmful interactive effects of widowhood and marital harmony on health, health service use, and health care costs. *The Gerontologist, 40*(3), 349–357.

Prins, J., Blanker, M., Bohnen, A., Thomas, S. & Bosch, J. (2002). Prevalence of erectile dysfunction: a systematic review of population-based studies. *International Journal of Impotency Research, 14*(6), 422–432.

Prochaska, J.O. (1979). *Systems of psychotherapy: A transtheoretical analysis.* Homewood, IL: Dorsety.

Prochaska, J.O. & Norcross, J. C. (2003). *Systems of psychotherapy: A transtheoretical analysis.* (5th ed.). Pacifica, CA: Brooks-Cole.

Quinn, M. J., & Tomita, S. K. (1997). *Elder abuse and neglect: Causes, diagnosis, and intervention strategies.* (2nd ed.). New York: Springer.

Raphael, S. (1997). Lesbian and Gay Elders. Paper presented to Conference of National Center on Elder Abuse, Long Beach, CA, June 1997. Cited in Cook-Daniels, Lovee: Lesbian, Gay Male, Bisexual & Transexual Elders: Elder Abuse Neglect Issues, *Journal of Elder Abuse & Neglect, 9*(2), 38.

Ragneskog, H., Gerdner, L., Josefsson, K., & Kihlgren, M. (1998). Probable reasons for expressive agitation in persons with dementia. *Clinical Nursing Research, 7*(2), 189–206.

Rapoport, M., van Reekum, R., Freedman, M., Streiner, D., Simard, M., Clarke, D., et al. (2001). Relationship of psychosis to aggression, apathy and function in dementia. *International Journal of Geriatric Psychiatry, 16*(2), 123–130.

Rashbaum, I. (2002). Rehabilitation and Cardiovascular Disease. *Geriatric Times, 3*(1).

Ray, W. A., Taylor, J A., Meador, K. G., Lichenstein, M. J., Griffin, M. R., Fought, M. L., et al. (1993). Reducing antipsychotic drug use in nursing homes: A controlled trial of provider education. *Archives of Internal Medicine, 153*(6), 713–721.

Ray, W. A., Thapa, P. B., & Gideon, P. (2000). Benzodiazepines and the risk of falls in nursing home residents. *Journal of Geriatric Society, 48*(6), 682–685.

Ready, R. G., Ott, B. R., Grace, J., & Cahn-Weiner, D. A. (2003). Apathy and executive function in mild cognitive impairment and Alzheimer's disease. *American Journal of Geriatric Psychiatry, II*(2), 222–228.

Reichman, W. (1994). Nondegenerative dementing disorders. In C. E. Coffey, & J. L. Cummings (eds.), *Textbook of geriatric neuropsychiatry,* (pp. 369–388). Washington, DC: American Psychiatric Press.

Renshaw, D. (1996). *Sexual disorders.* In J. Sadavoy, L. Lazarus, L. Janik et al. (eds.), *Comprehensive review of geriatric psychiatry, II.* New York: Guilford Press.

Resnick, B. (2002). Health promotion or destruction: Helping your older patients decide on alcohol. *Geriatric Times, 3*(4), 37–38.

Reynolds, C. III, Frank, E. Perel, J. M., Imber, S. D., Cornes, C., Miller, M., et al. (1999). Nortriptyline and interpersonal psychotherapy as maintenance therapies for recurrent major depression: A randomized controlled trial in patients older than 59 years. *Journal of the American Medical Association (JAMA), 281*(1), 39–45.

Robinson, K. (2000). *Older Americans 2000: Key indicators of well-being.* Hyattsville, MD. Federal Interagency Forum on Aging Related Statistics.

Roman, G. C., Tatemichi, T. K., Erkinjuntti, T., Cummings, J. L., Masdeau, J. C., Garcia, J., et al. (1993). Vascular dementia: Diagnosis criteria for research studies. Report of the NINDS-AIREN International Workshop. *Neurology, 43:* 250–260.

Rossouw, J., Anderson, G., Prentice, R., LaCroix, A., Kooperberg, Stefanik, M., et al. (2002). Risks and benefits of estrogen plus progestin in healthy postmenopausal women: Principal results From the Women's Health Initiative randomized controlled trial. *Journal of the American Medical Association (JAMA), 28,* 321–333.

Rothschild, J. M., Bates, D. M., & Leape, L. L. (2000). Preventable medical injuries in older patients. *Archives of Intern Medicine, 160*(18):2717–28.

Sajatovic, M. (2002). Treatment of bipolar disorder in older adults. International Journal of *Geriatric Psychiatry, 17*(9):865–873.

Samovar, L. A., & Porter, R. E. (2003). *Intercultural communication: A reader (with InfoTrac).* (10th ed.). Florence, KY: Wadsworth Publishing Company, Thompson Learning.

Samraj, G., & Kuritzky, L. (2002). Issues in essential geriatric hypertension. *Geriatric Times, 3*(2), 38–42.

Schaefer, D. C., & Cheskin, L. J. (1998). Constipation in the Elderly. *American Family Physician, 58*(4), 907–914.

Seshadri, S., Beiser, A., Selhub, J., Jacques, P., Rosenberg, I., D'Agostino, R., et al. (2003). Plasma homocysteine as a risk factor for dementia and Alzheimer's disease. *New England Journal of Medicine, 346*(7), 476–483.

Schofield, I., & Dewing, J. (2001). The care of older people with a delirium in acute care settings. *Nursing Older People, 13*(1), 21–25, quiz 26.

Shea, C., Mahoney, M. & Lacey, J. (1997). Breaking through the barriers to domestic violence intervention. *American Journal of Nursing, 97*(6):26–34.

Sheikh, J., & Yesavage, J. (1986). Geriatric Depression Scale (GDS): Recent evidence and development of a shorter version. *Clinical Gerontology: A guide to assessment and intervention,* 165–173, New York: The Haworth Press.

Simon, H. (2003). Alcoholism. UC Davis health systems well-connected report: Retrieved on January 9, 2003 from: http://www.ucdmc.uc davis.edu/ucdhs/health/a-z/56Alcoholism/index.html

Simon, G., vonKorff, M., Piccinelli, M., Fullerton, C., & Ormel, J. (1999). An international study of the relation between somatic symptoms and depression. *New England Journal of Medicine,* (18), 341, 1329–1335.

Simor, A. E., Bradley, S. F., Strausbaugh, L. J., Crossley, K., & Nicolle, L. E. (2002). Clostridium difficile in long-term-care facilities for the elderly. *Infection Control Hospital Epidemiology, 23*(11), 696–703.

Slotwiner-Nie, P., & Brandt, L. (2001). Infectious diarrhea in the elderly. *Gastroenterology Clinic of North America, 30*(3), 625–635.

Small, G. (1997), Recognizing and treating anxiety in the elderly. *Journal of Clinical Psychiatry, 58*(suppl 3), 41–47.

SMARxT Coalition. (2003). *Facts about older adults and medicine in the United States.* Retrieved on January 9, 2003, from: http://www.smartcoalition.org/about.htm

Sorkin, D., Rook, K., & Lu, J. (2002). Loneliness, lack of emotional support, lack of companionship, and the likelihood of having a heart condition in an elderly sample. *Annuals of Behavioral Medicine, 24*(4), 290–298.

Social Security Administration. (2000). Income of the population 55 or older, *Social Security Administration Publication No. 13–11 8 7 1.* Washington DC: Social Security Administration.

Sourial, R., McCusker, J., Cole, M., & Abrahamowicz, M. (2001). Agitation in demented patients in an acute care hospital: prevalence, disruptiveness, and staff burden. *International Psychogeriatrics, 13*(2), 183–97.

Spratley, E., Johnson, A., Sochalski, J., Fritz, M. & Spencer, W. (2000). The registered nurse population: Findings from the National Sample Survey Of Registered Nurses. Rockville, MD: U.S. Department of Health and Human Services, Health Resources and Service Administration, Bureau of Health Professions, Division of Nursing.

Specht, J. Lyon, S., & Maas, M. (2002). Patterns and treatment of urinary incontinence on special care units. *Journal of Gerontological Nursing, 28*(5), 13–21.

Spector, A., Orrell, M., Davies, S., & Woods, B. (2001). Reality orientation for dementia. (Cochrane review). In: The Cochrane Library, 1, 2001. Oxford Update Software.

Stanley, M., & Beare, P. (1995). *Gerontological nursing.* Philadelphia: FA. Davis Co.

Starr, D. (2002). Tips for everyday clinical practice: Documenting informed consent. *The Clinical Advisor, 5*(11/12), 104.

Stegbauer, C., Mojica, T. R., & Bailey, P. P. (2000). Hallucinations in the vision-impaired elderly: The Charles Bonnet syndrome. *The Nurse Practitioner, 25*(8), 74–76.

Stekler, J., & Elmore, J. (2002). Cervical Cancer Screening: Who, when, why? *The Clinical Advisor, 5*(10), 107–115.

Stotland, N. (2002). Menopause: social expectations, women's realities. *Archives of Women Mental Health, 5*(1), 5–8.

Strain, L., Grabusic, M., Searle, M. S., & Dunn, N. J. (2002). Continuing and ceasing leisure activities in later life: A longitudinal study. *The Gerontologist, 42*(2), 217–223.

Strawbridge, W. J., Wallhagen, M. I., & Cohen, R. P. (2002) Successful aging and well-being: Self-rated compared with Rowe and Kahn. *The Gerontologist, 42*(6), 727–733.

Stolley, J. M., & Buckwalter, K. C., Fjordbak, B., & Bush, S. (1991). Iatrogenesis in the elderly. Drug-related problems. *Journal of Gerontological Nursing, 17*(9), 12–17.

Stone, R. G. (1996). Warner: Tacoma, WA: University of Puget Sound, http://otpt.ups. edu/Gerontological_Resources/Gerontology_ Manual/06a-Theories_Aging(VIII).html

Stupay, S., & Sivertsen, L. (2000). Herbal and nutritional supplement use in the elderly. *The Nurse Practitioner, 25*(9), 56–58, 61–62, 64.

Substance Abuce & Mental Heath Services Administration (SAMHSA). (2001). National Household Survey on Drug Abuse, h t t p : / / w w w . s a m h s a . gov/oas/nhsda/2k1nhsda/vol1/toc.htm

Suhayda, R., & Walton, J. C. (2002). Preventing and managing dehydration. *Medsurg Nursing, 11*(6), 267–278.

Sullivan-Marx, E. M. (2001). Achieving restraint-free care of acutely confused older adults. *Journal of Gerontological Nursing, 27*(4), 57–61.

Swanson, J. (2001). Falls cause 90 percent of America's 350,000 hip fractures. *American Academy of Orthopedic Surgeons.* Retrieved on January 15, 2003 from: http://www.newswise. com/articles/2001/1/HIPFALL.OSR.html

Talerico, K. A., Evans, L. K., & Strumpf, N. E. (2002). Mental Health corralates of aggression in nursing home residents with dementia. *Gerontologist, 42*(2), 169–177.

Teaster, P. B. (2000). A Response to the Abuse of Vulnerable Adults: The 2000 Survey of State Adult Protection Service. Washington, DC: National Center on Elder Abuse.

Teno, J. M., S., Wetle, T., & Mor, V. (2001). Persistent pain in nursing home residents. *Journal of the American Medical Association (JAMA), 285*(16), 2081.

Teresi, J., Abrams, R., Holmes, D., Ramirez, M., & Eimicke, J. (2001). Prevalence of depression and depression recognition in nursing homes. *Social Psychiatry Epidemiology, 36*(12), 613–620.

Thomas, P., Clement, J., Hazif-Thomas, C., & Leger, J. (2001). Family, Alzheimer's disease and negative symptoms. *International Journal of Geriatric Psychiatry, 16*(2), 192–202.

Thomas, D. R., Zdrowski, C. D., Wilson, M. M., Conright, K., Lewis, C., Tariq, S., et al. (2002). Malnutrition in sub-acute care. *American Journal of Clinical Nutrition, 75*(2), 308–313.

Tichawa, U. (2002). Creating a continuum of care for elder individuals. *Journal of Gerontological Nursing, 28*(1), 46–52.

Tractenberg, R. E., Weiner, M. F., & Thal, L. J. (2002). Estimating the prevalence of agitation in community-dwelling persons with Alzheimer's disease. *Journal of Neuropsychiatry: Clinical Neuroscience, 14*(1), 11–18.

Travis, S. S., Bernard, M. , Dixon, S., McAuley, W., Loving, G., & McClanahan, L. (2002). Obstacles to palliation and end-of-life care in a long-term care facility. *The Gerontologist, 42*(3), 342–349.

Tremethick, M. (2001). Alone in a crowd: A study of social networks in home health and assisted living. *Journal of Gerontological Nursing 27*(5), 42–47.

U.S. Census Bureau. (2000). Population projections of the United States by age, sex, race, Hispanic origin, and nativity: 1999–2001. Washington, DC: U.S. Census Bureau.

U.S. Department of Health and Human Services (DHHS). (1999). Changes in Elderly Disability rates and the implications for healthcare utilization and cost: Executive Summary. Retrieved July 19, 2003. http://aspe.hhs.gov/daltcp/reports/hcutlces.htm

U.S. Department of Health and Human Services. Mental Health: A report of the Surgeon General: Executive summary. Rockville, MD: U.S. Department of Health and Human Services, Substance Abuse and Mental Health Services Administration, Center for Mental Health Services, National Institutes of Health, National Institute of Mental Health.

U.S. Department of Health and Human Services. (1990). The Health Benefits of Smoking Cessation. Public Health Service, Center for Disease Control, Center for Disease Prevention and Health Promotion, Office on Smoking Health. DHHS Publicatin No (CDC), 90–846.

U.S. Department of Health and Human Services. (2002). Tobacco intervention and prevention source: Tips to stop smoking. Washington, DC. National Center For Chronic Disease Prevention and Health Promotion

U.S. Department of Health and Human Services Centers for Medicare & Medicaid Services (DHHS, CMMS). (2002). *Guide to choosing a nursing home.* Publication No. CMS - 02174.

U.S. Department of Justice. (2003). *Americans with Disabilities Act.* Retrieved on May 20, 2003, from: http://www.usdoj.gov/crt/ada/adahom1.htm

Unwin, B. K., Davis, M. K., & Leeuw, J. B. (2000) Pathological Gambling. *American Family Physician, 61*(3), 741–749.

Van Houten B. (2002), BHI pursues physician referrals with innovative new program. *The Hearing Review, 9*(2), 26, 28, 60.

Van Wynen, E. A. (2001). A key to successful aging: Learning-style patterns of older adults. *Journal of Gerontological Nursing, 27*(9), 6–15.

Vap, P,. & Dunaye, T. (2000). Pressure ulcers risk assessment in long-term care nursing. *Journal of Gerontological Nursing, 26*(6), 37–45.

Walker, Z., & Stevens, T. (2002). Dementia with Lewy bodies: clinical characteristics and diagnostic criteria. *Journal of Geriatric Psychiatry & Neurology, 15*(4),188–194.

Wallston, B., & Wallston. K. (1978). Locus of control and health: A review of the literature. *Health Education Monographs,* Spring, 6(2), 107–117.

Weaver, A. J., Flannelly, L. T., & Flannelly, K. J. (2001). A review of research on religious and spiritual variables in two primary gerontological nursing journal: 1991 t o 1997. *Journal of Gerontology Nursing, 27*(9), 47–54.

Wehren, L. E. (2002). Osteoporosis increases mortality risk in men. *Geriatric Times, 3*(4), 27–30.

Wendland, B., Greenwood, C., Weinberg, I., & Young, K. (2003). Malnutrition in institutionalized seniors: The iatrogenic component. *Journal of American Geriatric Society, 51*(1), 85–90.

White, J. V., Dwyer, J. T., Posner, B.M., Ham, R. J., Lipschitz, D. A., et al. (1992). Nutrition screening initiative. Development and implementation of the public awareness checklist and screening tools. *Journal of the American Dietetic Association, 92*(2),163–167.

Willard, S., & Dean, L. (2000). AIDS in the elderly. *Advance for the Nurse Practitioner, 7*(7), 54–58.

Won, A., Lapane, K., Gambassi, G., Bernabei, R., Mor, Z., & Lipsitz, L. (1999). Correlates and management of nonmalignant pain in the nursing home: SAGE study group. Systematic assessment of geriatric drug use via epidemiology. *Journal of American Geriatric Society, 47*(8), 936–342.

Wunderlich, G., & Kohler, P. (2001). *Improving the quality of long term care.* Washington DC: National Academy Press.

Yardley, L., & Smith, H. (2002). A prospective study of the relationship between feared consequence of falling and avoidance of activity in community-living older people. *The Gerontologist, 42*(1), 17–23.

Zanocchi, M., Ponzetto, M., Spada, S., Risso, R., Aimar, T., et al. (1999). Sleep disorders in the aged. *Minerva Med., 90*(11–12), 421–427.

Zimberg, S. (1996). Treating alcoholism: An age-specific intervention that works for older patients. *Geriatrics, 51*(10), 45–51.

Zembrzuski, C. (2000). Nutrition and hydration. *Journal of Gerontological Nursing, 26*(12), 6–7.

INDEX

PRETEST KEY

Nursing Care of the Older Adult

Question	Answer	Chapter
1.	B	1
2	A	2
3	C	2
4	D	3
5	A	4
6	C	4
7	B	5
8	A	5
9	B	6
10	A	6
11	D	7
12	C	8
13	A	9
14	B	9
15	C	10
16	D	10
17	A	11
18	B	12
19	C	13
20	A	14

Notes

Notes

Western Schools® offers over 1,400 hours to suit all your interests – and requirements!

Advanced Level Courses

Nurse Anesthesia
— Common Diseases ....20 hrs
— Common Procedures ....21 hrs
— Drugs...17 hrs
Obstetric and Gynecologic Emergencies
— Obstetric Emergencies ....22 hrs
— Gynecologic Emergencies ....22 hrs
Practical Guide to Moderate Sedation/Analgesia...31 hrs
Geropsychiatric and Mental Health Nursing ....40 hrs
Palliative Practices: An Interdisciplinary Approach
— Issues Specific to Palliative Care ....20 hrs
— Specific Disease States and Symptom
        Management ....24 hrs
— The Dying Process, Grief, and Bereavement...22 hrs
Practice Guidelines for Pediatric Nurse Practitioners.46 hrs
The 12-Lead ECG in Acute Coronary Syndromes ..42 hrs

Clinical Conditions/Nursing Practice

A Nurse's Guide to Weight Control
        for Healthy Living....................................25 hrs
Airway Management with a Tracheal Tube ....1 hr
Asthma: Nursing Care Across the Lifespan ....28 hrs
Auscultation Skills: Breath and Heart Sounds .... hrs
Cardiovascular Nursing: A Comprehensive
        Overview ....32 hrs
Care at the End of Life...3 hrs
Chest Tube Management ....2 hrs
Death, Dying & Bereavement ....30 hrs
Healing Nutrition ....24 hrs
Hepatitis C: The Silent Killer ....2 hrs
HIV/AIDS ....1, 2, or 4 hrs
Holistic & Complementary Therapies ....1 or 18 hrs
Humor in Healthcare: The Laughter Prescription..20 hrs
Managing Obesity and Eating Disorders ....30 hrs
Orthopedic Nursing: Caring for Patients with
        Musculoskeletal Disorders ....30 hrs
Pain Management: Principles and Practice............30 hrs
Pharmacologic Management of Asthma...................1 hr
Seizures: A Basic Overview ....1 hr
The Neurological Exam...1 hr
Wound Management and Healing...........................30 hrs

Critical Care/ER/OR

Ambulatory Surgical Care ....20 hrs
Case Studies in Critical Care Nursing: A Guide for
        Application and Review ....46 hrs
Principles of Basic Trauma Nursing (2nd ed.) ......30 hrs

Geriatrics

Alzheimer's Disease: A Complete Guide for Nurses ..25 hrs
Home Health Nursing ....30 hrs
Nursing Care of the Older Adult ....30 hrs
Psychosocial Issues Affecting Older Adults ....16 hrs

Infectious Diseases/Bioterrorism

Avian Influenza ....1 hr
Biological Weapons ....5 hrs
Bioterrorism & the Nurse's Response to WMD ......5 hrs
Bioterrorism Readiness: The Nurse's Critical Role .. 2 hrs
Infection Control Training for Healthcare Workers ..4 hrs
Influenza: A Vaccine-Preventable Disease ....1 hr
SARS: An Emerging Public Health Threat ....1 hr
Smallpox...2 hrs
West Nile Virus ....1 hr

Oncology

Cancer in Women..30 hrs
Cancer Nursing: A Solid Foundation for Practice ..30 hrs
Chemotherapy Essentials: Principles & Practice ..15 hrs

Pediatrics/Maternal-Child/Women's Health

Attention Deficit Hyperactivity Disorders
        Throughout the Lifespan...............................30 hrs
Diabetes in Children ....30 hrs
End-of-Life Care for Children and
        Their Families ....2 hrs
Manual of School Health..30 hrs
Maternal-Newborn Nursing....................................30 hrs
Menopause: Nursing Care for Women
        Throughout Mid-Life ....25 hrs
Pediatric Nursing: Routine to Emergent Care........30 hrs
Pediatric Pharmacology ....10 hrs
Pediatric Physical Assessment................................10 hrs
Women's Health: Contemporary
        Advances and Trends ....30 hrs

Professional Issues/Management/Law

Documentation for Nurses.......................................24 hrs
Medical Error Prevention: Patient Safety ....2 hrs
Nursing and Malpractice Risks:
        Understanding the Law ....30 hrs
Ohio Law: Standards of Safe Nursing Practice ....1 hr
Supervisory Skills for Nurses ....30 hrs
Surviving and Thriving in Nursing ....30 hrs
Understanding Managed Care ....30 hrs

Psychiatric/Mental Health

Antidepressants ....1 hr
Antipsychotics ....1 hr
Anxiolytics and Mood Stabilizers............................1 hr
Basic Psychopharmacology......................................5 hrs
Depression: Prevention, Diagnosis, and Treatment...25 hrs
IPV (Intimate Partner Violence):
        A Domestic Violence Concern ....1 or 3 hrs
Psychiatric Principles & Applications for
        General Patient Care ....30 hrs
Psychiatric Nursing: Current Trends
        in Diagnosis and Treatment ....30 hrs